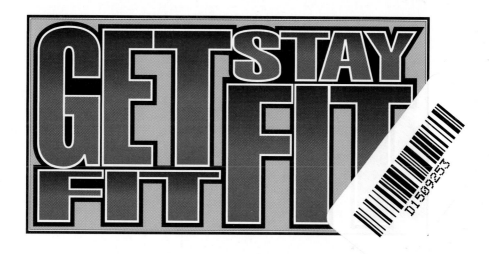

WILLIAM E. PRENTICE, PH.D., P.T., A.T.C.

Professor, Coordinator of the Sports Medicine Specialization,
Department of Exercise, and Sport Science
Clinical Professor, Division of Physical Therapy,
Department of Medical Allied Health Professions
Associate Professor, Department of Orthopaedics
School of Medicine
The University of North Carolina
Chapel Hill, North Carolina

Second Edition

Boston Burr Ridge, IL Dubuque, IA Madison, WI New York San Francisco St. Louis
Bangkok Bogotá Caracas Lisbon London Madrid
Mexico City Milan New Delhi Seoul Singapore Sydney Taipei Toronto

McGraw-Hill Higher Education

A Division of The **McGraw-Hill** *Companies*

GET FIT STAY FIT, SECOND EDITION

Published by McGraw-Hill, an imprint of The McGraw-Hill Companies, Inc., 1221 Avenue of the Americas, New York, NY 10020. Copyright © 2001, 1996 by The McGraw-Hill Companies, Inc. All rights reserved. No part of this publication may be reproduced or distributed in any form or by any means, or stored in a database or retrieval system, without the prior written consent of The McGraw-Hill Companies, Inc., including, but not limited to, in any network or other electronic storage or transmission, or broadcast for distance learning.

Some ancillaries, including electronic and print components, may not be available to customers outside the United States.

This book is printed on acid-free paper.

1 2 3 4 5 6 7 8 9 0 DOC/DOC 0 9 8 7 6 5 4 3 2 1 0

ISBN 0–07–232906–8

Vice president and editor-in-chief: *Kevin T. Kane*
Executive editor: *Vicki Malinee*
Senior developmental editor: *Michelle Turenne*
Senior marketing manager: *Pamela S. Cooper*
Project manager: *Mary Lee Harms*
Senior production supervisor: *Mary E. Haas*
Coordinator of freelance design: *Rick D. Noel*
Cover designer: *Mary Sailer*
Interior designer: *Kathleen Theis*
Cover image: *©FPG International, image number SP2161, Women with weights*
Senior supplement coordinator: *Candy M. Kuster*
Compositor: *Carlisle Communications, Ltd.*
Typeface: *10/12 Palatino*
Printer: *R. R. Donnelley & Sons Company/Crawfordsville, IN*

Library of Congress Cataloging-in-Publication Data

Prentice, William E.
    Get fit, stay fit / William E. Prentice.—2nd ed.
      p. cm.
    Includes index.
    ISBN 0–07–232906–8
    1. Physical fitness.   2. Exercise.   3. Health.   I. Title.

RA781 .P67   2001
613.7—dc21
                          00–036124
                          CIP

www.mhhe.com

PREFACE

If you believe what you hear, see, and read in the media, you would think that every person in America has become a "fitness junkie." It is true that millions of people exercise in some way, shape, or form on a somewhat consistent basis. But the fact is, that for the vast majority of Americans the thought of going out and "exercising" never even crosses their minds. Through TV and videos, on the internet, in magazines or newspapers, our society is constantly bombarded by images that suggest the importance of being physically fit and healthy. It seems that people in your generation, in contrast to all the previous ones, are finally starting to realize that there really is a reason for living a healthy lifestyle and for incorporating regular exercise into that lifestyle.

Get Fit: Stay Fit is a text designed to tell you not only how you can go about getting yourself fit, but also why it is to your advantage to make fitness and exercise a regular part of your lifestyle. It begins by discussing the basic principles of fitness that apply to any type of exercise program, and then explains how being fit relates to a healthy lifestyle. Specific techniques and guidelines for developing cardiorespiratory endurance, for improving muscular strength and endurance, for increasing flexibility, and for maintaining appropriate body weight and composition are described in detail so that you can put together a personalized fitness program based on your individual needs. This book also provides recommendations and suggestions on selecting and using the exercise equipment available to help you get fit, as well as tips for making your exercise program as safe and free of injury as possible.

FEATURES

- Practical application chapters are dedicated to Starting your own fitness program (3), Becoming a wise consumer (9), and Practicing safe fitness (10). These chapters cut through the confusion and provide essential information on how to start up, equip yourself, and safely execute an individual fitness program.
- Special boxes—Fit Lists, Health Links, and Safe Tips—highlight, summarize, and provide quick reference to important information.
- Lab Activities assist in evaluating a number of personal measures of fitness as well as providing guidelines for increased health.
- Key terms are in color and are defined in boxes to help build a working vocabulary of concepts, terms, and principles necessary for understanding, beginning, and maintaining any fitness program.
- Chapter pedagogy also includes chapter objectives, key terms, definition boxes, bulleted summaries, and suggested readings to enhance the learning process.
- The Appendix includes an extensive Food Composition Table which provides the nutritive value of commonly used foods.

NEW TO THIS EDITION

- *New exercise trends:* Discussions of new trends such as elliptical training and kick boxing allow the student to make informed choices while assembling a fitness program, becoming a fitness consumer, and continuing with a fitness regimen.

- *Fluid replacement:* The author discusses recent research on fluid replacement and emphasizes the importance of fluids during exercise.
- *Supplements:* The author presents the most current information on the effects and hazards of creatine and herbal supplements to enable students to make informed decisions.
- *Safety:* All exercise safety information and illustrations have been updated to provide proper fitness techniques for a safe and effective fitness program.
- *Photographs:* More than 150 photographs illustrate a range of fitness levels to provide an excellent visual guide to the proper execution of exercises, stretches, and activities.
- *Web Sites:* Each chapter contains a list of reviewed websites relevant to the chapter topic. Using the power of the World Wide Web as a resource, the student will be able to obtain further information to take his or her studies beyond the classroom.
- *References:* An updated and expanded list of references provides a significant resource for students as well as instructors for further study of key issues and topics.

ANCILLARIES

- *Computerized Test Bank:* Microtest contains 300 multiple choice, true-false, fill-in, and short essay test questions which accompany the text. These are in IBM and Macintosh formats and are available to qualified adopters.
- *Fitness and Wellness Super Site:* This site includes additional resources for instructors and students, including additional lab activities. For more information from textbooks to technology, visit the site at this address: *www.mhhe.com/hper/physed/fitness-wellness.*
- *FitSolve II Software:* This software encourages students to evaluate their fitness behaviors and learn problem-solving skills by designing and implementing their own fitness programs. The colorful graphics and easy point-and-click data entry system allows students to focus on content and important concepts. The software provides many assessment activities students can use to evaluate their fitness level, such as the 1.5-mile run; the Rockport Fitness Walking Test; muscle, endurance, and flexibility tests; and body measurement analyses.
- *HealthQuest CD-ROM: HealthQuest* is designed to help students explore the behavioral aspects of health and fitness through a state-of-the-art interactive CD-ROM. Students will be able to assess their current health and fitness status, determine their health risks, and explore options and make decisions to improve the behaviors that impact their health and fitness.

ACKNOWLEDGMENTS

In revising *Get Fit: Stay Fit,* my editors have been instrumental in the development of the second edition, and have provided a great deal of help and support. The reviewers provided many constructive recommendations about content and organization. Their input and suggestions have been greatly appreciated and are reflected throughout the text. They include the following:

Steve Carney
James Madison University

Pete DiLorenzo
Floyd College

Mary Ann Erickson
Fort Lewis College

Judy Peel
North Carolina State University

Linn Stranak
Union University

Kenneth E. Weatherman
Floyd College

And finally, as always, this is for my wife Tena and our boys, Brian and Zach, who each day make my life more worthwhile.

By writing this book, I have tried to provide you with all the details you need to know about getting yourself fit and to stress the importance of developing a healthy lifestyle. But the bottom line is that, to get fit, you need to stop reading about it and start doing it. There is no better time than now!

William E. Prentice

BRIEF CONTENTS

CONTENTS

CHAPTER 1

GETTING FIT
WHY SHOULD YOU CARE?

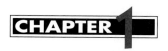

OBJECTIVES

After completing this chapter, you should be able to do the following:

- Give several reasons why being fit should be important to you.
- Discuss the physical, social, and psychological benefits of being fit.
- List the component parts of physical fitness.
- Determine your reasons for wanting to become physically fit.

So, you've finally decided it's time to get fit. Why is that? People have many different reasons and motivations for beginning a physical activity program. Are you interested in improving your overall health and well-being? Are you concerned about the way you look to your friends? Are you tired of being a couch potato? Are you interested in fitness primarily because you are required to take this fitness class? Whatever your motivation happens to be, consistently engaging in physical activities can make you physically fit, and can have many positive benefits on your style of living.

Key Terms

physical fitness
health-related components
skill-related components
cardiorespiratory endurance
flexibility
muscular strength
muscular endurance
body composition
atherosclerosis
caloric intake
caloric expenditure
speed
power
agility
reaction time
coordination
balance

WHY SHOULD YOU CARE ABOUT BEING PHYSICALLY ACTIVE?

Have you noticed that it is virtually impossible to go through a day without being exposed to something involving **physical fitness**? We eat, sleep, go to class, and some of us even try to include some form of exercise in our busy schedules. Fitness information comes from many sources. "Experts" give advice on television or radio and in magazines, books, and newspapers. Even our friends and classmates are willing to give opinions on the best ways to work out or on how to lose weight. Furthermore, the image of the attractive, healthy, physically active person is used to market everything—clothing, food, cosmetics, health care products, sports equipment, weight loss programs—the list goes on. People of all ages and backgrounds are deciding to take responsibility for their own physical and emotional well-being by becoming physically active.

Our society is characterized by a fast-paced lifestyle, with obligations and stresses that affect our physical and emotional fitness. One of the most obvious reasons for becoming physically active is the benefit you may derive from a healthy lifestyle that includes proper exercise and nutrition.

Physical fitness is not entirely dependent on exercise. Desirable health practices also play an important role. Physical fitness affects the total person, including intellect, emotional stability, physical conditioning, and stress levels. The road to physical fitness includes proper medical care, eating the right foods in the right amounts, appropriate physical activity that is adapted to individual needs and physical limitations, satisfying work, healthy play and recreation, and proper amounts of rest and relaxation.

Engaging in physical activity to get yourself fit allows you to satisfy your needs regarding mental and emotional stability, social consciousness and adaptability, spiritual and moral fiber, and physical health consistent with your heredity. Being fit means that the various systems of your body are healthy and function efficiently to enable you to engage in activities of daily living, as well as recreational pursuits and leisure activities, without unreasonable fatigue.

THE PHYSICAL BENEFITS OF BEING PHYSICALLY ACTIVE

Human beings are designed to be active creatures. Although changes in civilization have resulted in a decrease in the amount of activity needed to accomplish the basic tasks associated with living, the human body has not changed. Therefore, it is important to be aware of the requirements for good health and recognize the importance of vigorous physical activity in your life. If you do not, your health, productivity, and effectiveness are likely to suffer. The accompanying Health Link on page 3 lists 10 physical benefits associated with physical activity.

THE SOCIAL REWARDS OF BEING PHYSICALLY ACTIVE

If you are not willing to participate in physical activities that help keep you fit, you may be depriving yourself of the social outlets, companionship, and feelings inherent in such activities. Participation in physical activity provides an opportunity for socializing. Physical fitness affects the entire person, and rich dividends

---

physical fitness: the various systems of your body are healthy and function efficiently to enable you to engage in activities of daily living, as well as recreational pursuits and leisure activities, without unreasonable fatigue

Health Link

Benefits of Being Physically Active

1. Regular, vigorous activity increases muscle size, strength, and power and develops endurance for sustaining work and resisting fatigue.
2. Exercise strengthens the heart muscle and improves the efficiency of the vascular system in delivering oxygenated blood to the working tissues and in using it.
3. Exercise improves the functioning of the lungs by deepening the respiration process.
4. Exercise helps to keep the digestive and excretory organs in good condition.
5. Muscular exercise enhances nerve-muscle coordination.
6. Exercise helps a person to maintain a healthy body weight by reducing the percentage of total body weight that is made up of fat tissue.
7. Exercise contributes to improved posture and appearance through the development of proper muscle tone, greater joint flexibility, and a feeling of well-being.
8. Physical activity generates more energy and thus contributes to greater individual productivity for both physical and mental tasks.
9. The person who is fit has more strength, energy, and stamina; an improved sense of well-being; better protection from injury (because strong, well-developed muscles safeguard bones, internal organs, and joints and keep moving parts limber); and improved cardiorespiratory function.
10. It is often the case that people who become physically active will pay more attention to such things as proper nutrition, rest, and relaxation and may also drink less alcohol and stop smoking because they do not want to undo the benefits gained through physical activity. They are likely to be committed to engaging in health-promoting, rather than health-harming, behavior.

come to the person who concentrates on the development of the body as well as the mind.

THE PSYCHOLOGICAL BENEFITS OF BEING PHYSICALLY ACTIVE

Many people use regular exercise, especially of a recreational nature, as a means of mental relaxation. Exercise can play a significant role in reducing stress. It diverts attention from stress-producing thoughts to a more relaxing and positive focus. Exercise may also help us to feel better about ourselves and to feel that we are more capable of handling potential stress-producing situations.

THE BENEFITS OF EXERCISE IN THE AGING PROCESS

At this point in your life, chances are that your physical health is fine. However, a fact which we wish we could change, but unfortunately cannot, is that aging begins immediately at birth and involves a lifelong series of changes in physiological and performance capabilities. These capabilities increase as a function of the growth process throughout adolescence, peak sometime between the ages of 18 and 30 years, then steadily decline with increasing age. Interestingly, this decline may be caused by the sociological constraints of aging as much as by biological effects. It is possible for you to maintain a relatively high level of physical function if you maintain an active lifestyle.

In most cases, after age 30, qualities such as muscular endurance, coordination, and strength begin to decrease. Furthermore, as we age, recovery from vigorous exercise requires a longer amount of time. Regular physical activity, however, tends to delay and in some cases prevent the appearance of certain degenerative processes. If you were active as a child, became fit as a teenager, and continue to stay fit throughout your life, it is very likely that you will have greater strength, flexibility, and cardiorespiratory health and a lower percentage of body fat than if you chose a more sedentary lifestyle.

WHAT COMPONENTS OF FITNESS ARE IMPORTANT TO YOU?

Engaging in physical activities can have a positive effect on many different physical attributes. For the vast majority of people in our society, regardless of age, the focus should be on those components of fitness which are concerned with the development of qualities necessary to function efficiently physically and to maintain a healthy lifestyle. Those fitness components include cardiorespiratory endurance, muscular strength, muscular endurance, flexibility, and body composition. Collectively, they are referred to as health-related components. The Fit List following summarizes the fitness components.

Cardiorespiratory endurance is the ability to persist in a physical activity requiring oxygen for physical exertion without experiencing undue fatigue (Figure 1-1). If you go out and run 2 miles or swim 2000 yards, you are displaying cardiorespiratory endurance. The functioning of the heart, lungs, and blood vessels is essential for distribution of oxygen and nutrients and removal of wastes from the body. For performance of vigorous activities, efficient functioning of the heart and lungs is necessary. The more efficiently they function, the easier it is to walk, run, work, and concentrate for longer periods. Exercise of this nature involves the heart, the vessels supplying blood to all parts of the body, and the oxygen-carrying capacity of the blood.

Muscular strength is the ability or capacity of a muscle or muscle group to exert force against

Fit List

Fitness Components

Health-related Components

- Cardiorespiratory endurance
- Flexibility
- Muscular strength
- Muscular endurance
- Body composition

Skill-related Components

- Speed
- Power
- Agility
- Coordination
- Balance
- Reaction time

health-related components: components of a healthy lifestyle, including muscular strength, muscular endurance, cardiorespiratory endurance, flexibility, and body composition

cardiorespiratory endurance: the ability to persist in a physical activity requiring oxygen for physical exertion without experiencing undue fatigue

muscular strength: the ability or capacity of a muscle or muscle group to exert force against resistance

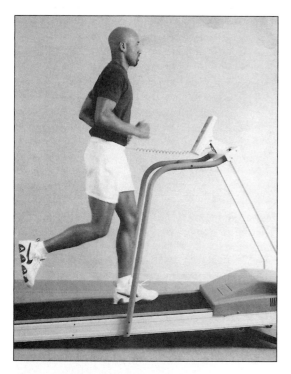

Figure 1-1. Cardiorespiratory Endurance.
Perhaps the most essential fitness component for both good health and skill-related performance.

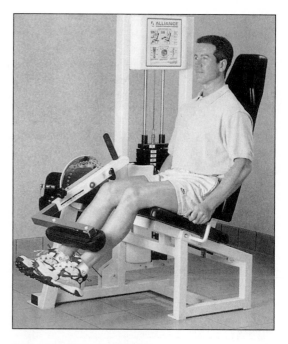

Figure 1-2. Muscular Strength.
The ability to generate force against resistance.

resistance (Figure 1-2). It refers to a muscle's ability to exert maximal force in a single effort. Strength is needed in all kinds of work and in physical activity, and strong muscles provide better protection of body joints, resulting in fewer sprains, strains, and muscular difficulties. Furthermore, muscle strength helps in maintaining proper posture and provides greater endurance, power, and resistance to fatigue.

Muscular endurance is the ability of muscles to perform or sustain a muscle contraction repeatedly over a period of time (Figure 1-3).

Muscular endurance is closely related to muscular strength. If you are strong, you will be more resistant to fatigue because relatively less effort will be required to produce repeated muscular contraction.

Flexibility is the ability to move your arms, legs, and trunk freely throughout a full, nonrestricted, pain-free range of motion (Figure 1-4). It may be improved by engaging regularly in stretching. Flexibility is important for performance in most active sports; it is also important for maintaining good posture. Flexibility is also essential in carrying on many daily activities and can help to prevent muscle strain and muscular problems such as backaches.

muscular endurance: the ability of muscles to perform or sustain a muscle contraction repeatedly over a period of time

flexibility: the ability to move your arms, legs, and trunk freely throughout a full, nonrestricted, pain-free range of motion

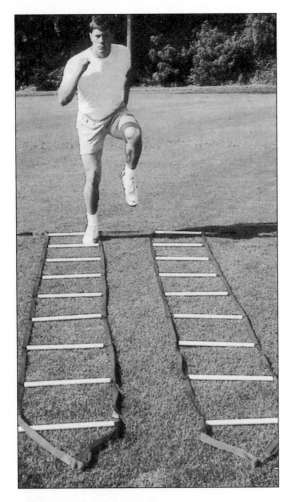

Figure 1-3. Muscular Endurance.
The ability to perform muscular contractions re-peatedly over a period of time.

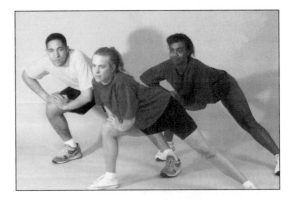

Figure 1-4. Flexibility.
The ability to move freely through a full range of motion.

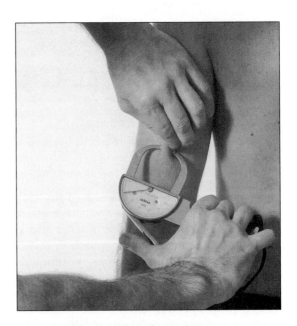

Figure 1-5. Measuring Body Composition.
Exercise reduces the percentage of total body weight that is fat tissue.

Body composition refers to the different types of tissues that make up your body. These primarily include bones, muscles, tendons, ligaments, skin, and fat (Figure 1-5). Body composition particularly refers to the percent-age of fat in the body relative to the percentage of all the other tissues. An excess of fat in the body is unhealthy because it causes the body to expend more energy for movement, and it may reflect a diet in which an individual is consuming more calories than he or she needs.

The demand on the cardiorespiratory system is greater when the percentage of body fat is high. Furthermore, it is believed that obesity contributes to degenerative diseases such as high blood pressure and **atherosclerosis**. Obesity can also result in psychological maladjustments and may shorten life. A balance between caloric intake and caloric expenditure is necessary to maintain proper body fat content. Adequate exercise, therefore, is effective in controlling body fat. **Caloric intake** is the total number of calories consumed in a 24-hour period regardless of the type of foods ingested. **Caloric expenditure** is the number of calories burned off in a 24-hour period from basal metabolism and exercise.

Other components of fitness, called **skill-related components**, are also important for any physically active person. These components deal more with performance in sports and other physical activities than with basic physical health and include speed, power, coordination, balance, and agility.

Speed is the ability to perform a particular movement very rapidly. It is a function of distance and time (Figure 1-6). Speed is an impor-

tant component for successful performance in many competitive athletic situations.

Power is the ability to generate great amounts of force against a certain resistance in a short period (Figure 1-7). Power is a function of both strength and speed. The ability to drive a golf ball, hit a softball, or kick a ball a long distance requires some element of power.

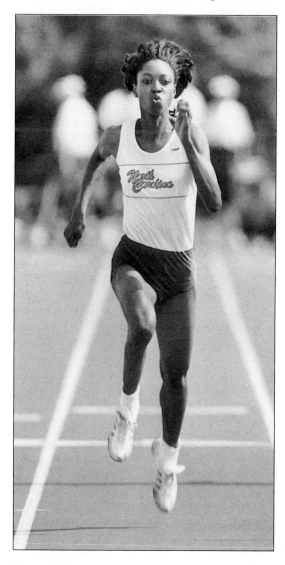

Figure 1-6. Speed.
An important component in many competitive athletic situations.

body composition: the percentage of fat in the body relative to the percentage of all the other tissues

atherosclerosis: a process by which fatty plaques are deposited along arterial walls

caloric intake: the number of calories consumed in the diet

caloric expenditure: the number of calories expended through basal metabolism and exercise

skill-related components: fitness components associated with athletic performance, including speed, power, coordination, balance, and agility

speed: the ability to perform a particular movement very rapidly. It is a function of distance and time

power: the ability to generate great amounts of force against a certain resistance in a short period of time

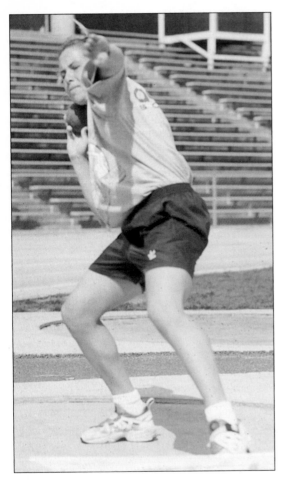

Figure 1-7. Power.
The ability to generate large amounts of force rapidly.

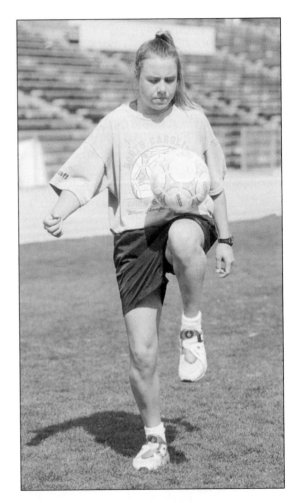

Figure 1-8. Neuromuscular Coordination.
The ability to integrate the senses with motor function to produce coordinated movement.

Coordination is the ability to integrate the senses—visual, auditory, and proprioceptive (knowing the position of your body in space)—with muscle function to produce smooth, accurate, and skilled movement (Figure 1-8).

Balance is the ability to maintain some degree of equilibrium while moving or standing still (Figure 1-9).

Agility is the ability to change or alter—quickly and accurately—the direction of body movement during activity. Agility to a large extent depends on coordination. Agility may

coordination: the ability to integrate the senses with muscle function to produce smooth, accurate, and skilled movement

balance: the ability to maintain some degree of equilibrium while moving or standing still

agility: the ability to change or alter—quickly and accurately—the direction of body movement during activity

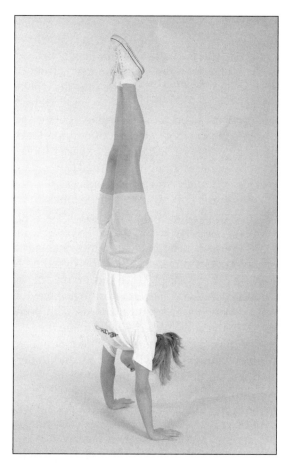

Figure 1-9. Balance.
The ability to maintain equilibrium when moving or stationary.

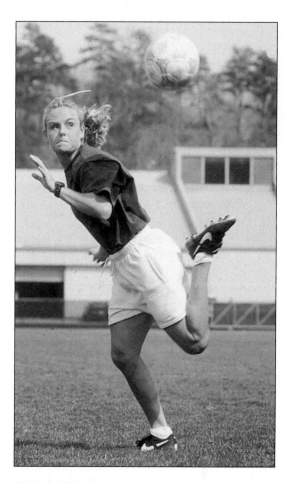

Figure 1-10. Agility.
The ability to change direction of movement quickly and accurately.

be improved with increased flexibility and muscular strength (Figure 1-10).

Reaction time is the time required to produce an appropriate and accurate physiological or mechanical response to some external stimulus.

reaction time: the length of time required to react to a stimulus

DETERMINING YOUR REASONS FOR WANTING TO BE FIT

Perhaps the most important thing that you have learned by this point in your life is that people are different. These differences are evident in all aspects of our being. Certainly, each person has his or her individual reasons for choosing to engage in physical activity. Before you begin your personal fitness program, it may be helpful to determine your personal reasons for wanting to get fit and your present level of activity.

Whatever your motivation for starting an individualized fitness program, you should first consider exactly what it is that you are trying to accomplish. The exercise program you choose should be one that results in the development of the desired fitness component(s). This means that activities selected should be specific to goals. For example, if your goal is increasing stamina or endurance, this may be achieved effectively by engaging in activities such as running, swimming, skating, or cycling—all activities that maximize the use of the circulatory system. Lab Activity 1-1 will help you to determine your individual reasons for wanting to become physically fit.

DETERMINING YOUR PRESENT LEVEL OF PHYSICAL FITNESS

Before you begin any type of fitness program, it is essential for you to establish some baseline information relative to your existing levels of fitness. It is important to appraise your daily schedule regularly to determine if you are devoting the proper amount of time to keeping yourself fit. Lab Activity 1-2 will help you determine your current levels of fitness activity. There is little question that incorporating consistent, regularly scheduled exercise into your lifestyle may be difficult, especially in light of existing demands on your time.

HOW LONG WILL IT TAKE YOU TO GET FIT?

There is no shortcut to fitness; it takes time. You should not expect results in a matter of hours or even days. After a month of appropriate activity on a regular basis, some improvement should be noted, depending on what your physical condition was when you started. After an extended period of gradual improvement, you may reach a plateau at which you experience no improvement but instead seem to stay at the same level of fitness. This is a natural phenomenon. In time, with regular workouts, improvement will occur; after several months, the desired results will be attained. Make a commitment to your fitness program and keep at it; you will feel better, and this will in turn motivate you to continue. Once you have attained a desirable physical fitness level, you will be strongly motivated to maintain this level through regular workouts.

Any physical fitness program requires effort to produce results. Too often, people look for the easy way to achieve their goals. Steam baths, sauna baths, fitness machines, massages, and gimmicks such as body wraps or fad diets may be relaxing or produce short-term effects, but it is necessary to exert effort to achieve the lasting benefits of physical fitness. The body must do the work. You can't sit and be fit!

The purpose of the chapters that follow is to provide you with knowledge about and understanding of the various aspects of fitness. They are designed to show the importance of its essential ingredients. They will explain how you can assess, develop, and maintain your fitness. Finally, they will show you how to plan, develop, and implement a personalized physical activity program based on your individual interests.

SUMMARY

- Being fit means that the various systems of your body are healthy and function efficiently to enable you to engage in activities of daily living, as well as recreational pursuits and leisure activities, without unreasonable fatigue.
- Being physically active produces various physiological, social, and psychological benefits.
- Engaging in regular exercise throughout your lifetime can delay many of the degenerative processes associated with aging.
- Most people should focus on those components of fitness which are concerned with maintaining a healthy lifestyle, in-

cluding cardiorespiratory endurance, muscular strength, muscular endurance, flexibility, and body composition.

- Other components of fitness are more closely related to skill of performance in sports and other physical activities than to good health; such components include speed, power, coordination, balance, agility, and reaction time.
- Before starting a personal training program, it is helpful to examine your attitude toward physical fitness and your reasons for wanting to be physically fit.
- There is no short-cut to becoming physically fit. It requires time, hard work, and determination.

SUGGESTED READINGS

ACSM ©1998. *Fitness Book.* Champaign, IL: Human Kinetics.

Almond, L., and S. McGeorge. 1998. Physical activity and academic performance. *British Journal of Physical Education* 29(2):8–12.

CDC. 1977. Guidelines for school and community programs: promoting lifelong physical activity. CAHPERD Journal/Times 60(2):7–12.

Curtis, J. E., and S. J. Russell, eds. 1997. *Physical activity in human experience: interdisciplinary perspectives.* Champaign, IL: Human Kinetics Publishers.

Greenwood Parr, M., and J. Oslin. 1998. Promoting lifelong involvement through physical activity. Journal of Physical Education, Recreation and Dance 69(2).

Nieman, D.C. ©1998. *The exercise-health connection.* Champaign, IL: Human Kinetics.

Okely, T., J. Patterson, and M. Booth. 1998. Promoting physical activity—rationale and guidelines for promoting physical activity in schools. *Journal of Physical Education—New Zealand* 31(3):3–5.

Pate, R. 1998. Physical activity for young people. *President's Council on Physical Fitness and Sports Research Digest* 3(3):1–6.

President's Council on Physical Fitness and Sports. 1998. Physical activity and aging: implications for health and quality of life in older persons. *President's Council on Physical Fitness and Sports Research Digest* (3/4):1–6.

Taylor, W. C., S. N. Blair, S. S. Cummings, C. C. Wun, and R. M. Malina, 1999. Childhood and adolescent physical activity patterns and adult physical activity. *Medicine and Science in Sports and Exercise* 31(1):118–23.

Weir, A. 1998. Physical activity and health: a literature review. *Sports Exercise and Injury* 4(2/3):97–101.

SUGGESTED WEBSITES

American College of Sports Medicine
ACSM promotes and integrates scientific research, education, and practical applications of sports medicine and exercise science to maintain and enhance physical performance, fitness, health, and quality of life.
http://www.acsm.org

American Council of Exercise
The American Council on Exercise (ACE) is committed to promoting active, healthy lifestyles and their positive effects on the mind, body, and spirit.
http://www.acefitness.org/

FitnessWorld Homepage
This website features health and fitness information for both professionals and enthusiasts.
http://www.fitnessworld.com/

FitnessLink
FitnessLink is a fitness information resource for news, articles, and tips on health, fitness, sport, diet, and exercise, and it provides links to hundreds of quality fitness websites.
http://www.fitnessLink.com

National Institute for Fitness and Sport
NIFS is a nonprofit organization committed to enhancing human health, physical fitness, and athletic performance through research, education, and service.
http://www.nifs.org

Nutrition and Fitness Software by NutriStrategy
This diet and exercise software helps you meet your nutrition and fitness goals. This site features nutrient information, weight training exercises, charts on calories burned during exercise, and facts about the health benefits of physical activity.
http://www.nutristrategy.com

Lab Activity 1-1

Importance of Physical Fitness

Name_____ Section_____ Date_____

PURPOSE   To determine how important it is for you to engage in a physical fitness activity.

PROCEDURE   Determine how important each of the following is to you. Check the appropriate box for each item. Then total your checked responses, multiply by the appropriate weighted factor (1–5), and add together.

Factor	Extremely Important 5	Very Important 4	Important 3	Not So Important 2	Of Little Concern 1
Lose weight	☐	☐	☑	☐	☐
Feel better	☐	☐	☑	☐	☐
Lessen the risk of heart attack	☐	☐	☑	☐	☐
Have a better self-image	☐	☐	☐	☑	☐
Be more successful in sports	☐	☐	☑	☐	☐
Have more strength	☐	☐	☑	☐	☐
Relieve stress	☐	☐	☐	☑	☐
Increase efficiency for study, work, and other responsibilities	☐	☐	☐	☑	☐
Help my sleep pattern	☐	☐	☐	☑	☐
Reduce tension	☐	☐	☐	☑	☐
Increase energy	☐	☐	☑	☐	☐
Have a better looking figure	☐	☐	☑	☐	☐
Contribute to my health	☐	☐	☑	☐	☐
Have a greater resistance to illness and disease	☐	☐	☑	☐	☐
Improve cardiorespiratory function	☐	☐	☑	☐	☐
Increase flexibility	☐	☐	☐	☑	☐
Improve my posture and appearance	☐	☐	☑	☐	☐
Improve my outlook on life	☐	☐	☑	☐	☐
Increase my social outlets	☐	☐	☐	☑	☐
Outlet for frustration/anger	☐	☐	☐	☑	☐
Total	—	—	—	—	—

13

After considering each item, analyze your basic motivation for becoming involved in some fitness activity.

"Extremely important" $\dfrac{}{\text{Total}} \times \dfrac{5}{\text{factor}} = \underline{}$

"Very important" $\dfrac{}{\text{Total}} \times \dfrac{4}{\text{factor}} = \underline{}$

"Important" $\dfrac{}{\text{Total}} \times \dfrac{3}{\text{factor}} = \underline{}$

"Not so important" $\dfrac{}{\text{Total}} \times \dfrac{2}{\text{factor}} = \underline{}$

"Of little concern" $\dfrac{}{\text{Total}} \times \dfrac{1}{\text{factor}} = \underline{}$

Sum Total _____

INTERPRETATION

Total Score

85–100	Physical fitness has extreme importance to you.
70–84	You believe being physically fit is very important.
50–69	Physical fitness is important but not a very high priority.
35–49	You do not believe physical fitness has as much importance in your life as it does for others.
20–34	You are not concerned about being physically fit.

Based on this assessment, to what extent do you believe physical fitness is important?

Lab Activity 1-2

Name _____   Section _____   Date _____

PURPOSE   It is important to regularly appraise your daily schedule to determine if you are devoting the proper amount of time to keeping fit.

PROCEDURE   For this activity, keep a daily record for one week using the form that follows.

	Mon.	Tues.	Wed.	Thurs.	Fri.	Sat.	Sun.
Physical Activity Type of activity							
Duration (min)							
Intensity 3 = High 2 = Moderate 1 = Mild							
Time of Day							
Recreational Activity Type of Activity							
Duration (min)							
Health Requirements (i.e., sleeping, eating) Type of Activity							
Duration (hrs)							

What was the total number of hours that you engaged in physical activity during the week?
_____

Did you choose to engage in the same type of physical activity each day?_____

What was the average length of time that you participated in a physical activity during each session?_____

What was your best estimate of the average intensity of the physical activity during each session?
_____

What was the best time of day for you to engage in physical activity?
_____

Was it at the same time every day?

_____

The American College of Sports Medicine recommends that you engage in physical activity at least 3 times per week at a moderate intensity level for a minimum of 20 minutes per session. Are you meeting these minimal recommendations?_____

If not, how can you change your lifestyle to fit time in in order to meet these recommendations?

_____

_____

_____

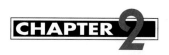
CREATING A
HEALTHY LIFESTYLE

OBJECTIVES

After completing this chapter, you should be able to do the following:

- Discuss the importance of creating a healthy style of living and how fitness fits into this lifestyle.
- Identify risk factors present in your lifestyle that may predispose you to coronary artery disease.
- Explain how unhealthy lifestyle practices may contribute to the development of cancer.
- Discuss the impact of stress on the healthy lifestyle and identify stress management techniques.
- Explain why alcohol, drugs, and tobacco are considered deterrents to fitness.
- Explain how sexually transmitted infections may interfere with a healthy lifestyle.

WHY SHOULD YOU BE CONCERNED ABOUT YOUR LIFESTYLE?

Being physically active is critical to a healthful style of living but is no more important for total well-being than is

Key Terms

stress management

coronary artery disease

cancer

sexually transmitted infections

hyperlipidemia

lipoproteins

coping

relaxation techniques

drug abuse

anabolic steroids

alcoholism

tobacco use

stress

your social, emotional, mental, or spiritual stability. Fitness can affect each of these components in either a positive or a negative manner.

Choosing a healthy lifestyle encourages you to prevent illness by improving your positive well-being in various ways, including (1) developing yourself physically, (2) expressing your emotions effectively, (3) having good relations with those persons around you, (4) being concerned about your decision-making abilities, and finally (5) paying attention to ethics, values, and spirituality. All these aspects of self are interwoven into the fabric of your being. One component affects the others, and you are only as strong as your weakest link. The bottom line in your effort to create a healthy style of living is to achieve a balance between all of the components, with no more emphasis on any single component than on the others.

Those who adhere to this approach believe it is the responsibility of the individual to work toward achieving a healthy lifestyle and thus realize an optimal sense of well-being. A healthy lifestyle should reflect the integration of such components as regular and appropriate physical activity, **stress management**, and elimination of controllable risk factors such as alcohol, smoking, and drug abuse. Unhealthy lifestyles ultimately may be associated with diseases such as **coronary artery disease, cancer,** or **sexually transmitted infections**.

This chapter focuses on various lifestyle choices or practices which potentially interfere with or are deterrents to achieving a healthy lifestyle and, in particular, physical fitness.

stress management: involves techniques that attempt to reduce both the quantity and the quality of stress in your life

coronary artery disease: disease that results from the accumulation of fatty deposits (atherosclerotic plaque) within the coronary arteries

cancer: a collection of abnormal cells that tends to invade and ultimately take over normal tissue

sexually transmitted infections: infectious diseases that can be contracted through sexual contact

HOW CAN YOU PREVENT CORONARY ARTERY DISEASE?

Half of all people who die in the United States each year die of coronary artery disease (CAD). The lifestyle you choose plays a major role in determining whether you develop CAD. Coronary artery disease results from the accumulation of fatty deposits (atherosclerotic plaque) within the coronary arteries (Figure 2-1). The coronary arteries supply blood to the heart muscle, which functions properly only when provided with a steady blood supply. The deposition of fatty plaque often begins early in life, and the continued, gradual deposition of plaque can lead to a significant narrowing of the coronary arteries, or *atherosclerosis*. The partial or complete blockage of one or more of the major coronary arteries can lead to a condition called *myocardial ischemia*, in which the heart muscle fails to receive an adequate supply of oxygen. This can produce symptoms such as chest pain (angina pectoris) and, if severe, can precipitate a heart attack. A heart attack can occur suddenly and without warning. The factors that ultimately lead to a cardiac arrest are present early in life but mostly go undetected until they manifest as a potentially life-threatening heart attack.

Among the cardiovascular diseases, coronary artery disease has the highest incidence of occurrence. Other cardiovascular diseases include hypertension, stroke, congenital heart disease, rheumatic heart disease, peripheral heart disease, and congestive heart failure.

RISK FACTORS

Coronary artery disease is related to personal lifestyle health habits known as **risk factors**. These risk factors cannot be labeled as causes but are instead characteristics that increase the probability of one's having CAD. The risk factors are summarized in the HEALTH LINKS on page 20.

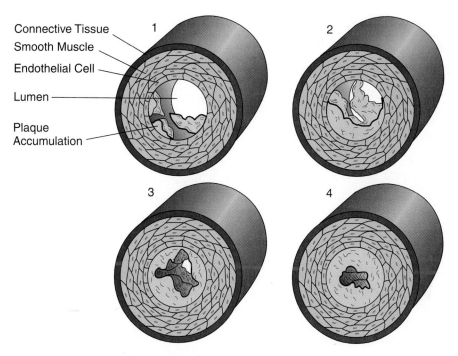

Figure 2-1. The Development of Atherosclerosis.
(1) Normal coronary artery. (2) Beginning stages of atherosclerosis; fatty plaque is deposited in vessel walls. (3) Advanced stage of atherosclerosis. (4) Completely blocked coronary artery.
Modified from Hahn D, Payne W: Focus on health, St Louis, 1991, Mosby.

Risk factors may be divided into those *risk factors* that cannot be changed, *risk ractors* that can be changed, and *contributing risk factors* whose significance and prevalence have yet to be precisely determined. Some of them can be changed, treated, or modified, and some cannot. Each of these risk factors is related to CAD in an additive fashion; the greater the number of risk factors present, the greater the likelihood of developing CAD. Also, each of these factors is, at least in part, a function of individual lifestyles and behavior patterns. This observation holds out hope that it may be possible to prevent premature CAD through modification of the risk factors. With the exception of age, sex, race, and heredity, each of the other risk factors can be altered through lifestyle modification.

▶ Risk Factors that Cannot be Changed

Family History. A history of CAD in the family is considered a predisposing risk factor when parents or siblings experienced evidence of the atherosclerotic disease process before the age of 55 to 60 years.

Age. As age increases, so do the chances of a person's having some type of CAD.

Gender. Males typically exhibit a higher incidence of CAD than females.

Race. African Americans have more severe hypertension than whites.

▶ Risk Factors that Can be Changed

Cigarette smoking. Of all the risk factors listed, perhaps none is as great a risk factor as cigarette smoking. It should be noted that all

Health Link

Risk Factors for Coronary Artery Disease

Risk Factors that Cannot be Changed

Family History
Age
Gender
Race

Risk Factors that Can be Changed

Cigarette smoking
Hypertension
High blood-cholesterol level
Physical inactivity

Contributing Risk Factors

Obesity
Diabetes
Stressful living

cigarette smokers have a much higher risk than nonsmokers. Recently it has also been shown that individuals exposed to second-hand smoke (the smoke from a cigarette that enters the environment) are also at higher risk for coronary artery disease and lung cancer.

Hypertension. Blood pressure is the pressure that the blood exerts against the inner wall of the arteries. Individuals with chronic high blood pressure are three to four times more likely to develop CAD and seven times more likely to develop a stroke than those with normal blood pressure.

High Blood Cholesterol Level. Cholesterol is a fatty substance transported in the bloodstream, and if present in excessive amounts, it adheres to the walls of the arteries. This contributes to the deposition of atherosclerotic plaque. Thus serum cholesterol levels are directly related to the incidence of CAD. The higher the serum cholesterol level, the greater the risk of CAD.

Lipoproteins are carriers of cholesterol. Low-density lipoprotein (LDL) is believed to deposit cholesterol in to the arterial wall, whereas high-density lipoprotein (HDL) seems to be able to remove the cholesterol deposited by LDL from the arterial walls. Thus the more HDL present, the better off you are, because it appears to be an anti-risk factor. Research has shown that individuals who engage in regular physical activity can increase HDL levels.

Physical Inactivity. Those individuals who lead a relatively sedentary style of living are more likely to suffer from CAD and are less likely to survive a heart attack than are those who maintain an active lifestyle. Recent evidence indicates that individuals who expend a minimum of 2000 calories of energy a week in physical activity, significantly reduce death rates from heart disease when compared with those who do not exercise.

▶ Contributing Risk Factors

Obesity. Obesity is related to CAD only in that people who are obese tend to have higher blood pressures as well as **hyperlipidemia**. Also, obese individuals are more likely to develop a form of diabetes. Obesity reduces the ability to engage in exercise, thus impacting on another risk factor—physical inactivity. All of these are risk factors for CAD.

Diabetes. Diabetes that has an onset in adulthood produces abnormalities in lipoproteins, which seems to accelerate atherosclerosis. Also, diabetics frequently have a weight problem which places additional stress on the cardiovascular system.

hyperlipidemia: an excessively high level of fat in the blood.

lipoproteins: a compound of fat and protein that carries cholesterol.

stress: the responses that occur in the body when the internal balance or equilibrium of the body systems is disrupted

Health Link

American Cancer Society's Cancer Warning Signals

Change in bowel or bladder habits
A sore that does not heal
Unusual bleeding or discharge
Thickening or lump in breast or elsewhere
Indigestion or difficulty in swallowing
Obvious change in wart or mole
Nagging cough or hoarseness

Modified from the American Cancer Society, *Cancer facts and figures*, New York, 1989, The Society.

Stressful Living. **Stress** increases blood pressure thus forcing the heart to work harder.

EFFECTS OF EXERCISE AND DIET ON RISK FACTORS

As physical activity levels increase, the number of deaths attributed to CAD decrease. These findings are consistent for both men and women. Even moderate levels of physical fitness that are attainable by most adults appear to provide some protection against early death.

Like exercise, diet can affect many of the risk factors identified. There is little doubt that adopting a healthful style of living, which incorporates good exercise and dietary habits, has the greatest influence in reducing the incidence of CAD.

WHAT IS CANCER?

Cancer is the second leading cause of death in adults, falling behind coronary artery disease. Cancer is a condition in which cellular behavior becomes abnormal. The cells no longer perform their normal functions. In general, cancer cells do not multiply at an increased rate. Instead, whatever causes the cancer alters the cell's genetic makeup and changes the way the cell functions. This abnormal cell then divides, forming additional cancer cells, and over a period of time this tumor, or collection of abnormal cells, tends to invade and ultimately take over normal tissue.

Tumors are either benign or malignant. Benign tumors typically pose only a small threat to tissue and tend to remain confined in a limited space. Malignant tumors, however, are cancerous, grow out of control, and spread within a specific tissue. Unfortunately, malignancies can invade surrounding tissues and spread via the blood and lymphatic systems (metastasize) throughout the entire body, thus making it difficult to control the cancer.

Malignancies are classified according to the types of tissues in which they occur as well as according to the rate at which they affect the tissue. Although different types of cancer cells share similar characteristics, each is separate and distinct. Some types are relatively easy to cure, whereas others are difficult to cure and even life threatening. Skin cancer is the most common type of cancer; fortunately, it is one of the easiest to detect and cure.

Males and females have a different incidence in other types of cancers. In the male, the highest incidence of cancer is in the prostate, followed closely by lung, colon/rectal, and urinary tract cancers and leukemias/lymphomas. In the female the highest incidence is found in the breast, followed by colon/rectal, lung, and uterine cancers and leukemias/lymphomas.

The precise causes of cancer are not easily identified. Researchers have identified more than 100 types of cancer with genetic origins. Certain cancers appear to occur along family lines. The onset of most cancer has also been attributed to certain environmental factors, including viruses, exposure to ultraviolet light, radiation, alcohol use, and certain chemicals, including tobacco. A fatty diet has also been linked to cancer. Probably a combination of heredity and environmental factors is responsible for the development of cancer.

The American Cancer Society has identified warning signs of cancer, which are listed in the Health Link box above. Unquestionably, early detection and treatment of cancer markedly improve the patient's chances of beating the disease.

EFFECTS OF EXERCISE AND DIET ON CANCER

Physical activity has been associated with a reduced risk of certain types of cancer. Moderate exercise has been shown to produce certain enzymes that reduce the formation of free radicals formed with incomplete oxidation of nutrients. These free radicals enhance the risk of chronic illnesses including cancer. However, some researchers are concerned that excessive exercise may potentially reduce the body's ability to produce these enzymes, thus increasing the chances of free radical-based cellular changes, including cancer.

Eating a healthy diet also has the potential to reduce the risk of cancer. The American Cancer Society recommends the following dietary precautions:

- Reduce total fat intake
- Eat more high-fiber foods
- Eat foods rich in Vitamins A and C
- Include vegetables in your diet (broccoli, brussels sprouts)
- Avoid smoked, salt-cured foods
- Limit alcohol consumption
- Avoid obesity

WHAT IS THE EFFECT OF STRESS ON A HEALTHY LIFESTYLE?

It is important for the health-conscious, physically active individual to understand the potential effect of stress on the body. Stress has been linked to many diseases. It may also interfere with performance of daily tasks or the attainment of one's goals. Most importantly, poorly managed stress greatly reduces the quality of one's life.

The term stress comes from the Latin word stringere, meaning "to draw tight." The term refers to the responses that occur in the body as a result of what is called a stressor, or stimulus. Stress occurs when the internal balance or equilibrium of the body systems is disrupted.

Everyone experiences stress, and some stress is needed to perform the daily tasks of life and, more importantly, to stimulate growth and development. Stress can be beneficial. However, too much stress, especially when it exists for a prolonged period and is unrelieved, can result in physical and mental illness. Stress is caused or triggered by stressors that may be physical, social, or psychological and negative or positive in nature. Human reactions to positive stressors are called eustress; that is, stress that is beneficial. The term distress describes detrimental responses or negative stressors. Often, only a fine line distinguishes whether a situation or action causes eustress or distress. For example, moderate physical training is a stressor that can make you stronger and more fit. However, if you do too much too soon, it can produce distress in the form of soreness or injury.

Sometimes the difference between eustress and distress is only a matter of interpretation; do you interpret the stressor as a threat or a challenge? Although we may habitually respond in ways that seem automatic and beyond our control, we can choose to examine the way we think and then work on changing counterproductive thinking or beliefs.

Stress should not, however, be considered solely a physiological phenomenon. Stress has also been viewed from a psychological or cognitive perspective. Current research suggests that the stress response is not a simple biological response. It is an interrelated process that includes the presence of a stressor, the circumstances in which the stressor occurs, the interpretation of the situation by the person, that person's typical reaction, and the resources the person has available to deal with the stressor.

For example, some people may find downhill skiing fun and exciting. They look forward to taking winter vacations to ski the slopes.

Other people may have tried to ski, but their dislike of cold weather and fear of injury make skiing a distressing activity. Therefore the stress response in a given situation depends on the individual's perceptions. Individuals under stress usually exhibit certain warning signs and symptoms that may vary from person to person. The Health Link box to the right lists the potential signs of stress.

THE PSYCHOLOGICAL OR COGNITIVE RESPONSE TO STRESS

Once the stress process is initiated by the presence of a stressor, psychological or thought processes that determine how the stressor is perceived take over. An individual's perceptions of a particular situation can cause a response that may vary from arousal to anxiety. The degree to which a particular situation elicits an emotional response depends greatly on how the individual views the situation and how well prepared he or she feels to handle the situation.

THE PHYSIOLOGICAL RESPONSE TO STRESS

Every organ system in the body is affected by the stress response. The physiological response to stress follows a three-stage pattern of alarm, resistance, and exhaustion. There are two regulatory systems in the body that govern the stress response: the nervous system and the endocrine system. Differences between the nervous and endocrine systems are found in terms of how quickly they respond to a stressor and how long their responses are sustained. The endocrine system secretes hormones that prepare the body to deal with a stressful situation. These hormones may remain in the bloodstream for several weeks. The endocrine system's response to stress endures, whereas the nervous system's response is short-lived. This suggests that the endocrine system is more important to inves-

Health Link

Signs of Stress

Irritability and depression
Heart palpitations
Dryness of throat and mouth
Impulsive behavior
Inability to concentrate
Feelings of weakness or dizziness
Crying
Anxiety
Emotional tension
Nervous tics
Vomiting
Easily startled by small sounds
Nervous laughter
Trembling hands
Stuttering or other speech problems
Insomnia
Breathlessness
Sweating
Frequent urination
Diarrhea and indigestion
Migraine headaches
Premenstrual tension or missed menstrual cycles
Pain in back
Increased smoking
Loss of appetite
Nightmares
Fatigue

Information from Selye H: The stress of life, New York, 1976, McGraw-Hill.

tigate for any connection between stress and disease.

During the alarm stage, the body undergoes physiological changes that are collectively referred to as the fight-or-flight syndrome (e.g., increased heart rate, blood pressure, respiratory rate). These physiological changes are primarily a nervous system response to prepare the body for vigorous muscular action. In the resistance stage, the body adjusts to stress and appears to return to its normal state of internal balance. If stress persists for a long time, exhaustion sets in. The person becomes less able to resist stress. Sustained stress can affect various body systems so that illness and even death may result.

▶ Exercise and Stress Reduction

Engaging in physical activity is widely used as a means for reducing or alleviating stress. Many people who exercise report the feeling of a "high" both during and immediately following exercise. This euphoric feeling may be attributed to the release of opiate-like chemicals called endorphins in the brain. Consistent exercise also lowers both resting blood pressure and cholesterol, both of which can help to minimize the insidious damage caused by stress.

PERSONALITY AND STRESS

In identifying people who are at risk for developing cardiovascular disease, researchers believed that there was a connection between behavior pattern and risk of heart disease. People were classified as being either "type A" or "type B" personalities. The type A person is always "on the go," never satisfied with his or her level of achievement, appears tense, suffers from a sense of time urgency, and is competitive and impatient. In contrast, the type B person is more easy-going and relaxed, more patient, and satisfied with his or her level of achievement. The type A person was believed to have a higher risk of developing cardiovascular disease. However, recent research suggests that only those individuals who have hostile or angry behavior patterns are at risk. Therefore, identifying the sources of anger and hostility in these people and helping them with behavior modification may allow them to cope more effectively with stress.

COPING WITH STRESS AND STRESS MANAGEMENT

Life is filled with many challenges, some of which represent potential obstacles in the path of your career and life goals. **Coping** is an attempt to effectively manage or control stress so that it does not dominate your life. By coping with stress, you use techniques that alter the physiological and psychological consequences of stress. Some of these methods show short-term usefulness but are ultimately harmful because the source of the stress has not been properly handled. Examples of negative or harmful ways of coping with stressful situations include overeating or starvation or increasing consumption of alcohol, tobacco, or caffeine.

Other people cope by employing various defense mechanisms, which serve to protect the ego. These mechanisms preserve harmony within a person and provide some sense of adequacy. For example, a commonly used defense mechanism is projecting blame for failure on someone or something else. Defense mechanisms are not necessarily the most effective way to deal with stress. They may bolster the ego, but they can also circumvent managing real problems.

Various methods of coping are beneficial because they allow people to achieve self-fulfillment. People learn to manage conflicts, sources of pressure, and frustration without experiencing harm to their bodies.

It is important for you to develop and incorporate into your lifestyle any techniques that will help you effectively reduce stress. The Fit List on page 25 identifies some general guidelines for reducing stress. Lab Activity 2-1 will help you become more aware of your response to stress and how you cope with stress.

> **coping:** an attempt to effectively manage or control stress by using techniques that alter the physiological and psychological consequences of stress

Fit List

General Guidelines for Stress Reduction

- Try not to be a perfectionist. Instead, perform and work within your capabilities.
- Spend your time in ways other than trying to befriend those persons who don't want to experience your love and friendship.
- Enjoy the simple things of life.
- Strive and fight only for those things that are really worthwhile.
- Accent the positive and the pleasant side of life.
- On experiencing a defeat or setback, maintain your self-confidence by remembering past accomplishments and successes.
- Do not delay tackling the unpleasant tasks that must be done; instead, get at them immediately.
- Evaluate people's progress on the basis of their performance.
- Recognize that leaders, to be leaders, must have the respect of their followers.
- Adopt a motto that you will live in a way that will earn your neighbor's love.
- Try to live so that your existence will be useful to society.
- Clarify your values.
- Take constructive action to eliminate a source of stress.

Other Suggestions

- Maintain good physical and mental health.
- Accept what you cannot change.
- Serve other people and some worthy cause.
- Share worries with someone you can trust.
- Pay attention to your body.
- Balance work and recreation.
- Improve your qualifications for the realistic goals you aspire to.
- Avoid reliance on things such as drugs and alcohol.
- Don't be narcissistic.
- Manage your time effectively.
- Laugh at yourself.
- Get enough rest and sleep.
- Don't be too hard on yourself.
- Improve your self-esteem.

Information from Selye H: The stress of life, New York, 1976, McGraw-Hill, and Selye H: Stress without distress, New York, 1974, Signet.

Stress management involves more than simply reducing the total quantity of stress in your life; it also means being able to change the quality of stress in your life. Uncontrolled stress can result in physical and psychological disorders that pose a real threat to well-being. To manage stress effectively you must realize that you are responsible for your own emotional and physical well-being. Your perception of events (but not the events themselves) is under your control. You do not need to allow other people's behavior to affect your ability to maintain a relatively stable emotional and physical condition. Besides using physical activity, learning to control thought processes can be an effective method of managing stress. Collectively referred to as relaxation techniques, these methods have been demonstrated to be helpful.

► **Relaxation Techniques**

Relaxation is essentially a mental phenomenon concerned with the reduction of tensions that could originate from muscular activity but are more likely to result from psychological responses to our hectic lifestyles. **Relaxation techniques** may be broadly classified as either muscle-to-mind techniques, which control the level of stimulation going to the brain from the muscles (progressive relaxation, massage, and biofeedback), or mind-to-muscle techniques, which control the level of stimulation along the nerve pathways coming from the brain to the muscles (yoga, meditation, imagery, and autogenic training). The Fit List to the right summarizes these relaxation techniques.

Progressive Relaxation. Progressive relaxation involves alternately tensing (5 to 10

relaxation techniques: techniques for reducing tensions that could originate from muscular activity but are more likely to result from psychological responses to hectic lifestyles

Fit List

Relaxation Techniques

Muscle-to-mind techniques

- Progressive relaxation
- Massage
- Biofeedback

Mind-to-muscle techniques

- Yoga
- Meditation
- Imagery
- Autogenic training

seconds) and relaxing (45 seconds) the muscles, moving through the body in a systematic fashion to tense and relax all major muscle groups. Concentrate first on the large muscle groups in the arms, legs, trunk, and neck. Then ease tension in the forehead, eyes, face, and even the throat through a program of progressive relaxation. The program teaches the person to relax his or her whole body to the point of negative exertion. The result is a release of tension, which is an antidote to fatigue; the result is also an inducement to sleep.

Massage. Massage can be useful as a stress-reducing technique, as it induces relaxation. You can massage your neck, face, head, and shoulders, or massage also can be done by another person. To many, touch is a useful form of nonverbal communication and can be reassuring.

Biofeedback. Biofeedback is a common form of stress management and relaxation therapy. Its main goals are to teach concentration, relaxation, awareness, and self-control. A machine monitors various body functions and relays the information to the subject in the form of either sounds or lights. Biofeedback helps people to become aware of tensions they had not previously perceived and learn to reduce them, eventually without relying on the monitoring machines.

Yoga. Yoga uses several positions for the body through which the practitioner may progress, beginning with the simplest and moving to the more complex. The purpose of the various positions is to increase mobility and flexibility of the body. Slow, deep, diaphragmatic breathing can help in alleviating stress and also help to lower blood pressure and heart rate. Deep breathing has a calming effect on the body. It also increases production of endorphins, the body's own natural, morphinelike pain-killing substances.

Meditation. Meditation uses mental-focusing exercises to control or concentrate one's attention. In most forms, meditation involves sitting quietly for a certain period, usually 15 to 20 minutes, and concentrating on a single word or image while breathing slowly and rhythmically to produce decreases in respiratory rate, heart rate, blood pressure, and muscle tension.

Imagery. Imagery can be used as a means of relaxation to cope with stressful situations. Images are pictures formed within the mind. The procedure is to sit relaxed, close your eyes, and concentrate on a particular image. With practice, you can learn to project your own body image into this picture and ultimately to perform various tasks within the mind, learning to cope with all possible variations of a situation that may be stress-producing before confronting the situation in real life.

Autogenic Training (Hypnosis). Autogenic training involves a series of specific exercises and autohypnosis that are designed to achieve a deep mental and physical state of relaxation.

WHAT LIFESTYLE HABITS ARE DETERRENTS TO FITNESS?

Physical fitness involves more than exercise. To be physically fit means that a person must develop lifestyle habits that exclude negative practices such as drinking excessive amounts of alcohol, abusing other drugs, and smoking.

DRUG ABUSE

Drug abuse differs from drug use and drug misuse. Drug use refers to the taking of any drug for medical purposes. Drug misuse refers to the irresponsibility that many individuals show in the use of drugs. People who ignore medical advice about proper use of a prescribed drug or lend prescriptions to others are displaying a misuse of drugs. Drug abuse may be defined as the use of drugs for nonmedical reasons; that is, with the intent of getting "high"—altering mood or behavior.

After time, the body builds a tolerance to the usual level of certain drugs. Therefore, after abusing one of these drugs for a certain period, a person no longer gets the same "high" unless the dosage is increased. This is one reason that chronic drug abusers continually need to increase their number of "fixes" or doses of a drug.

Habituation is defined as psychological dependence as a result of continued use. People can be habituated to the use of alcohol, cigarettes, or drugs. They can become habituated to almost anything if they feel that it is helping them. In other words, drug abuse can become a habit if the individual feels psychologically that it is helping him or her in some way.

The term addiction means physical dependence. An addicted individual's body (1) needs a drug to function, (2) builds a tolerance to that drug, and (3) in most cases suffers from withdrawal symptoms. Withdrawal symptoms are the unpleasant physical problems that occur when the drug is taken away.

drug abuse: the use of drugs for nonmedical reasons; that is, with the intent of getting "high"—altering mood or behavior

Drugs are most commonly abused because of their effects on mood and behavior. For example, a drug may produce a feeling of euphoria, often called a "high." These drugs are often referred to as psychoactive or psychotropic drugs. However, certain drugs, when abused, can distort the personality to such a degree that the individual may become dangerous to self or society. Research has indicated that most individuals who abuse psychoactive drugs have the type of personality that is often impressionable, escapist, or fragile. Persons with stronger personalities may experiment with drugs but are less likely to become dependent on them because the drugs do not satisfy their needs.

▶ Recreational Drugs

Obviously, there are many drugs of abuse in our society. Among the more common "recreational" drugs are marijuana and cocaine.

Marijuana. When used in small doses, marijuana produces a "high" feeling and sense of relaxation lasting for several hours after use. The immediate effects of use are relaxation and feelings of heightened awareness of visual, auditory, and tactile sensations. It also causes impairment of coordination, performance, perception, attention, and short-term memory. Problems associated with long-term use include restlessness, irritability, loss of motivation, sleep disturbances, and possible damage to the lungs.

Cocaine. Cocaine has become one of the most popular drugs of abuse during recent years. Cocaine is a stimulant with effects of short duration. Cocaine use produces immediate feelings of euphoria, excitement, decreased sense of fatigue, and heightened sexual drive. Cocaine may be snorted, taken intravenously, or smoked ("free-based"). Crack is a rocklike crystalline form of cocaine that is heated in a small pipe and then inhaled, producing an immediate rush. The initial effects are extremely intense, and because they are pleasurable, strong psychological dependence is developed rapidly by users, regardless of whether they can afford this expensive habit.

Long-term effects include nasal congestion and damage to the membranes and cartilage of the nose if snorted, bronchitis, loss of appetite leading to nutritional deficiencies, convulsions, impotence, and cocaine psychosis with paranoia, depression, hallucinations, and disorganized mental function. An overdose can cause abnormal heart rhythms, which can result in death.

▶ Anabolic Steroids

The unfortunate use of anabolic steroids by persons attempting to develop high levels of strength is becoming commonplace (strength training itself is discussed in Chapter 5). **Anabolic steroids** are organic compounds that contain primarily sterols and sex hormones (testosterone). These drugs are prescribed and used therapeutically in the treatment of diseases in which protein synthesis is an essential component of the healing process. Athletes use the drug for increasing lean body weight, muscle mass, and strength. Often these drugs are obtained by body builders through mail order advertisements in magazines or through illegal channels.

Considerable research has taken place in this area, and results are at best conflicting. Anabolic steroids do increase muscle size and strength when taken in conjunction with an intense weight-training program over a period of 1 to 2 months. However, it has also been proposed that prolonged use of anabolic steroids may result in harmful side effects

anabolic steroids: organic compounds that primarily contain sterols and sex hormones and are used for increasing lean body weight, muscle mass, and strength

such as liver dysfunction and cancer, sterility, reduced testicular function and loss of sexual interest, headaches, nausea, acne, baldness, unpredictable aggressive behavior, increased blood pressure and risk of coronary heart disease, kidney tumors, and so on. For this reason, using anabolic steroids for the purpose of strength improvement cannot be recommended and has in fact been banned by the International Olympic Committee.

Despite the uncertainty about the long-range effects of these drugs, anabolic steroid use is a continuing problem affecting many persons involved with heavy weight training at all levels.

ALCOHOL ABUSE

The consumption of alcohol in our American society is commonplace. The reasons that some people abstain, drink moderately, or imbibe heavily have never been completely answered. The studies seem to indicate that alcohol serves to meet individual need patterns. It is felt that situations and environmental conditions that produce tension and insecurity may cause some to resort to drinking.

People who are uncomfortable and lack poise at social gatherings use drinking as a social lubricant. The alcohol gives them courage and helps them feel at ease. Unfortunately, some people have failed to develop wholesome interpersonal relationships. Alcohol provides a temporary means of escape from those experiences that frustrate and worry them. Drinking does not solve the problem but instead offers a temporary means of escape from reality. Although there are some conflicting views as to its cause, there appears to be agreement that some of the causes are psychological. Some psychologists believe that individuals who are emotionally disturbed, have compulsive personalities, or exhibit obsessive-compulsive behavior are more prone to alcoholism.

▶ What Is Alcoholism

Alcoholism is called a disease because an alcoholic is sick, totally dependent on the substance and the abuse of it. The National Council on Alcoholism defines an alcoholic as "a person who is powerless to stop drinking, and whose drinking seriously alters his normal living pattern." Many persons may ask, "Why do some people become alcoholics while others in the same situation or environment do not?" Why is it that only 10 to 15 percent of the more than 100 million drinkers become alcoholics? These are valid questions for which there are no absolute answers. There are many potential alcoholics who do not become alcoholics. Unfortunately, alcoholism is a chronic condition that does not go away. It is progressive and incurable as long as the alcoholic keeps on drinking. If he or she stops drinking, the disease can be arrested. But most experts believe that the alcoholic cannot drink again. Otherwise that person will be right back where he or she was when the decision was made to stop drinking. Alcoholics are sensitive to alcohol and all other sedatives. The brain of an alcoholic produces a substance called THIQ, which is extremely addicting. Years of abstinence will not eliminate the ability to produce THIQ. It is always present and renders the alcoholic powerless to quit once he or she begins drinking.

▶ What Are the Effects of Alcohol?

Alcohol is classified as a drug that depresses the central nervous system. Alcohol is absorbed from the digestive system into the bloodstream very rapidly. Factors that affect how rapidly absorption takes place include the number of drinks consumed, the rate of consumption,

alcoholism: a disease in which a person is powerless to stop drinking and drinking seriously alters his or her normal living pattern

alcohol concentration of the beverage, and the amount of food in the stomach. Some alcohol is absorbed into the blood through the stomach, but the greater part is absorbed through the small intestine. Alcohol is transported through the blood to the liver, where it can be metabolized at a rate of 2/3 ounce per hour. An excess causes an increase in the level of alcohol circulating in the blood. As blood alcohol content (BAC) levels continue to increase, predictable signs of intoxication appear. At 0.1 percent the person loses motor coordination, and from 0.2 to 0.5 percent the symptoms become progressively more profound and perhaps even life threatening. Intoxication persists until the remainder of the alcohol can be metabolized by the liver. There is no way to accelerate the liver's metabolism of alcohol ("sober-up"); it just takes time.

▶ Alcohol Related Diseases

Alcohol consumption can directly or indirectly cause numerous physical problems. Gastritis, an inflammation of the stomach, can result from excessive alcohol consumption. Alcoholics suffer from malnutrition because they lose interest in food and are unable to purchase proper foods. Also, alcohol provides considerable calories but lacks important nutrients.

Alcohol is poisonous to cells. The most common cause of liver disorders, cirrhosis (a scarring and hardening of liver tissue), is a result of chronic alcoholism. Over the years there has been some linkage of alcohol to cancer, especially cancer of the liver, larynx, esophagus, and tongue. These represent only a few of the diseases caused when excessive amounts of alcohol are consumed for extended periods of time.

How can you tell whether you currently have or are developing a drinking problem? You must identify the warning signs that let you know that the potential for such a problem exists. The Health Link Box following will give you some idea of the warning signs.

Health Link

Warning Signs for Excessive Alcohol Use

Do you:
- Drink more frequently than you did a year ago?
- Drink more heavily than you did a year ago?
- Plan to drink, sometimes days in advance?
- Gulp or "chug" your drinks, perhaps in a contest?
- Set personal limits on the amount you plan to drink but then consistently disregard these limits?
- Drink at a rate greater than two drinks per hour?
- Encourage or even pressure others to drink with you?
- Frequently want a nonalcoholic beverage but then end up drinking an alcoholic drink?
- Drive your car while under the influence of alcohol or ride with another person who has been drinking?
- Use alcoholic beverages while taking prescription or over-the-counter medications?
- Forget what happened while you were drinking?
- Have a tendency to disregard information about the effects of drinking?
- Find your reputation fading because of alcohol use?

TOBACCO USE

The number of deaths caused by **tobacco use** is alarming, and the impact of tobacco use on health care cost is almost mind-boggling. The United States government is currently waging an all-out war against tobacco. Over the years many steps have been taken to educate the nation's 53 million smokers about the dangers of tobacco. Yet millions of Americans continue to smoke.

▶ Why Do People Smoke?

The pleasure derived from smoking may be due as much to the social ritual that is associated with it as to the physiologic effects. Certainly, many young people who begin to smoke do so because they regard it as symbolic of adulthood. It has been suggested that the habit-forming nature of tobacco is to a large extent psychologically and socially determined. As millions of smokers know, smoking is a habit that becomes more difficult to break the more and the longer one smokes. It is known that nicotine is physically addictive. Although a smoker does not suffer the harsh withdrawal symptoms typical of certain addictive drugs, nervousness and irritability are commonly experienced when smoking is stopped.

▶ What Is In Tobacco Smoke?

The major components of tobacco smoke are carbon monoxide, nicotine, and tars, all of which have harmful effects on the body. The more deeply the smoker inhales and the shorter the length to which the cigarette is smoked, the more nicotine is absorbed.

Nicotine. Nicotine, a colorless, oily compound, is extremely poisonous in concentrated form. Nicotine affects the body in a variety of

ways. Small doses have a stimulating effect upon various brain centers. It constricts the blood vessels of the skin, resulting in a clammy, pallid appearance and a reduction of skin temperature. Nicotine also increases the blood pressure and the heart rate. It has a numbing effect on the taste receptors of the tongue, hence the loss of interest in food by many heavy smokers. Beginning smokers may experience some slight toxic effects such as nausea and vomiting, but, as the smoker builds up a tolerance, these generally disappear.

Carbon Monoxide. Approximately 1 percent of cigarette smoke is composed of carbon monoxide. A highly poisonous gas, carbon monoxide is also a component of automobile exhaust. Many individuals are killed each year by the inhalation of this gas in closed areas such as garages. The carbon monoxide in cigarette smoke reduces the oxygen carrying capacity of the red blood cells and therefore causes a reduction of oxygen in the body. This is one of the reasons why smokers complain of "shortness of breath" after mild exercise.

Tar. Tobacco tar is a dark, sticky substance that can be condensed from cigarette smoke. It is the substance discussed in advertisements concerning "low tar and nicotine." Tar is extremely toxic and is carcinogenic (causing cancerous lesions) on test animals. The chemicals in cigarette tar are believed to contribute to the development of lung cancer.

▶ Passive Smoke

There are dangers associated with the passive inhalation of smoke ("second hand") by nonsmokers. Both smokers and nonsmokers are exposed to smoke containing carbon monoxide, nicotine, ammonia, and cyanide. Obviously smokers inhale the greater quantity of contaminated air. However, it has been estimated that for each pack of cigarettes smoked, the nonsmoker, sharing a common air supply, will inhale the equivalent of three to five cigarettes. According to a review of passive smoking research, passive smoking may be responsible for as many as 15,000 premature deaths among exposed nonsmokers. It is also true that significant numbers of individuals exposed to passive smoke develop nasal symptoms, eye irritation, headaches, cough, and in some cases allergies to smoke. For these reasons and others, many state, local, and private sector policies have been established that restrict or ban smoking in public areas. There is little doubt that passive smoking poses a significant health threat to the nonsmoker.

▶ Smokeless Tobacco

Unfortunately, the use of smokeless chewing tobacco has seen a tremendous increase in recent years. Once a pinch or pouch of chewing tobacco is placed "between the cheek and gum," nicotine is absorbed through the mucous membranes, and within a short period of time the level of nicotine in the blood is equivalent to that of a cigarette smoker. The user of chewing tobacco experiences the nicotine effects without exposure to the tar and carbon monoxide associated with a burning cigarette. Certainly the use of smokeless tobacco has eliminated many of the risks associated with cigarette smoking. However, inadvertently swallowed saliva contains carcinogens that must be eliminated through the digestive and urinary systems, thus predisposing the user to the risks of cancer. Additionally, the use of chewing tobacco increases the risk of periodontal disease in the gums, destroys the enamel on teeth, and causes the development of white blotches on the mucous membranes of the mouth, which are thought to be associated with development of cancer in the mouth.

▶ Curbing the Use of Tobacco

Many steps have been taken to caution the nation's 53 million smokers about the dangers of tobacco. A warning from the U.S. Surgeon General is printed on each package of cigarettes. Television commercials for cigarettes have been banned. Group therapy sessions have been organized to help people stop smoking. Patches that deliver nicotine through the skin are often prescribed along with group sessions to help smokers "kick the habit." Special cigarette holders and filter tips have been devised to cut down on tar and nicotine. Many public buildings have been designated as nonsmoking areas. Municipalities are acting to ban smoking altogether in public places. In many states it is illegal to sell tobacco products to individuals under 18 years of age. Yet millions of Americans, including many college students, continue to smoke. Many adults belong to the hard core group of smokers who will never quit the habit. However, a major focus is educational efforts to prevent young people from choosing to begin to smoke.

WHAT ARE THE EFFECTS OF SEXUALLY TRANSMITTED INFECTIONS?

Sexually transmitted infections (STIs) are infectious diseases that are contracted through sexual contact. Any of the STIs can be transmitted through sexual contact (including vaginal and anal intercourse and oral-genital contact) with an infected partner who may or may not show any signs or symptoms. STIs may be caused by bacteria or viruses. Bacterial infections such as gonorrhea, syphilis, and chlamydia can be cured in most cases with antibiotics. Serious health problems are prevented if these infections are diagnosed and treated early. Unfortunately, viral infections causing herpes, genital warts, and human immunodeficiency virus (HIV) are much more difficult to treat. In some cases, no cure exists for these viral infections. Most importantly, some of these diseases have the potential to cause serious, long-term health problems and even death.

The current trend is to emphasize prevention through "safe sex" practices and treatment of STIs rather than to focus on the ethics of sexual behavior. The Safe Tip following provides some guidelines for practicing "safe sex."

Safe Tip

Precautions for "Safe" Sex

- Form a monogamous relationship and learn to communicate effectively with your partner.
- Use latex condoms.
- Learn the common symptoms of STIs.
- Include STI testing as part of your regular medical examination.
- Never mix alcohol and drugs with sexual activity.
- Choose lower risk sexual activities.

Modified from the American College Health Association: What are sexually transmitted diseases? Rockville, MD, 1988, The Association.

The American College Health Association states the following:

Everyone who is sexually active can get or transmit an STI. It does not matter if you are rich or poor, gay or straight. It is not who you are that makes you vulnerable to a sexually transmitted infection—it is what you do. Reduce your risk by protecting yourself.

Practicing safer sex may help you to avoid contracting an STI.

HIV

Some special consideration must be given to the human immunodeficiency virus (HIV). HIV is a virus that can be transmitted from person to person through contact with different body fluids (i.e., blood, semen, vaginal fluid). Within approximately 6 weeks of exposure to the virus, antibodies to HIV can be detected through a blood test. Unfortunately, in some cases the symptoms do not become evident for up to 10 years after exposure. AIDS is a disease caused by the human immunodeficiency virus. AIDS is an acronym for acquired immunodeficiency syndrome. A syndrome is a collection of signs and symptoms that are recognized as the effects of an infection. HIV destroys a person's immune system so it cannot battle other infections. A person who has AIDS has no protection against even the simplest infections and thus is extremely vulnerable to developing various illnesses, even cancers that cannot be stopped. Tests that detect the presence of HIV cannot predict when or if the individual will show the symptoms of AIDS. About 50 percent of those infected develop AIDS within 10 years of becoming infected. Those individuals who develop AIDS generally die within 2 years after the symptoms appear.

It has been estimated that one in 250 people in the United States is infected with HIV. Approximately one of every 100 adult males between the ages of 20 and 49 is HIV positive. Estimates suggest that 650,000 to 900,000 Americans are now living with HIV, and at least 40,000 new infections occur each year. According to the Centers for Disease Control, as of December 1997, 641,086 Americans have been reported with AIDS. At least 385,000 of them have died. In 1996, an estimated 242,000 people were living with AIDS, an increase of almost 12 percent over 1995. The World Health Organization estimates that worldwide there are 10 to 12 million adult carriers of the virus with 40 million estimated by the year 2000.

Even though some drug therapy may extend patients' lives, there is currently no available treatment to cure those with AIDS. Much work is being done to find a preventive vaccine and an effective treatment. Presently, antiviral drugs such as azidothymidine (AZT) have slowed replication of the virus and improved survival prospects.

Initially, symptoms of AIDS are similar to those of the flu: night sweats, fevers, chills, excessive tiredness, sore throat, and persistent cough. The person may become free of symptoms for a while, but many instead proceed to develop full-blown AIDS. With AIDS, the individual develops various life-threatening infections; most patients die within a few years.

HIV is transmitted by intimate sexual contact or by exposure to infected blood or other body fluids. You cannot get the virus simply by being around someone or touching someone infected with HIV. The virus enters the body through damaged skin or membranes. You can dramatically reduce your chances of contracting HIV by making careful choices about sexual activity, such as by knowing your sexual partner, using condoms during any type of sexual contact, avoiding injury to body tissues that results in bleeding during sex, and not mixing alcohol or drugs with sex. Drugs tend to cloud your judgment about sexual behavior. Also, avoid contact with the blood of others, and do not abuse intravenous (IV) drugs, since the other dominant way this virus is spread is through the sharing of IV drug needles by addicts.

CREATING A HEALTHY LIFESTYLE: YOUR PERSONAL RESPONSIBILITY

Some people today think of health as the responsibility of doctors, hospitals, clinics, insurance companies, and the government. It is important to realize, however, that health cannot be purchased or the responsibility relegated to some other person or agency. Health is an obligation on the part of each individual, and it is erroneous to equate more health services with better health. Instead, individuals must take responsibility for their own health.

The decisions that people make relative to their lifestyle have an effect on their health. They are the ones who decide what to eat and when and whether to exercise, drink, engage in drug abuse, smoke, or see a doctor. Thus the decisions they make leave an imprint on their health and well-being. In many cases people who become sick have only themselves to blame.

The call to attain the optimal level of health for ourselves and our loved ones is a lifetime challenge. No one can do the job for us, nor should they. This is a responsibility each person should assume to the extent he or she is able, with pride and conviction. Lab Activity 2-2 will help you determine whether you are living a healthy lifestyle.

SUMMARY

- Creating a healthy lifestyle incorporates aspects of intellectual, physical, social, emotional, and spiritual health in a manner that allows you to enjoy the highest level of health and well-being possible.

- Coronary artery disease (CAD) accounts for half of all the deaths in the United States each year. The major risk factors which cannot be changed that predispose a person to CAD are family history, age, gender and race. Risk factors that can be changed include cigarette smoking, hypertension, lack of physical activity and high blood-cholesterol levels. Obesity, diabetes, and stressful living would be considered contributing risk factors.

- Cancer is the second leading cause of death in adult Americans. Early detection and treatment are critical for reducing the likelihood of death.

- Everyone experiences stress, and some stress is needed to perform the daily tasks of life and for growth and development. Stress involves physiological and psychological responses.

- Coping skills to ward off stress are those procedures which allow a person to deal with reality in a positive way. Several relaxation techniques for coping with stress exist, including the progressive relaxation technique, biofeedback, yoga, breathing exercises, meditation, imagery, massage, and autogenic training.

- It is important to recognize that using alcohol, tobacco, or other drugs is a deterrent to health and wellness.

- Sexually transmitted infections (STIs) are extremely common and have a negative impact on wellness. AIDS and other STIs are life-threatening diseases.

• Creating a healthy style of living is a personal responsibility.

SUGGESTED READINGS

American Cancer Society. 1999. *1999 cancer facts and figures.* Atlanta: American Cancer Society.

American Heart Association. 1998. *Primary prevention of coronary heart disease: guidance from Framingham.* Dallas: American Heart Association.

Cox, M.H. 1997. Exercise for coronary artery disease: a cornerstone of comprehensive treatment. *Physician and sports medicine* 25(12):27–32, 34.

Haveson, R. 1998. Meet the alcohol abuse problem head on. *NCAA sports sciences education newsletter.*

Iven, V.G. 1998. Recreational drugs. *Clinics in sports medicine* 17(2):245–59.

Merz, C.N., A. Rozanski, and J.S. Forrester. 1997. The secondary prevention of coronary artery disease. *American Journal of Medicine* 102(6):572–81.

Nieman, D.C. © 1998. *The exercise-health connection.* Champaign, IL: Human Kinetics.

Page, R.M., J. Hammermeister, A. Scanlan, and L. Gilbert. 1998. Is school sports participation a protective factor against adolescent health risk behaviors? *Journal of Health Education* 29(3):186–92.

Payne, W., and D. Hahn. 1998. *Understanding your health.* St. Louis: WCB/McGraw-Hill.

Schnirring, L. 1997. Pact may help stifle smokeless tobacco use. *Physician and sportsmedicine* 25(8):46–47.

Shephard, R.J., and P.N. Shek, 1998. Associations between physical activity and susceptibility to cancer: possible mechanisms. *Sports medicine* 26(5):293–315.

Simons-Morton, B.G., L. Donohew, and A.D. Crump. 1997. Health communication in the prevention of alcohol, tobacco, and drug use. *Health education and behavior* 23(5):544–54.

Stainback, R.D. 1997. *Alcohol and sport.* Champaign, IL: Human Kinetics.

Wann, D.L. Tobacco use and sport fandom. 1998. *Perceptual and motor skills* 83(3):878.

Wells, C.L. Physical activity and cancer prevention: focus on breast cancer. 1999. *American College of Sports Medicine's Health and Fitness Journal* 3(1):13–18.

Zuzanek, J., J.P. Robinson, and Y. Iwasaki. 1998. The relationships between stress, health, and physically active leisure as a function of life-cycle. *Leisure sciences* 20(4):253–75.

SUGGESTED WEBSITES

ACSH: Tobacco
The American Council on Science and Health has been a leader in restoring scientific fact and context to health issues, in exposing both overstated and understated risks. This page covers tobacco, including what the warning label doesn't tell you.
http://www.acsh.org/tobacco/index.html

American Cancer Society
This is the official web site of the American Cancer Society. The site provides information on all types of cancer, cancer research, therapy, support groups, and local community resources for cancer patients and their families.
http://www.cancer.org/index_4up.html

American College Health Association
ACHA provides health information, facts, and guidance for college students.
http://www.acha.org/home.htm

American Heart Association
This site is dedicated to providing you with education and information on fighting heart disease and stroke.
http://www.americanheart.org/

CDC's TIPS: Tobacco Information and Prevention Source
The Centers for Disease Control and Prevention (CDC) presents the Tobacco Information and Prevention Source (TIPS). This website is maintained by the CDC's Office on Smoking and Health, which is a division of the National Center for Chronic Disease Prevention and Health Promotion (US Gov't website). Information covering tobacco-related issues and statistics is presented. There are also sections dedicated to youth.
http://www.cdc.gov/tobacco/

Health Education Alliance for Life and Longevity
This site presents 10,000+ hand-picked resources that sort the wheat from the chaff on alternative

medicine, Y2K, vitamins, herbs, natural product recommendation, and resource lists. Marketing coop, wellness author features, and Citizen's Action and Freedom of Choice in Medicine updates are also featured.
http://www.heall.com

National Institute on Drug Abuse
The mission of the National Institute on Drug Abuse (NIDA) is to lead the nation in bringing the power of science to bear on drug abuse and addiction.
http://www.nida.nih.gov/

National Wellness Institute—
NationalWellness.org
Search the Wellness Resource Directory! The National Wellness Institute helps professionals interested in wellness and health promotion.
http://www.wellnesswi.org/index.htm

Stress Management and Relaxation Central
Take control of your stress response and learn to relax, yet retain alertness and energy.
http://www.futurehealth.org/stresscn.htm

The National Wellness Association
NWA is the Membership Division of the National Wellness Institute. NWA is a non-profit professional membership organization that serves professionals working in all areas of wellness and health promotion.
http://www.nationalwellness.org

The Sexually Transmitted Disease (STD) Online Guide
This site presents detailed photographs and education on sexually transmitted diseases (STDs), including herpes, chlamydia, gonorrhea, trichomonas, vaginal warts (genital HPV), HIV and AIDS, and much more.
http://www.afraidtoask.com/std.html

Tobacco BBS—Resources on Tobacco, Smoking, Cigarettes
Tobacco BBS presents tobacco issues, tobacco and smoking-related news, addresses, tobacco history, quitting, and a great quote-of-the-day section.
http://www.tobacco.org/

Wellness Institute
This site provides the community with services that promote health, prevent illness and disability, and restore wellness of body, mind, and spirit.
http://www.wellnessinstitute.mb.ca/

4Addictions—A Guide to Addictions from 4Anything
Get the support and information you need. Here you can anonymously learn all about addictions to alcohol, drugs, tobacco, food, sex, and other things. You can find support groups and counseling, prevention organizations, or just someone to talk to.
http://www.4addictions.com/

Lab Activity 2-1

Name _____ Section _____ Date _____

PURPOSE   To manage stress effectively, you need to learn about your unique patterns of stress: what factors promote it, how you experience it, and how you cope with it. Understanding your patterns and becoming more aware of early signs of stress are important first steps in managing stress.

This personal inventory will help you become more aware of your responses to stress, life events that may impact your stress level, and how you cope with stress. There are no right or wrong answers; instead, the scoring system is designed to give a general indication of stress levels and to help you focus on those unhealthy responses that could be changed through improved stress management techniques.

PROCEDURE   1. Circle the appropriate response for each question.

2. Total your score.

Response	Never	Rarely	Some-times	Often	Very Often
Physical Responses to Stress					
1. I have frequent headaches.	N	R	S	O	A
2. I get stomachaches or experience discomfort.	N	R	S	O	A
3. My back aches.	N	R	S	O	A
4. I have stiffness in my shoulders or upper back.	N	R	S	O	A
5. My blood pressure is elevated.	N	R	S	O	A
6. I get palpitations or a rapid heartbeat.	N	R	S	O	A
7. I get short of breath and breathe rapidly.	N	R	S	O	A
8. I feel dizzy or shaky.	N	R	S	O	A
9. I'm fatigued, tired, or unrested.	N	R	S	O	A
10. I feel "wound up" and tense inside.	N	R	S	O	A
Total Number O's and A's Circled: _____					_____
Behavioral Responses to Stress					
1. I eat compulsively or too fast.	N	R	S	O	A
2. I light up a cigarette.	N	R	S	O	A
3. I drink alcohol or use mood-altering drugs.	N	R	S	O	A
4. I grind my teeth.	N	R	S	O	A
5. I clench my fists.	N	R	S	O	A
6. I pace, walk rapidly, or rush.	N	R	S	O	A

Continued

37

Response	Never	Rarely	Some-times	Often	Very Often
7. I tap my feet.	N	R	S	O	A
8. I sleep a lot or have trouble falling asleep.	N	R	S	O	A
9. I sulk and don't talk to people.	N	R	S	O	A
10. I snap back or get angry with others.	N	R	S	O	A
Total Number O's and A's Circled: _____					_____
Cognitive (Thinking) Responses to Stress					
1. I can't concentrate on what I'm doing.	N	R	S	O	A
2. I forget things or I get confused.	N	R	S	O	A
3. My thoughts seem to race.	N	R	S	O	A
4. This isn't where I want to be in my life.	N	R	S	O	A
5. I worry a lot.	N	R	S	O	A
6. I have recurring, troublesome thoughts.	N	R	S	O	A
7. I can't turn off my thoughts at night and relax.	N	R	S	O	A
8. I have trouble sleeping because of things on my mind.	N	R	S	O	A
9. Things must be perfect.	N	R	S	O	A
10. I must do it myself.	N	R	S	O	A
Total Number O's and A's Circled: _____					_____
Emotional (Feelings) Responses to Stress					
1. I feel depressed, sad, and unhappy.	N	R	S	O	A
2. I can't say no without feeling guilty.	N	R	S	O	A
3. I feel worthless, disappointed in myself and life.	N	R	S	O	A
4. I don't get a sense of accomplishment most days.	N	R	S	O	A
5. I feel trapped.	N	R	S	O	A
6. I can't seem to share my feelings with my family/friends.	N	R	S	O	A
7. I feel exploited, used by others.	N	R	S	O	A
8. I'm afraid of things that didn't used to bother me.	N	R	S	O	A
9. I feel cynical and disenchanted.	N	R	S	O	A
10. I feel agitated, irritated, short-tempered, impatient.	N	R	S	O	A
Total Number O's and A's Circled: _____					_____

Scoring Interpretation

Total the number of circled responses in the columns indicating frequent reactions to stress (O: Often and A: Always). Those reactions will most likely be the first to alert you that you are experiencing excessive stress.

Notice which category (physical, behavioral, cognitive, or emotional) has the most O's and A's. For example, if you have more frequent reactions in the physical category, you may want to become aware of those tension spots and learn about relaxation or biofeedback techniques to reduce stress.

By simply becoming aware of your signs of stress, you'll be taking a major step toward better managing your stress level.

Lab Activity 2-2

Health Style: A Self-Test

Name _____ Section _____ Date _____

PURPOSE All of us want good health. But many of us do not know how to be as healthy as possible. Health experts now describe lifestyle as one of the most important factors affecting health. In fact, it is estimated that as many as seven of the ten leading causes of death could be reduced through common-sense changes in lifestyle. That's what this brief test, developed by the Public Health Service, is all about. Its purpose is simply to tell you how well you are doing to stay healthy. The behaviors covered in the test are recommended for most Americans. Some of them may not apply to persons with certain chronic diseases or handicaps, or to pregnant women. Such persons may require special instructions from their physicians.

PROCEDURE
1. Circle the appropriate response for each question.

2. Add the total number of points for each section.

Behavior	Almost Always	Sometimes	Almost Never
Tobacco Use			
If you *never smoke* or use tobacco products, enter a score of 10 for this section and go to the next section on Alcohol and Drugs.	10	0	0
1. I avoid smoking cigarettes and chewing tobacco.	2	1	0
2. I smoke only low tar and nicotine cigarettes or I smoke a pipe or cigars.	2	1	0
		Smoking Score: _____	
Alcohol and Drugs			
1. I avoid drinking alcoholic beverages *or* I drink no more than 1 or 2 drinks a day.	4	1	0
2. I avoid using alcohol or other drugs (especially illegal drugs) as a way of handling stressful situations or the problems in my life.	2	1	0
3. I am careful not to drink alcohol when taking certain medicines (for example, medicine for sleeping, pain, colds and allergies) or when pregnant.	2	1	0
4. I read and follow the label directions when using prescribed and over-the-counter drugs.	2	1	0
		Alcohol and Drugs Score: _____	
Eating Habits			
1. I eat a variety of foods each day, such as fruits and vegetables, whole grain breads and cereals, lean meats, dairy products, dry peas and beans, and nuts and seeds.	4	1	0

Continued

Behavior	Almost Always	Sometimes	Almost Never
2. I limit the amount of fat, saturated fat, and cholesterol I eat (including fat in meats, eggs, butter, and other dairy products, shortenings, and organ meats such as liver).	2	1	0
3. I limit the amount of salt I eat by cooking with only small amounts, not adding salt at the table, and avoiding salty snacks.	2	1	0
4. I avoid eating too much sugar (especially frequent snacks of stick candy or soft drinks).	2	1	0
		Eating Habits Score: _____	
Exercise Habits			
1. I maintain a desired weight, avoiding overweight and underweight.	3	1	0
2. I do vigorous exercises for 15–30 minutes at least 3 times a week (examples include running, swimming, brisk walking).	3	1	0
3. I do exercises that enhance my muscle tone for 15–30 minutes at least 3 times a week (examples include yoga and calisthenics).	2	1	0
4. I use part of my leisure time participating in individual, family, or team activities that increase my level of fitness (such as gardening, bowling, golf, and baseball).	2	1	0
		Exercise/Fitness Score: _____	
Stress Control			
1. I have a job or do other work that I enjoy.	2	1	0
2. I find it easy to relax and express my feelings freely.	2	1	0
3. I recognize early and prepare for events or situations likely to be stressful for me.	2	1	0
4. I have close friends, relatives, or others whom I can talk to about personal matters and call on for help when needed.	2	1	0
5. I participate in group activities (such as church and community organizations) or hobbies that I enjoy.	2	1	0
		Stress Control Score: _____	
Safety			
1. I wear a seat belt while riding in a car.	2	1	0
2. I avoid driving while under the influence of alcohol and other drugs.	2	1	0
3. I obey traffic rules and the speed limit when driving.	2	1	0
4. I am careful when using potentially harmful products or substances (such as household cleaners, poisons and electrical devices).	2	1	0
5. I avoid smoking in bed.	2	1	0
		Safety Score: _____	

What Your Scores Mean to YOU

Scores of 9 and 10: Excellent! Your answers show that you are aware of the importance of this area to your health. More importantly, you are putting your knowledge to work for you by practicing good health habits. As long as you continue to do so, this area should not pose a serious health risk. It's likely that you are setting an example for your family and friends to follow. Since you got a very high test score on this part of the test, you may want to consider other areas where your scores indicate room for improvement.

Scores of 6 to 8: Good. Your health practices in this area are good, but there is room for improvement. Look again at the items you answered with a "Sometimes" or "Almost Never." What changes can you make to improve your score? Even a small change can often help you achieve better health.

Scores of 3 to 5: Fair. Your health risks are showing! Would you like more information about the risks you are facing and about why it is important for you to change these behaviors? Perhaps you need help in deciding how to successfully make the changes you desire. In either case, help is available.

Scores of 0 to 2: Poor. Obviously, you were concerned enough about your health to take the test, but your answers show that you may be taking serious and unnecessary risks with your health. Perhaps you are not aware of the risks and what to do about them. You can easily get the information and help you need to improve, if you wish. The next step is up to you.

What am I doing to become as healthy as possible? _____

_____

What steps can I take to feel better? _____

_____

_____

What changes do I need to make in my lifestyle? _____

_____

_____

_____

YOU Can Start Right Now!
In the test you just completed, there were numerous suggestions to help you reduce your risk of disease and premature death. Here are some of the most significant.

Avoid Cigarettes and Other Tobacco Products Cigarette smoking is the single most important preventable cause of illness and early death. It is especially risky for pregnant women and their unborn babies. Persons who stop smoking reduce their risk of getting heart disease and cancer. So if you're a cigarette smoker, think twice about lighting that next cigarette. If you choose to continue smoking, try decreasing the number of cigarettes you smoke and switching to a low tar and nicotine brand. If you chew, stop the habit.

Follow Sensible Drinking Habits Alcohol produces changes in mood and behavior. Most people who drink are able to control their intake of alcohol and to avoid undesired, and often harmful, effects. Heavy, regular use of alcohol can lead to cirrhosis of the liver, a leading cause of death. Also, statistics clearly show that mixing drinking and driving is often the cause of fatal or crippling accidents. So if you drink, do it wisely and in moderation. **Use care in taking drugs.** Today's greater use of drugs—both legal and illegal—is one of our most serious health risks. Even some drugs prescribed by your doctor can be dangerous if taken when drinking alcohol or before driving. Excessive or continued use of tranquilizers (or "pep pills") can cause physical and mental problems. Using or experimenting with illicit drugs such as marijuana, LSD, heroin, cocaine, and PCP may lead to a number of damaging effects or even death.

Eat Sensibly Overweight individuals are at greater risk for diabetes, gallbladder disease, and high blood pressure. So it makes good sense to maintain proper weight. But good eating habits also mean holding down the amount of fat (especially saturated fat), cholesterol, sugar, and salt in your diet. If you must snack, try nibbling on fresh fruits and vegetables. You'll feel better—and look better, too.

Exercise Regularly Almost everyone can benefit from exercise—and there's some form of exercise almost everyone can do. (If you have any doubt, check first with your doctor.) Usually, as little as 15–30 minutes of vigorous exercise three times a week will help you have a healthier heart, eliminate excess weight, tone up sagging muscles, and sleep better. Think how much difference all these improvements could make in the way you feel!

Learn to Handle Stress Stress is a normal part of living: everyone faces it to some degree. The causes of stress can be good or bad, desirable or undesirable (such as a promotion on the job or the loss of a spouse). Properly handled, stress need not be a problem. But unhealthy responses to stress—such as driving too fast or erratically, drinking too much, or prolonged anger or grief—can cause physical and mental problems. Even on a very busy day, find a few minutes to slow down and relax. Talking over a problem with someone you trust can often help you find a satisfactory solution. Learn to distinguish between things that are "worth fighting about" and things that are less important.

Be Safety Conscious Think "safety first" at home, at work, at school, at play, and on the highway. Buckle seat belts, and obey traffic rules. Keep poisons and weapons out of the reach of children, and keep emergency numbers by your telephone. When the unexpected happens, be prepared.

Where Do You Go From Here?

Start by asking yourself a few frank questions: Am I really doing all I can to be as healthy as possible? What steps can I take to feel better? Am I willing to begin now? If you scored low in one or more sections of the test, decide what changes you want to make for improvement. You might pick that aspect of your lifestyle where you feel you have the best chance for success and tackle that one first. Once you have improved your score there, go on to other areas.

If you already have tried to change your health habits (to stop smoking or exercise regularly, for example), don't be discouraged if you haven't yet succeeded. The difficulty you have encountered may be due to influences you've never really thought about—such as advertising—or to a lack of support and encouragement. Understanding these influences is an important step toward changing the way they affect you.

There's Help Available In addition to personal actions you can take on your own, there are community programs and groups (such as the YMCA/YWCA or the local chapter of the American Heart Association) that can assist you and your family to make the changes you want to make. If you want to know more about these groups or about health risks, contact your local health department or the address below. There's a lot you can do to stay healthy or to improve your health—and there are organizations that can help you. Start a new HEALTHSTYLE today!

National Health Information Clearinghouse
PO Box 1133
Washington, DC 20013-1133
1-800-336-4797

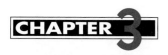
STARTING YOUR OWN
FITNESS PROGRAM

OBJECTIVES

After completing this chapter, you should be able to do the following:

- Determine your present level of fitness.
- Identify the seven principles of a fitness program.
- Discuss the importance of the warm-up and cool-down periods.
- Determine your individual goals for your fitness program.
- Identify precautions for beginning a fitness program.

A t this point, you should have some idea about why you need to get fit. Your individual reasons and motivations have been identified in Chapter 1. Beginning a fitness program is simple. In addition, you can do several things to ensure that your program is successful and yet fun and enjoyable.

Key Terms

overload
progression
consistency
specificity
SAID principle
warm-up
cool-down

WHAT ARE THE SEVEN PRINCIPLES OF A FITNESS PROGRAM?

Regardless of the type of physical activity in which you choose to participate, certain principles should be incorporated into every program. These principles and guidelines apply to anyone who is physically active. Paying attention to these seven principles will help to create an effective yet safe environment for physical activities. The Fit List on the following page summarizes these principles.

Fit List

The Seven Basic Principles of a Fitness Program

- Fun and enjoyable
- Overload
- Progression
- Consistency
- Specificity
- Individuality
- Safety

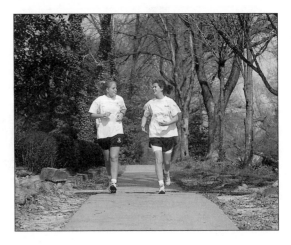

Figure 3-1.
An exercise program should be fun and enjoyable.

THE PROGRAM MUST BE FUN AND ENJOYABLE

Enjoying yourself may be one of the most critical factors for a successful fitness program over the long run. The activity you select must be one that you enjoy and that provides motivation to continue for a lifetime (Figure 3-1). For example, a quick look at the streets on a sunny day will show that running is a popular form of physical activity. There is no question that a running program eventually will result in significant improvement in cardiorespiratory endurance. Personally, I hate to run and would prefer to do any other activity. If I were to select running as my fitness activity because it is "in" and not because I enjoy doing it, then chances are that I would not stick with it for long. You should enjoy getting into good physical condition, and a successful fitness program will be considered fun rather than work.

Motivation plays an important role in your ability to stick with an exercise program. You should select the type of activity that will allow you to do two things: (1) achieve the ultimate goals of physical fitness improvement that you have established for yourself, and (2) maintain your interest and motivation for a long time (weeks, months, even years). The Fit List on page 45 provides some suggestions that can make your program fun and enjoyable.

OVERLOAD

To achieve the greatest benefits from an exercise program, you should recognize the principle of **overload** (Figure 3-2). For a physical component of fitness to improve, the system must work harder than it is used to working. The system must experience stress so that over a period of time it will improve to the point where it can easily accommodate additional stress. The **SAID principle** (an acronym for **s**pecific **a**daptation to **i**mposed **d**emands) states that when the body is subjected to stresses and overloads of varying intensities, it

overload: exercising at a higher level than normal

SAID principle: when the body is subjected to stresses and overloads of varying intensities, it will gradually adapt, over time, to overcome whatever demands are placed on it

Fit List

Suggestions for Making Physical Activity Fun

Some students find physical activity dull. Here are some ways to make it more inviting.
- Exercise to music.
- Exercise with classmates.
- Keep your program simple.
- Instill variety into activity: for example, dancing, hiking, tennis, and swimming.
- Reward yourself when fitness goals are met.
- Don't become upset when goals are not met and benefits are not immediate.
- Keep a record of things such as your weight and the distance you jog.
- Take a break whenever you wish.
- Plan the program to fit into your daily life.

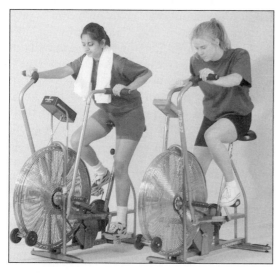

Figure 3-2.
To see improvement you must use the principle of overload.

will gradually adapt, over time, to overcome whatever demands are placed on it. Even though overload is a critical factor for getting fit, the stress must not be great enough to produce damage or injury. The body needs to have

a chance to adjust to the imposed demands. Therefore overload is a gradual increase in the frequency, duration, or intensity of the physical activity that is a part of the fitness program. This is one of the most critical factors in any activities program. For example, if you are on a jogging program to improve cardiorespiratory endurance and you go out and run 1 mile in 15 minutes, the cardiorespiratory system will be able to accommodate this distance and intensity very easily. However, if the long-range goal of your fitness program is to run the New York Marathon, it is foolish to believe that you could finish a race of this distance and intensity by running only one 15-minute mile a day. If you gradually overload the system by running farther at a faster pace, you will force the cardiorespiratory system to work more efficiently to keep up with increased physical demands. In weight training, adding more weight and decreasing the number of sets and repetitions will help in developing muscular strength. Therefore, by overloading the system over a long period, one should expect to produce significant improvement in that system's ability to handle a stressful exercise session.

PROGRESSION

A little today and a little more tomorrow is a good principle to follow in any fitness program. You should start gradually and add a little each day. The rate of **progression** should be within your capabilities to adapt physically. In other words, the workout should gradually become a little longer or more intense until you reach the desired level of physical fitness. There comes a time in many fitness programs when *improving* fitness levels becomes less important than *maintaining* fitness levels. Progression is closely related to overload. Without overloading the system, progression does not occur. Progression is also important for motivation. Interest level in an activity remains high as long as you continue to see improvement in your physical ability. Even though weight increases may be minimal in strength training, a progression of even 1 pound is often enough to maintain interest and motivation.

CONSISTENCY

One of the biggest problems with beginning a fitness program is finding time during the day to fit in an hour or so of activity. This is particularly true for students who have many demands on their time. Nevertheless, it is important to select a specific period for exercising each day and stick to it.

The best time of day for you to exercise is whenever you have the time and are motivated to do so. The important point is to set aside some time for a fitness program and make it part of your daily routine for **consistency**. The least desirable times are probably after a meal, when activity may make you uncomfortable, and just before bedtime, when the activity has been so invigorating that it is difficult to fall asleep. The number of days per week you are involved with a specific activity will vary depending on several personal factors. However, it is recommended that you try to work out at least 3 days per week to see minimal improvement.

SPECIFICITY

The type of physical changes that occur is directly related to the type of training undertaken. To realize the maximum gains desired, activities and programs should be selected and designed with **specificity** to achieve this aim. Once again, according to the SAID principle, a particular physical system will respond and adapt over time to whatever specific demands are placed on it. For example, to develop flexibility in a specific joint, stretching exercises must be incorporated that progressively lengthen the muscles and tendons that surround that joint.

INDIVIDUALITY

When you become involved in a fitness program, it is important to remember that no two persons are exactly the same. People have different ideas about their goals for a fitness program, motivation, and state of physical fitness. A fitness program for one person will not necessarily satisfy the needs of another person. Furthermore, not all people involved in similar activities will progress at the same rate, nor will they be able to overload their systems to the same degree. Exercise is good, but it must be adapted to individual needs and abilities. Just as a medical prescription must be related to a person's health needs, so should a physical fitness prescription. A person's exercise prescription needs to be based on his or her objectives, needs, functional capacity, and interests.

progression: gradually increasing the level and intensity of exercise

consistency: engaging in fitness activities on a frequent and regular basis

specificity: the type of physical changes that occur are directly related to the type of training used

Also, stress levels vary among individuals. It is important to consider the degree to which stress affects you and how it may interfere with your fitness program. Actually, some people tend to view physical activity as an outlet to release the stress that builds up during a day.

SAFETY

Another factor to consider when planning a fitness program is safety. The purpose of your fitness program should be to improve selected components of fitness through physical exercise. Unfortunately, injuries often occur as the result of poorly planned activity programs. The rule of thumb to follow is to start out slowly and progress according to your own capabilities. Adhering to the rule "train—don't strain" can certainly reduce the likelihood of injury. If you are unsure of how to get started or perhaps of how quickly to progress in a personal fitness program, seek professional advice from persons with some expertise in fitness.

SHOULD YOU DO A WARM-UP ROUTINE BEFORE YOU EXERCISE?

It is important for you to **warm up** before you begin any type of workout for several reasons. The warm-up routine increases body temperature, stretches ligaments and muscles, and increases flexibility. Warm-up routines have been found to be important in preventing injury and muscle soreness. It appears that muscle injury can result when vigorous exercises are not preceded by a related warm-up routine. A good, short warm-up routine can also be an effective

> **warm-up:** designed to increase body temperature, stretch ligaments and muscles, and increase flexibility

motivator. If you get satisfaction from warming up, you probably will have a stronger desire to participate in an activity. By contrast, a poor warm-up routine can lead to fatigue and boredom, limiting your attention and ultimately resulting in a poor program. Also, there is some evidence that a good warm-up routine may improve certain aspects of performance.

The function of the warm-up routine is to prepare your body physically for a workout. Most professionals view the warm-up period as a precaution against unnecessary muscle injury and possible muscle soreness. The purpose is to gradually stimulate the cardiorespiratory system to a moderate degree. This produces an increased blood flow to exercising muscles and results in an increase in muscle temperature.

Moderate activity speeds up your metabolism, producing an increase in your body temperature. Furthermore, an increase in the temperature of muscle allows the muscle to stretch to a greater degree without fear of injury.

A good warm-up routine should begin with 2 or 3 minutes of slow walking, light jogging, or cycling to increase your metabolism and warm up the muscles. Breaking into a light sweat is a good indication that the muscle temperature has increased (Figure 3-3). At that point you should begin stretching, concentrating on the muscles you will use during the activity. For example, if you are going to swim, it makes sense for you to spend time stretching the muscles around the shoulder. Conversely, if you are going to walk or jog, you should stretch the leg muscles. The total warm-up routine should last no longer than 10 to 15 minutes, and you should begin your activity immediately following the warm-up routine.

The type and length of workout in which you choose to engage are determined by your reasons for engaging in a fitness program and by the goals you have established for yourself. Thus the workout will differ significantly between individuals. Recommendations for

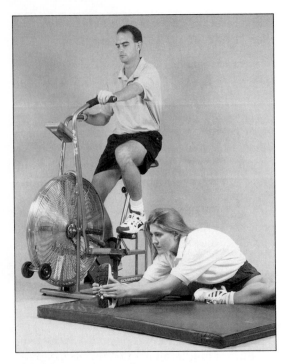

Figure 3-3.
A warm-up routine should begin with an activity to increase body temperature, followed by stretching.

workouts to accomplish specific fitness goals are presented throughout the text.

After a vigorous workout, a **cool-down** period is essential. The cool-down period prevents pooling of blood in the arms and legs, thus maintaining blood pressure and enabling the body to cool and return to a resting state. The cool-down period should last about 5 to 10 minutes. During the cool-down period, you should engage in stretching activities as was done during the warm-up routine. Some people feel that stretching during the cool-down period is more effective in pre-

> **cool-down:** prevents pooling of blood and enables the body to cool and return to a resting state

venting injury than is stretching during the warm-up routine. Although the value of warm-up routine and workout periods is well accepted, the importance of a cool-down period is often ignored. Again, experience and observation indicate that people who stretch during the cool-down period tend to have fewer problems with muscle soreness after strenuous activity.

WHAT ARE THE GOALS OF YOUR FITNESS PROGRAM?

When designing an individualized physical fitness program, you must first decide what it is you are trying to accomplish and then select those specific components of fitness which ultimately help you to reach your goal. For example, the goals of fitness improvement for a person who plays Frisbee occasionally on weekends will differ considerably from those of a person preparing to compete in varsity soccer. Most people who are not athletes should be more concerned with fitness components related to good health such as cardiorespiratory endurance, flexibility, muscular strength, muscular endurance, and body composition. Improvement in these five specific areas enhance a person's ability to perform daily tasks without undue fatigue, as stated in our definition of physical fitness.

On the other hand, the soccer player must be concerned not only with the components that have been mentioned above but also with components such as strength, speed, power, balance, and agility. If he or she does not include activities in the training regimen that specifically address these various skill-related fitness components, chances are that he or she will be unsuccessful in a competitive situation.

The Fit List following recommends several activities that may help you develop each of the health-related components of fitness. Please note that several activities are recommended under more than one fitness component—thus

Fit List

Activities to Improve Various Components of Fitness

Muscular Strength

- Swimming
- Weight training
- Judo
- Calisthenic exercises (e.g., push-ups, leg raises, bench step-ups, flutter kicks)
- Gymnastics
- Karate
- Cycling
- Racquetball
- Backpacking
- Rock climbing
- Rapelling

Muscular Endurance

- Jogging
- Running
- Swimming
- Weight training
- Rowing
- Cycling
- Cross-country skiing
- Backpacking
- Dancing
- Ice skating
- Mountain climbing
- Fencing
- Handball
- Hiking
- Calisthenics
- Rock climbing
- Downhill skiing
- Snowboarding

Cardiorespiratory Endurance

- Aerobic dancing
- Skipping rope
- Running
- Jogging
- Swimming
- Cross-country skiing
- Cycling
- Backpacking
- Handball
- Hiking
- Rock climbing
- Rowing
- Kick boxing
- Rollerblading/In-line skating
- Spinning

Flexibility

- Calisthenics
- Gymnastics
- Judo
- Karate
- Swimming
- Modern dancing
- Static stretching
- Kick boxing
- Rock climbing

Body Composition

- Jogging
- Running
- Walking
- Swimming
- Cycling
- Aerobic exercise
- Cross-country skiing
- Skipping rope
- Kick boxing

the benefits of those activities accrue to several components of fitness simultaneously.

HOW SHOULD YOU EXERCISE?

It has been well documented that engaging in regular, moderate-intensity physical activity will result in substantial health benefits. Based on this concept, it is recommended that everyone should try to accumulate a minimum of 30 minutes of physical activity on most days—ideally, every day. This 30-minute total does not have to consist solely of what has traditionally been considered exercise, i.e., walking, swimming, cycling, etc. It can involve a series of short bouts of physical activity that may include more intermittent activities such as walking up or down stairs, doing lawnwork or gardening, or cleaning the house which collectively accumulate to a total of at least 30 minutes of moderate-intensity physical exercise.

This most recent recommendation relative to the quantity and quality of exercise is substantially less formal than what has been recommended in the past. An exercise bout of 20 to 60 minutes duration at an intensity of 60 to 90 percent of maximum heart rate performed three or more times per week was, for years, the recommended standard for promoting good health and preventing disease. Recent research has indicated that many health benefits can be achieved by engaging in moderate-intensity physical activities not typically associated with formal exercise. The total amount of activity appears to be more critical to improving health than the specific manner in which the activity is performed.

WHERE DO YOU BEGIN?

Just as you are never too sedentary to begin a fitness program, you are also never too old. It is wise to start a fitness program early in life, but all of us can benefit from exercise no matter when we begin. Long-term success in staying with an exercise program undoubtedly has some basis in your underlying motivation for beginning such a program in the first place.

PRECAUTIONS IN BEGINNING A FITNESS PROGRAM

For most high school and college students, chances are that overall health is pretty good. In the normal healthy individual, there is virtually no reason to expect that participation in any type of fitness activity will pose a threat to health or well-being. Generally, exercise is considered a safe activity for most individuals. Nevertheless, it is always a good idea to assess your medical history by identifying any preexisting medical conditions that should be considered before beginning an exercise program. This is especially true for anyone over 30 years of age. If your medical history identifies any health-related problem, it is advisable to consult appropriate medical personnel before engaging in any type of activity. Lab Activity 3-1 will help you to assess your current medical history and may indicate a reason for you to seek additional medical advice.

Paying attention to the principles and guidelines of fitness as detailed earlier in this chapter can markedly reduce your chances of suffering injuries associated with exercise. Many of the injuries that occur with exercise can be eliminated by an awareness of the way you exercise, by "listening" to what your body is telling you through aches and pains.

READY TO BEGIN?

At this point you have been given the basic guidelines and considerations for beginning a fitness program. The chapters that follow will provide you with knowledge about and understanding of the various aspects of fitness. The chapters are designed to show the importance of fitness's essential ingredients, and they will explain how you can assess, develop, and maintain fitness. Finally, the rest of this text will demonstrate how to plan, develop, and implement a personalized fitness program based on your individual interests. Lab Activity 3-2 will help you begin planning your physical activity program.

SUMMARY

- Before starting a personal training program, it is helpful to examine your attitude toward physical fitness, reasons for wanting to be physically fit, and present level of activity.
- The basic considerations of any training and conditioning program should include the following principles: the program should be fun and enjoyable; overload; progression; consistency; specificity; individuality; and safety.
- The three basic elements of any training and conditioning program include a warm-up routine, the workout or conditioning activity, and the cool-down period.
- As a precaution, before you begin an exercise program, you should complete a medical history questionnaire to identify any problems.

SUGGESTED READINGS

American College of Sports Medicine. 1998. *ACSM fitness book,* 2nd edition. Champaign, IL: Human Kinetics.

American College of Sports Medicine. 1995. *Guidelines for graded exercise testing and exercise prescription.* Baltimore: Williams and Wilkins.

American College of Sports Medicine. 1990. Position stand on recommended quantity and quality of exercise for developing and maintaining cardiorespiratory and muscular fitness in healthy adults. *Medicine and science in sports and exercise* 22:265–74.

Bouchard, C., R. Shepard, and T. Stephens. 1994. *Physical activity fitness and health.* Champaign, IL: Human Kinetics.

Dick, F. W. 1997. *Sports training principles,* 3rd edition. London: A. and C. Black Publishers, Ltd.

Do you really need to warm up? 1998. *Penn State sport medicine newsletter* 6(12):4–5.

Franks, B. D., and E. T. Howley. 1998. *Fitness leader's handbook,* 2nd edition. Champaign, IL: Human Kinetics.

Pate, R. et al. 1995. Physical activity and public health: A recommendation from the Centers for Disease Control and Prevention and the American College of Sports Medicine. *Journal of the American Medical Association* 273(5):402–7.

Prentice, W. 1999. *Fitness and wellness for life,* 6th edition. St. Louis: WCB/McGraw-Hill.

Stewart, I. B., and G. G. Sleivert. 1998. The effect of warm up intensity on range of motion and anaerobic performance. *Journal of Orthopedic and Sports Physical Therapy* 27(2):154–61.

SUGGESTED WEBSITES

Aerobics and Fitness Association of America
AFAA, the world's largest fitness educator, links members, consumers, corporate subscribers, and allied professionals throughout the world with a revolutionary group of dynamic fitness services. Whether you're looking for aerobics certification, a personal trainer, or just some fitness facts, this is the place to be.
http://www.afaa.com/

**American Alliance for Health, Physical
 Education, Recreation, and Dance**
This site is sponsored by the national organization of physical education, health, and fitness professionals.
http://www.aahperd.org

Health: Fitness
Search the contents of 2,000,000 reviewed sites available on the internet.
http://gocrawl.com/web/Health/Fitness/

The Fitness Zone
This site includes an extensive collection of articles, tips, and recommendations for engaging in a fitness program.
http://www.fitnesszone.com/

The Internet's Fitness Resource

The primary purpose of this site is the dissemination of information on exercise and nutrition. IFR offers a comprehensive listing of fitness related sites as well as the Fitness Instructor FAQ, the Fitness Plan, guest editorials, fitness classifications and more.
http://www.netsweat.com/

www.fitness.com

Fitness.com includes everything about fitness: chat, discussion board, links, shopping.
http://www.fitness.com/e_index.htm

Lab Activity 3-1

Medical History Questionnaire

Name _____ Section _____ Date _____

PURPOSE   To determine whether your past medical history warrants further medical evaluation before beginning an exercise program.

PROCEDURE   Check the appropriate column below if you think you have or if you have ever been told you had any of the conditions listed below.

	Yes	No
Coronary heart disease	_____	_____
Chest pain (during rest or during exercise)	_____	_____
Pain in your shoulder and jaw	_____	_____
Irregular heartbeats	_____	_____
High blood pressure	_____	_____
Shortness of breath	_____	_____
Family history of heart disease	_____	_____
Rheumatic fever	_____	_____
High cholesterol levels	_____	_____
Respiratory problems	_____	_____
Chronic cough	_____	_____
Diabetes	_____	_____
Sickle cell anemia	_____	_____
Dizziness or loss of consciousness	_____	_____
Seizures or convulsions	_____	_____
Severe headaches	_____	_____
Obesity	_____	_____
Arthritis	_____	_____
Serious bone, joint, or muscle injury	_____	_____
Low back pain	_____	_____
Do you smoke cigarettes?	_____	_____
Are you using any prescription drugs?	_____	_____
Do you have any physical problems that are of concern to you?	_____	_____

If you have checked the yes column for any of the conditions listed, it is recommended that you consult your physician before engaging in a physical activity program.

The American College of Sports Medicine* and the American Medical Association have established the following guidelines and recommendations for medical evaluation before engaging in a physical activity program.

1. Any individual less than 35 years of age who has (1) no previous history of cardiovascular disease, (2) no known primary risk factors, and (3) undergone a medical evaluation within the past 2 years may generally begin a physical activity program without additional medical evaluation or clearance.
2. Any individual less than 35 years of age who exhibits (1) evidence of coronary heart disease or (2) a significant combination of risk factors should be examined and cleared medically before engaging in a physical activity program.
3. For all individuals over 35 years of age, medical evaluation and clearance are recommended before any major increase in physical activity levels.

*American College of Sports Medicine: Guidelines for exercise testing and prescription, Philadelphia, 1991, Lea & Febiger.

Lab Activity 3-2

Planning for a Physical Activity Program

Name _____ Section _____ Date _____

PURPOSE   To determine whether you have addressed the necessary considerations for beginning a physical activity program.

PROCEDURE   In the space provided, indicate your best response.

1. Based on your responses in Lab Activity 1-1, list the goals you wish to accomplish by engaging in a physical activity program. _____
_____
_____
_____
_____
_____

2. What are the components of fitness that you want to concentrate on to accomplish these goals? (muscular strength, flexibility, cardiorespiratory endurance, etc.) _____
_____
_____
_____

3. What are the physical activities that you most enjoy participating in that you think will be the most effective in accomplishing these goals? _____
_____
_____

4. When do you think will be the best time during the day for you to work out? _____
_____

5. How many days a week do you plan to engage in physical activity? _____
_____

6. Do you plan to work out on your own, or will you choose a workout partner? List the people with whom you might like to work out. _____
_____

7. How long do you think your warm-up, workout/activity, cool-down will take? _____
_____

8. What will your warm-up activity consist of? _____
_____
_____
_____

9. Briefly describe what you plan to do during your workout. (Specific exercises and instruction relative to the various health-related components of fitness will be covered in subsequent chapters.) _____
_____
_____
_____

10. What will your cool-down activity consist of? _____
_____
_____
_____

11. What things can you do to make your physical activity program safe and reduce the possibility of injury? _____
_____
_____
_____

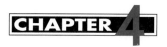
DEVELOPING CARDIORESPIRATORY FITNESS

OBJECTIVES

After completing this chapter, you should be able to do the following:

- Discuss the importance of cardiorespiratory endurance to overall fitness and health.
- Describe the differences between aerobic and anaerobic activity.
- Explain how maximum aerobic capacity determines your level of cardiorespiratory endurance.
- Describe the principles of continuous, interval, fartlek, and par cours training and the potential of each technique for improving cardiorespiratory endurance.
- Discuss specific aerobic activities that can be used to improve cardiorespiratory endurance.
- Identify methods for assessment of cardiorespiratory endurance.

Key Terms

aerobic activity
anaerobic activity
aerobic capacity
maximum aerobic capacity
stroke volume
cardiac output
fast-twitch muscle fibers
slow-twitch muscle fibers
target heart rate
rating of perceived exertion
continuous training
interval training
fartlek
par cours

WHY IS CARDIORESPIRATORY FITNESS IMPORTANT FOR YOU?

Of all the components of physical fitness listed in Chapter 1, none is more important than cardiorespiratory endurance, also referred to as cardiovascular endurance. Cardiorespiratory endurance is the ability to perform whole-body activities and continue movement for extended periods without undue fatigue. We rely on the cardiorespiratory system to transport and supply the oxygen needed by the various tissues within our bodies. It is the basic life-support system of the body. Without oxygen, the cells within the human body cannot function, and ultimately death occurs.

Everyone needs some degree of cardiorespiratory endurance to carry out normal daily activities. If you are engaged in exercise, the cardiorespiratory system must work harder to deliver enough oxygen to sustain that activity. Thus as the cardiorespiratory system becomes more efficient at supplying the needed oxygen, your level of cardiorespiratory fitness improves and you are likely to be more resistant to fatigue.

For the older individuals such as nontraditional college students, the health benefits of improving cardiorespiratory endurance may be more important than the fitness benefits.

Engaging in regular exercise will also improve your cardiovascular health and can greatly reduce your chance of heart disease. If you have low levels of cardiorespiratory endurance, your risk of developing heart disease is higher than normal.

Aerobic exercise is great for building cardiorespiratory fitness. An **aerobic activity** is one in which the intensity of the activity is low enough that the cardiovascular system can supply enough oxygen to continue the activity for long periods. An activity in which the intensity is so great that the demand for oxygen is greater than the body's ability to deliver oxygen is called an **anaerobic activity**. Short bursts of

muscle contraction, as in running or swimming sprints or lifting weights, use predominantly the anaerobic system. However, endurance events such as walking depend a great deal on the aerobic system. In most activities, both aerobic and anaerobic systems function simultaneously. Table 4-1 provides a comparison summary between aerobic and anaerobic activities.

The capacity of the cardiorespiratory system to carry oxygen throughout the body depends on the coordinated function of four components: (1) the heart, (2) the blood vessels, (3) the blood, and (4) the lungs. Improvement of cardiorespiratory endurance through exercise occurs because of an increase in the capability of each of these four components in providing necessary oxygen to the working tissues. A basic discussion of what occurs in the heart in

aerobic activity: an activity in which the intensity of the activity is low enough that the cardiovascular system can supply enough oxygen to continue the activity for long periods

anaerobic activity: an activity in which the intensity is so great that the demand for oxygen is greater than the body's ability to deliver oxygen

TABLE 4-1
Comparison of Aerobic versus Anaerobic Activities

	Mode	Relative Intensity	Performance	Frequency	Duration
Aerobic Activities	Continuous, long-duration, sustained activities	Less intense	60% to 85% of maximum range	At least 3 but no more than 6 times per week	20 to 60 minutes
Anaerobic Activities	Explosive, short-duration, burst-type activities	More intense	85% to 100% range	3 to 4 days per week	10 seconds to 2 minutes

response to training and exercise should make it easier for you to understand why the training techniques discussed later are effective in improving cardiorespiratory endurance.

HOW DOES EXERCISE AFFECT THE FUNCTION OF THE HEART?

The heart is the main pumping mechanism and circulates oxygenated blood throughout the body to the various tissues. The heart receives oxygen-poor blood from the venous system and then pumps the blood through the pulmonary vessels to the lungs, where carbon dioxide is exchanged for oxygen. The oxygen-rich blood then returns to the heart, from which it exits through the aorta to the arterial system and is circulated throughout the body, supplying oxygen to the tissues (Figure 4-1).

As you begin to exercise, your muscles use the oxygen at a much higher rate, and thus your heart must pump more oxygenated blood to meet this increased demand. Like any other muscle, the heart will adapt to the increased demands placed on it over a period of time. The heart is capable of adapting to this increased demand through three mechanisms, as listed below.

1. *Increased Heart Rate* As the intensity of the exercise increases, the heart rate also increases, reaching a plateau at a given level after about 2 to 3 minutes. At rest, the heart beats about 70 times per minute. The

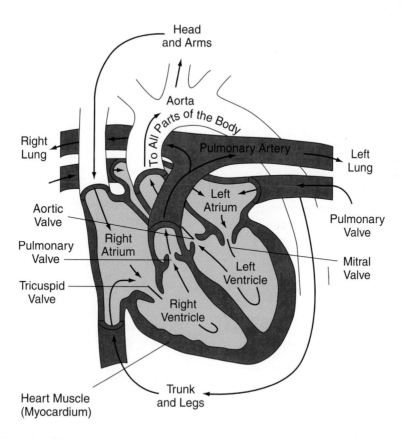

Figure 4-1. Anatomy of the Heart and Blood Flow.

maximal heart rate is different in everybody, but it can be estimated by subtracting the person's age (in years) from 220.

2. *Increased Stroke Volume.* The volume of blood being pumped out of the heart with each beat is called the **stroke volume**. At rest, the heart pumps out approximately 70 ml of blood per beat. During acute exercise, stroke volume increases. Stroke volume can continue to increase only to a point (about 110 ml/beat) at which there is simply not enough time between beats for the heart to fill up. The long term effects of exercise produce an increase in maximum stroke volume during exercise, particularly in individuals who are sedentary.

3. *Increased Cardiac output.* **Cardiac output** indicates how much blood the heart is capable of pumping in exactly 1 minute. It is determined by heart rate (the rate of pumping) and stroke volume (the quantity of blood ejected with each heart beat). Cardiac output is the primary determinant of the maximal rate at which oxygen can be used. Approximately 5 liters (L) of blood are pumped through the heart during each minute at rest. During exercise, cardiac output increases to approximately four times that experienced during rest (about 20L) in the normal individual and may increase as much as six times in the elite endurance athlete (about 30L). As your level of fitness improves, the heart becomes more efficient because it is capable of pumping more blood with each stroke and thus heart rate during exercise will be lower.

WHAT DETERMINES HOW EFFICIENTLY THE BODY IS USING OXYGEN?

The greatest rate at which oxygen can be taken in and used during exercise is referred to as **aerobic capacity,** or as your **maximum aerobic capacity.** Maximum aerobic capacity is measured in a laboratory to determine how much oxygen can be used during 1 minute of maximal exercise. It is most often presented in terms of the volume of oxygen used relative to body weight per unit of time (ml/kg/min). Normal maximal aerobic capacity for most men and women ages 15 to 25 years would fall in the range of 38 to 46 ml/kg/min. However, a world-class male marathon runner may have a maximum aerobic capacity in the 70 to 80 ml/kg/min range, and a female marathoner may have a 60 to 70 ml/kg/min range.

The performance of any activity requires a certain rate of oxygen utilization that is about the same for everybody. Generally, the greater the rate or intensity of the activity, the greater the oxygen demands. Each person has his or her own maximal rate of oxygen utilization, and his or her ability to perform an activity is closely related to the amount of oxygen required by that activity.

The maximal rate at which oxygen can be used is largely a genetically determined characteristic. Each person's maximal aerobic capacity falls within a given range. The more active you are, the higher the existing maximum aerobic capacity will be within that range. The less active you are, the lower your maximum

stroke volume: the volume of blood being pumped out of the heart with each beat

cardiac output: indicates how much blood the heart is capable of pumping in exactly 1 minute

aerobic capacity: the greatest rate at which oxygen can be taken in and used during exercise

maximum aerobic capacity: measured in a laboratory to determine how much oxygen can be used during 1 minute of maximal exercise

aerobic capacity will be in that range. Thus, by engaging in a training program, it is possible to increase your aerobic capacity to its highest limit within your range.

The range of maximal aerobic capacity that you inherit is mostly determined by the types of muscle fibers that you have. **Fast-twitch muscle fibers** (FT), or fast-contracting fibers, are not as dependent on the presence of oxygen for contraction and tend to tire very rapidly. Fast-twitch fibers are responsible for speed or power activities such as sprinting or weight lifting. **Slow-twitch muscle fibers** (ST) are slow-contracting fibers that require large amounts of oxygen for contraction and are more resistant to fatigue. Slow-twitch fibers are more useful in long-term, endurance activities such as marathon running or cross-country skiing. If you have a greater percentage of slow-twitch muscle fibers than fast-twitch fibers throughout your body, you will be able to use oxygen more efficiently and thus your maximum aerobic capacity will be higher.

Fatigue is closely related to the percentage of maximum aerobic capacity that a particular activity demands. It should be apparent that the greater the percentage of maximal aerobic capacity required during an activity, the shorter the time the activity may be performed. Fatigue partly occurs when insufficient oxygen is supplied to muscles. For example, Figure 4-2 presents two people, A and B. A has a maximum aerobic capacity of 50 ml/kg/min, whereas B has a maximum aerobic capacity of only 40 ml/kg/min. If both A

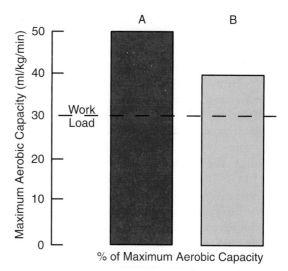

Figure 4-2. Fitness and Aerobic Capacity
Individual A should be able to work longer than can individual B as a result of lower use of maximum aerobic capacity.

and B are exercising at the same intensity, then A is working at a much lower percentage of maximum aerobic capacity than is B. Consequently, A should be able to sustain his or her activity over a much longer period. Everyday activities such as walking up stairs or running to catch a bus may be adversely affected if your ability to use oxygen efficiently is impaired. Thus improvement of cardiorespiratory endurance should be an essential component of any fitness program.

HOW DO YOU KNOW WHAT YOUR AEROBIC CAPACITY IS?

The most accurate technique for measuring aerobic capacity is done in a laboratory. It involves exercising a person on a treadmill or bicycle ergometer at a specific intensity and then monitoring heart rate and collecting samples of expired air using somewhat expensive and sophisticated equipment. Obviously, this is a somewhat impractical technique for the typical person. Therefore, what

fast-twitch muscle fibers: a type of muscle fiber used for speed or power activities such as sprinting or weight lifting

slow-twitch muscle fibers: a type of muscle fiber that is resistant to fatigue and is more useful in long-term endurance activities

we most often do is monitor the heart rate as a means of estimating a percentage of maximum aerobic capacity.

Monitoring heart rate is an indirect method of estimating oxygen uptake. In general, heart rate and oxygen uptake have a linear relationship, although at very low intensities as well as at high intensities this linear relationship breaks down (Figure 4-3). The greater the intensity of the exercise, the higher the heart rate. Because of this existing relationship, it should be apparent that the rate of oxygen utilization can be estimated by measuring the heart rate. The Lab Activities at the end of this chapter, which all monitor heart rates, are a means of estimating maximum aerobic capacity.

▶ Monitoring Heart Rate

There are several sites at which heart rate is easily measured. The most accurate site for measuring the pulse rate is the radial artery (located on the thumb side of the wrist joint). By placing your index and middle fingers on the thumb side of the wrist, you should be able to locate a strong pulse (Figure 4-4, *A*). Do not use your thumb to monitor pulse rate. Each pulse represents one heartbeat. You should count the number of beats that occur in 30 seconds and then multiply that number by 2 to give you an accurate heart rate. Heart rate should be monitored within 15 seconds after stopping exercise.

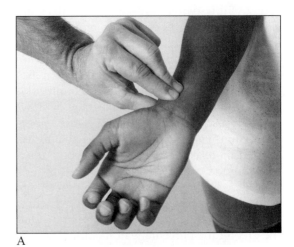

A

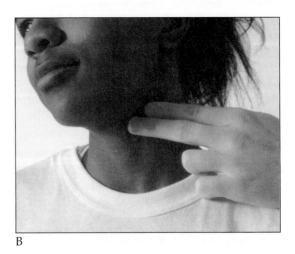

B

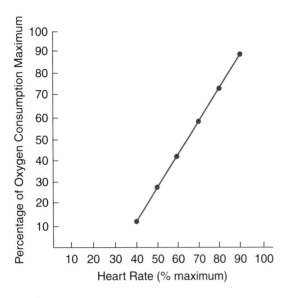

Figure 4-3. Maximal Heart Rate and Maximum Aerobic Capacity.
Maximal heart rate is achieved at about the same time as maximum aerobic capacity.

Figure 4-4. Measuring Pulse.
Measuring pulse rate at A, radial artery and B, carotid artery.

WHAT TRAINING TECHNIQUES CAN BE USED TO IMPROVE CARDIORESPIRATORY ENDURANCE?

Several methods can be used to improve cardiorespiratory endurance, including (1) continuous or sustained training, (2) interval training, (3) fartlek, and (4) par cours. The amount of improvement possible is largely determined by initial levels of cardiorespiratory endurance. The lower your endurance at the start, the more you will improve. Regardless of the training technique used for the improvement of cardiorespiratory endurance, one principal goal remains the same. You are trying to increase the ability of the cardiorespiratory system to supply a sufficient amount of oxygen to working muscles. Without oxygen, the body is incapable of producing energy for an extended period.

CONTINUOUS TRAINING

Continuous training is a technique that uses exercises performed at the same level of intensity for long periods. There are four considerations with continuous training:

- The type of activity
- The frequency of the activity
- The intensity of the activity
- The duration of the activity

▶ Type of Activity

The type of activity used in continuous training must be aerobic. Aerobic activities are any type that use large amounts of oxygen, elevate the heart rate, and maintain it at that level for an extended time. Aerobic activities generally involve repetitive, whole body, large-muscle movements performed over an extended time. Examples of aerobic activities are found in the Fit List below. The advantage of these aerobic activities as opposed to more intermittent activities, such as racquetball, squash, basketball, or tennis, is that it is easy to regulate the intensity of aerobic activities by either speeding up or slowing down the pace. Because we already know that the given intensity of the workload elicits a given heart rate, these aerobic activities allow us to maintain heart rate at a specified or target level. Intermittent activities involve variable speeds and intensities that cause the heart rate to fluctuate considerably. Although these intermittent activities will improve cardiorespiratory endurance, they are much more difficult to monitor in terms of intensity. It is important to point out that any type of activity, from gardening to aerobic exercise, can improve fitness and reduce the risks for developing several chronic diseases. Again, the fact that you enjoy a specific type of activity should be an important factor in your selection of one.

Fit List 4-1

Examples of Aerobic Fitness Activities

- Walking
- Jogging
- Running
- Swimming
- Cycling
- Stepping
- Aerobic dance exercise
- In-line skating
- Cross-country skiing
- Rowing

continuous training: a technique that uses exercises performed at the same level of intensity for long periods

▶ Frequency of Activity

To see at least minimal improvement in cardiorespiratory endurance, it is necessary for the average person to engage in no less than three sessions per week. If possible, you should aim for five sessions per week. A competitive athlete should be prepared to train as often as six times per week. Everyone should take off at least 1 day per week to give damaged tissues a chance to repair themselves.

▶ Intensity of Activity

The intensity of the exercise is also a critical factor, even though recommendations regarding training intensities vary. This is particularly true in the early stages of training, when the body is forced to make a lot of adjustments to increased workload demands.

Determining Exercise Intensity by Monitoring Heart Rate. The objective of aerobic exercise is to elevate your heart rate to a specified target rate and maintain it at that level during your entire workout. Because heart rate is directly related to the intensity of the exercise as well as to the rate of oxygen use, it becomes a relatively simple process to identify a specific workload (pace) that will make the heart rate plateau at the desired level. By monitoring heart rate, we know whether the pace is too fast or too slow to get the heart rate into a target range.

Heart rate can be increased or decreased by speeding up or slowing down your pace. It has already been indicated that heart rate increases proportionately with the intensity of the workload and will plateau after 2 to 3 minutes of activity. Thus you should be actively engaged in the workout for 2 to 3 minutes before measuring your pulse.

Several formulas allow you to easily identify a training **target heart rate**. To calculate a specific target heart rate, you must first determine your maximal heart rate. Exact determination of maximal heart rate (HR) involves exercising an individual at a maximal level and monitoring the HR using an electrocardiogram. This is

a difficult process outside of a laboratory. However, an approximate estimate of maximal HR for both young boys and girls is that maximal HR is thought to be about 220 beats per minute. However, maximal HR is related to age, and, as you get older, your maximum HR decreases. Thus a relatively simple estimate of your maximal HR would be Maximal HR = 220 − Age. For a 20-year-old individual, maximal heart rate would be about 200 beats per minute (220 − 20 = 200). If you are interested in working at 70 percent of your maximal rate, the target heart rate can be calculated by multiplying $0.7 \times (220 - \text{Age})$.

Another commonly used formula that takes into account your current level of fitness is the Karvonen equation.

Target HR = Resting HR* +
(0.6 [Maximal HR − Resting HR])

Resting heart rate generally falls between 60 and 80 beats per minute. A 20-year-old person with a resting pulse of 70 beats per minute, according to the Karvonen equation, would have a target training heart rate of 148 beats per minute (70 + 0.6 [200 − 70] = 148).

Regardless of the formula you use, the American College of Sports Medicine recommends that young healthy individuals train with a target heart rate in the 60 to 85 percent range when training continuously. Exercising at a 70 percent level is considered a moderate level because activity can be continued for a long period with little discomfort and still produce a training effect. In a highly trained individual it is not difficult to sustain a heart rate at the 85 percent level.

> **target heart rate:** a specific heart rate to be achieved and maintained during exercise

*True resting heart rate should be monitored with the subject lying down.

Determining Exercise Intensity Through Rating of Perceived Exertion (RPE). Rating of perceived exertion (RPE) can be used in addition to monitoring heart rate to indicate exercise intensity. During exercise, individuals are asked to rate on a numerical scale from 6 to 20 exactly how they feel relative to their level of exertion (Table 4-2). More intense exercise that requires a higher level of oxygen consumption and energy expenditure is directly related to higher subjective ratings of perceived exertion. Over a period of time, individuals can be taught to exercise at a specific RPE that relates directly to more objective measures of exercise intensity

rating of perceived exertion: a technique used to subjectively rate exercise intensity on a numerical scale

TABLE 4-2
Rating of Perceived Exertion

Scale	Verbal Rating
7	Very, very light
8	
9	Very light
10	
11	Fairly light
12	
13	Somewhat hard
14	
15	Hard
16	
17	Very hard
18	
19	Very, very hard
20	

Used with permission from Borg GA: Psychological ratings of perceived exertion, Med Sci Sports Exerc & Comm 14:377, copyright American College of Sports Medicine, 1982, Williams & Wilkins Publishing Company.

▶ Duration of Activity

The American College of Sports Medicine (ACSM) is a professional organization whose members include physicians, exercise physiologists, biomechanists, athletic trainers, and physical therapists. ACSM sets standards and guidelines for exercise. For minimal improvement to occur, you must participate in at least 15 minutes of continuous activity with the heart rate elevated to its working level. ACSM recommends engaging in 15 to 60 minutes of workout/activity with the heart rate elevated to training levels. Generally, the longer the duration of the workout, the greater the improvement in cardiorespiratory endurance. The competitive athlete should train for at least 45 minutes per session.

▶ Guidelines for Continuous Training

In summary, when using the continuous training method, the activity selected must be aerobic and should be enjoyable. To see minimal improvement in cardiorespiratory endurance, training must be done for 15 to 60 minutes, three to five times per week with the heart rate elevated to an intensity of no less than 60 percent of its maximal rate. As mentioned in Chapter 3, each training program should be designed to meet individual needs and abilities. The principle of overload states that you must stress the system if you are to see improvement and progress from one level to another. Everyone should begin slowly with the idea that he or she will progress as quickly as possible at his or her own rate. If you are able to perform an activity at a given level without undue stress and it seems that you are not being "challenged" at that particular level, you may progress to the next level. Remember, however, that beginning at a level that is too high will probably produce various musculoskeletal injuries that often cause setbacks in a training program.

All training programs are based on monitoring heart rate during some type of aerobic activity. Heart rate can be increased or decreased

TABLE 4-3

Guidelines For Continuous Training

Training Level	Frequency (Sessions per Week)	Duration (Minutes)	Intensity of Training Heart Rate (% Maximal Heart Rate)
Beginner	3	20	60%
Intermediate	4-5	30-45	70%-80%
Advanced	5-6	45-60	80%-90%

by altering the pace. The guidelines in Table 4-3 can be applied to beginning, intermediate, and advanced levels.

ADVANCED TRAINING METHODS

INTERVAL TRAINING

Unlike continuous training, **interval training** involves activities that are more intermittent. Interval training consists of alternating periods of relatively intense work with periods of active recovery. It permits you to perform much more work at a more intense workload over a longer period than you could if you were working continuously. It is most desirable in continuous training to work at an intensity of about 60 to 85 percent of maximal heart rate. Obviously, sustaining activity at a relatively high intensity over a 20-minute period would be extremely difficult. The advantage of interval training is that it allows work at this 80 percent or higher level for a short period, followed by an active period of recovery during which you may be working at only 30 to 45 percent of maximal heart rate. Thus the intensity of the workout and its duration can be greater than with continuous training.

interval training: alternating periods of relatively intense work with periods of active recovery

Most sports are anaerobic, involving short bursts of intense activity followed by a type of active recovery period (football, basketball, soccer, and tennis all qualify). Training with the interval technique allows you to be more sport specific during the workout. With interval training you can apply the overload principle by making the training period much more intense. Several important factors should be considered in interval training. The training period is the amount of time that continuous activity is actually being performed, and the recovery period is the time between training periods. A set is a group of combined training and recovery periods, and a repetition is the number of training/recovery periods per set. Training time or distance refers to the rate or distance of the training period. The training/recovery ratio indicates a time ratio for training versus recovery.

An example of interval training would be a soccer player running sprints. An interval workout would involve running ten 120-yard sprints in under 22 seconds, with a 1-minute recovery period (walking) between each sprint. During this training session the soccer player's heart rate would probably increase to 85 to 95 percent of maximal level during the sprint and should probably fall to the 35 to 45 percent level during the recovery period.

Inactive or sedentary individuals should exercise some caution when using interval training as a method for improving cardiorespiratory endurance. The intensity levels attained during the active periods may be too high for the inactive individual.

FARTLEK TRAINING

Fartlek is a training technique, a type of cross-country running, that originated in Sweden. Fartlek literally means "speed play." It is similar to interval training in that you must run for a specified period; however, specific pace and speed are not identified. The course for a fartlek workout should be some type of varied terrain including some level running, some uphill and downhill running, and some running around obstacles such as trees or rocks. The object is to put surges into a running workout, varying the length of the surges according to individual purposes. One big advantage of fartlek training is that because the pace and terrain are always changing, the training session is less regimented and allows for an effective alternative in the training routine. **When you really think about it, most people who jog or walk are really engaging in a fartlek-type workout.**

Again, if fartlek training is going to improve cardiorespiratory endurance, it must elevate the heart rate to at least minimal training levels (60 to 85 percent). Fartlek may best be used as an off-season conditioning activity or as a change-of-pace activity to counteract the boredom of a training program that uses the same activity day after day.

PAR COURS

Par cours is a technique for improving cardiorespiratory endurance that basically combines continuous training and circuit training.

fartlek: a type of workout that involves jogging at varying speeds over varying terrain

par cours: a technique for improving cardiorespiratory endurance that basically combines continuous training and circuit training

This technique involves jogging a short distance from one station to the next and performing the station's designated exercise according to directions on an instruction board located at that station. Par cours circuits provide an excellent means for gaining some aerobic benefits while incorporating some of the benefits of calisthenics. Typically, par cours circuits are found in parks or recreational areas within metropolitan areas.

GOOD AEROBIC ACTIVITIES FOR IMPROVING CARDIORESPIRATORY ENDURANCE

WALKING

If walking is your primary form of exercise, you're part of a large club that has become the fitness phenomenon of the new millenium. More than 60 million Americans now walk for exercise, making it the number one participation sport in the country.

There are several reasons why people are walking for fitness. It is, after all, an activity that can be pursued at almost any time, anywhere, with anyone, at no cost. Besides being fun, walking can expend a lot of energy. A walking regimen can be started easily at any age and can be worked into almost anybody's daily schedule. Although some techniques are better than others, walking demands little skill or practice. It does require a pair of comfortable shoes, but no other specialized clothing or equipment is really necessary. As long as you're in relatively good health, the activity presents few, if any, health hazards. As with any program involving your health, just check with your physician before you begin.

Walking's greatest value as a fitness activity is that you can just go out and walk. Like other physical activities, technique becomes a factor in developing a more effective program. In walking, the development of proper technique involves correct stride, arm swing, posture, and a steady pace. Although it's fun to experiment with techniques, it's by no means mandatory in walking. You know how to put one foot in front of the other, and there's no reason to complicate a simple activity.

RUNNING

For years now, running has been viewed by the American public as an important fitness activity. Within the last 15 years, millions of people have taken to the streets and now run or jog on a regular basis. And the running phenomenon doesn't seem to be restricted to any one segment of the population. Young children, college students, office personnel, laborers, elderly persons, people of all backgrounds and both sexes regularly put on their running shoes and go for a run.

Although many people run to control their weight and attain a healthful physical appearance, other people run for the other physiological benefits a running program offers. Many people report that running (or jogging) is relaxing and alleviates stress, tension, and depression. They express feelings of greater self-worth and enthusiasm toward life after a run. This euphoric feeling has been called a "runner's high," and most people agree that this is both a psychological and a physiological phenomenon.

As is the case with walking, the only equipment required is a pair of running shoes and some shorts. Running offers the advantages of low cost, flexibility of time, year-round availability, and a relatively high level of benefit in return for time and effort.

However, there are some disadvantages to running. Because the feet and legs are subjected to repetitive pounding on the running surface, overuse injuries are very likely. Most of these injuries involve the muscles, tendons, ligaments, and occasionally bones of the lower extremities. Proper running and training techniques and properly fitted running shoes can reduce the number of injuries associated with running.

SWIMMING

Like running, swimming is an excellent method of developing cardiorespiratory fitness. The physiological benefits of swimming are similar to those of running; however, several differences should be addressed. The first difference is that not only must the energy of the arms and legs be used to propel the body through the water, but some energy must also be expended to keep the body afloat. For these reasons, it has been estimated that the amount of energy required to swim a given distance is approximately four times as great as running an equal distance. Energy expenditure and heart rates vary with the type of stroke. For both trained and highly skilled swimmers swimming at any given speed, the breaststroke seems to require the greatest amount of energy, then the backstroke, and last the front crawl.

Swimming also eliminates several of the stresses and strains on the weight-bearing joints that are commonly experienced in running. Although the shoulder joint undergoes a significant amount of overuse-type stress, the ankle and knee joints are spared the trauma of the foot repeatedly banging into a hard surface.

A swimsuit and perhaps a pair of goggles for persons whose eyes are irritated by chlorine are all that is necessary to begin a swimming program. For many, the biggest drawback of using a swimming program for cardiorespiratory conditioning is the unavailability of a swimming pool.

AEROBIC DANCE EXERCISE

In today's terminology, the word aerobics is primarily used to refer specifically to aerobic dance exercise, which may well be the country's largest, most widespread, organized fitness endeavor. The growth in aerobic dance exercise during the past decade has been truly phenomenal. It is estimated that more than 30 million Americans, both males and females, now participate in aerobic dance exercise. Aerobics is a combination of choreographed fitness routines set to music. In other words, it is movement to music that contributes to physical fitness by improving cardiorespiratory endurance, strength, flexibility, and muscular endurance.

As a rapidly developing participation sport, aerobics is undergoing an evolutionary process. Different styles of aerobics have been advocated over the last few years.

High-impact aerobics. This is the more traditional form in which the cardiorespiratory conditioning component consists of running, jumping, and hopping movements set to music. High-impact aerobics has produced a significant number of musculoskeletal injuries as a result of the repetitive pounding of the lower extremities against a hard surface.

Low-impact aerobics. The impact to the lower extremities is reduced by eliminating excessive jumping and by keeping one leg slightly bent and in constant contact with the floor throughout the conditioning phase of the workout. Traveling movements rather than stationary steps are used, with an emphasis on maintaining proper body alignment at all times.

Aquatic aerobics. Aquatic aerobics are done in water to eliminate any jarring of the weight-bearing body parts while taking advantage of the water's resistance to movement during the conditioning component. Of all the types of aerobics, water aerobics will probably be the safest.

Step aerobics. "Stepping" uses a bench ranging between 4 and 8 inches high and slower music that makes it appropriate for all age groups. The intensity of the workout can be modified by changing the height of the bench.

Kick boxing. Kick boxing is the latest aerobic dance-type exercise. Kick boxing is an exercise technique that combines kicks from the ancient martial art of Tae Kwon Do with punches from boxing performed to high energy exercise music. It has become extremely popular in both health clubs and in home exercise videos.

Circuit aerobics. Circuit aerobics combines the use of resistance equipment with an advanced aerobic dance exercise class. Holding light hand weights or wearing banded wrist weights is a common practice in various forms of aerobic exercise. Addition of these light weights increases energy expenditure during activity. Approximately 30 minutes is devoted to aerobic dance and 30 minutes to resistance training at various stations.

CYCLING

Cycling is another aerobic activity that is excellent for improving cardiorespiratory endurance. It is also enjoyed by people of all ages, primarily because of the ease with which anyone can learn to ride without formal training. Like running and swimming, cycling produces some very desirable physiological responses in terms of strength, endurance, and weight control.

Bicycles come in thousands of different makes and models, with countless numbers of available accessories and options. The cost of purchasing a bicycle is not much more than that of buying a pair of good running shoes for the average person.

Perhaps the biggest problem with cycling is locating a safe place to ride. No matter how safety conscious you are on the bicycle, there is always a danger posed by traffic. For this reason, stationary exercise bikes, or ergometers, have become popular. The stationary bike allows you to gain all the cardiovascular benefits of cycling without having to worry about dealing with traffic safety. Additionally, you can exercise in privacy, regardless of outdoor conditions, and read, watch TV, or listen to music at the same time.

SPINNING

Spinning is a new exercise technique that is basically aerobic exercise performed on stationary exercise bikes. It is being recommended as a great work-out with no impact, thus minimizing chances of injury. Spinning usually involves a 40 to 45 minute workout. It is good for all levels in any class because you can get a very intense workout or a low-level workout in the same class depending on your fitness level and how hard you want to work. The workout is done to music, with the class instructor acting as a coach to work you through the routine. At this point spinning classes are found primarily in health clubs, although in the near future spinning clubs and videos will be increasingly available to the consumer.

IN-LINE SKATING

In-line skating, also called rollerblading, is another fitness and recreational activity that has quickly gained popularity throughout the United States. However, contrary to popular belief, skating is not a new activity. In-line skating is essentially "high-tech" rollerskating. A pair of rollerblades looks like ice skates that have had the blade replaced with a series of four to six small wheels. These wheels are made for gliding on hard, smooth surfaces. In-line skaters are capable of attaining speeds approaching 25 miles per hour. For this reason, pads must be worn to protect elbows, knees, and hands. It is also recommended that protective headgear, such as a cycling helmet, be worn to minimize the likelihood of injury.

The motions used with in-line skating are similar to those used in ice skating—pushing with the legs from side to side and using a side-to-side swinging motion of the arms for balance. In-line skating uses gross movements of both the arms and the legs, making it an excellent aerobic activity.

WHAT IS YOUR LEVEL OF CARDIORESPIRATORY ENDURANCE?

How fit is your cardiorespiratory system? Several tests have been developed to evaluate fitness levels. Most of these tests are based on the idea that cardiorespiratory endurance ca-

pacity is best indicated by the maximal aerobic capacity of the working tissues to use oxygen. We know from an earlier discussion that maximal aerobic capacity can be predicted or estimated by measuring heart rates at varying workloads. You can use Lab Activities 4-2 and 4-3 as tests to determine your specific levels of cardiorespiratory endurance. It must be remembered that each of these activities is based largely on one or both of the following factors: (1) the motivation of the person, and (2) the minimal level of cardiovascular endurance.

SUMMARY

- Cardiorespiratory endurance involves the coordinated function of the heart, lungs, blood, and blood vessels to supply sufficient amounts of oxygen to the working tissues.
- The best indicator of how efficiently the cardiorespiratory system functions is aerobic capacity, or the maximal rate at which oxygen can be used by the tissues.
- Heart rate is directly related to the rate of oxygen consumption. It is therefore possible to predict the intensity of the exercise in terms of a rate of oxygen use by monitoring heart rate.
- Aerobic exercise involves an activity in which the level of intensity and duration is low enough to provide a sufficient amount of oxygen to supply the demands of the working tissues.
- In anaerobic exercise the intensity of the activity is so high that oxygen is being used more quickly than it can be supplied; thus an oxygen debt is incurred that must be repaid before working tissue can return to its normal resting state.
- Continuous training for improving cardiorespiratory endurance involves selecting an activity that is aerobic in nature and training at least 3 times per week for a period of no less than 15 minutes with the heart rate elevated to 60 to 85 percent of maximal rate.
- Interval training involves alternating periods of relatively intense work followed by

periods of active recovery. Interval training allows performance of more work at a relatively higher workload than does continuous training.

- Fartlek makes use of jogging or running over varying types of terrain at changing speeds.
- Par cours is a training technique that combines continuous training with exercises done at stations along the course.
- Walking, running, swimming, aerobic dance exercise, cycling, and in-line skating are all excellent activities for improving cardiorespiratory endurance.

SUGGESTED READINGS

American College of Sports Medicine. 1995. *Guidelines for exercise testing and prescription.* Philadelphia: Lea and Febiger.

American College of Sports Medicine. 1990. The recommended quantity and quality of exercise for developing and maintaining cardiorespiratory and muscular fitness in healthy adults. *Medicine and science in sports and exercise* 22:265–74.

Banks, B. 1999. *The tae bo way.* New York: Bantam, Doubleday, Dell Publishing.

Billat, V.L. et al. 1999. Interval training at VO_{2max}: Effects on aerobic performance and overtraining markers. *Medicine and science in sports and exercise* 31(1): 156–63.

Borg, G.A. 1982. Psychophysical basis of perceived exertion. *Medicine and science in sports and exercise* 14:377.

Burfoot, A. 1998. The run/walk plan: A simple new training technique can increase your endurance and calorie-burning decrease injuries and maybe even help you get faster. *Runner's world* 33(4):46–48, 50–51.

Colwin, C. 1999. *Swimming dynamics: Winning techniques and strategies.* Lincolnwood, IL: Masters Press.

Joyce, D., C. Reid, and P. Vincent. 1999. *The complete book of cycling: equipment touring maintenance racing.* London: Hamlyn Books.

Liz, M., and M. Neporent. 1999. *Fitness walking for dummies.* Foster City, CA: IDG Books Worldwide.

McMahon, S. 1998. The relationship between aerobic fitness and both power output and subsequent recovery during maximal intermittent exercise. *Journal of Science and Medicine in Sport* 1(14): 219–27.

Nealy, W. 1998. *Inline: A manual for beginning to intermediate inline skating.* Birmingham, AL: Menasha Ridge Press.

Noakes, T.D. 1998. Maximal oxygen uptake: "Classical" versus "contemporary" viewpoints: A rebuttal. *Medicine and science in sports and exercise* 30(9):1381–98.

O'Connor, J. 1999. *Fitness on foot today: Walking, jogging, and running health sciences series.* Pacific Grove, CA: Brooks Cole Publishing Co.

Porcari, J.P. 1999. Pump up your walk. *American College of Sports Medicine's Health and Fitness Journal* 3(1): 10–17.

Pryor, E., and M. Kraines. 1999. *Keep moving: It's aerobic dance.* Mountain View, CA: Mayfield Publishing.

The walking workout. 1998. *IDEA: International Association of Fitness Professionals health and fitness source* 16(6):80.

SUGGESTED WEBSITES

Bicyclopedia
This site is a comprehensive encyclopedia which covers nearly everything about bikes and cycling.
http://pwp.starnetinc.com/olderr/bcwebsite/

Endurance Training: Increasing Your Aerobic Capacity
This site presents activities related to increased aerobic fitness.
http://www.ama-assn.org/insight/gen_hlth/trainer/aerobic.htm

International Dance Exercise Association
A membership organization for health and fitness professionals, IDEA brings you a virtual on-line library of late-breaking news, information, and research.
http://ideafit.com/

Runner's World Online
This site presents a beginner's program, marathon training, health, and fitness.
http://www.runnersworld.com/

Swimmersworld.com
This site features competitive swimming news and information.
http://www.swimmersworld.com/

The Cooper Institute for Aerobics Research
This nonprofit research and education organization is dedicated to preventive medicine and research.
http://www.cooperinst.org

Walking
This complete guide to walking for fitness, recreation, and competitive racewalking features new articles weekly, a comprehensive link library, chat, bulletin board, and newsletter.
http://walking.miningco.com/

Yeah! Walking
A global walking community features free e-mail, chats, message boards, links, and shopping.
http://www.yeahsports.com/dir/walking/

4Rollerblading
This is a guide to in-line skating from 4anything.com. It is essentially a directory of links.
http://www.4rollerblading.com/

Lab Activity 4-1

Calculating Target Heart Rate

Name _____ Section _____ Date _____

PURPOSE   To calculate a target heart rate range.

EQUIPMENT   Clock or watch

PROCEDURE   Count resting heart rate during a one-minute period. Then perform the following calculations.

220
−   _60_ age
=   _160_ maximum heart rate
=   _____ working heart rate
×   _.60_ intensity (60%)
=   _____
+   _____ resting heart rate
=   _____ lower limit of THR range

220
−   _____ age
=   _____ maximum heart rate
=   _____ working heart rate
×   _.85_ intensity (85%)
=   _____
+   _____ resting heart rate
=   _____ lower limit of THR range

Target Heart Rate Range = _____ bpm to _____ bpm

73

Lab Activity 4-2

1.5-Mile Test

Name   Section   Date

PURPOSE   To determine the level of cardiorespiratory endurance by recording the time required to complete a 1.5-mile measured distance course.

EQUIPMENT   1. Measured course of 1.5 miles, preferably on flat surface
                   2. Stopwatch

PROCEDURE   Subjects are instructed to cover the 1.5-mile distance as quickly as possible by either running, jogging, or walking.

TREATMENT OF DATA   1. Time required to cover the distance should be recorded to the nearest second.
                   2. Consult Table 4-4 to determine appropriate fitness category.

Sample Worksheet for 1.5-Mile Test

		Example
1. Record the time required to complete the 1.5-mile distance.	_20_	1. 11.00
2. Record your age classification.	_60_	2. Age 20
3. Record your sex	_F_	3. Man
4. Record your fitness category as indicated in Table 4-4.		4. Good

Continued

75

TABLE 4-4

1.5-Mile Run Standards for Moderately Fit* College Students†

Fitness Category		Time: Age 17-25	Time: Age 26-35
1. Superior	(females)	<10:30	<11:30
	(males)	<8:30	<9:30
2. Excellent	(females)	10:30-11:49	11:30-12:49
	(males)	8:30-9:29	9:30-10:29
3. Good	(females)	11:50-13:09	12:50-14:09
	(males)	9:30-10:29	10:30-11:29
4. Moderate	(females)	13:10-14:29	14:10-15:29
	(males)	10:30-11:29	11:30-12:29
5. Fair	(females)	14:30-15:49	15:30-16:49
	(males)	11:30-12:29	12:30-13:29
6. Poor	(females)	>15.49	>16.49
	(males)	>12:29	>13:29

From Draper DO, Jones G: Personal communication, 1991, Illinois State University.
*Moderately fit college students are not athletes but laypersons who engage in continuous aerobic activity lasting a minimum of 20 minutes, 3 times a week.
†Based on data collected n = 427 females, 511 males.

Lab Activity 4-3

Cooper's 12-Minute Walking/Running Test

Name _____ Section _____ Date _____

PURPOSE   To determine the level of cardiorespiratory endurance of college students during a 12-minute running or walking activity.

EQUIPMENT   1. Measured running course, preferably a track
2. Stopwatch

PROCEDURE   During a 12-minute period the subject attempts to cover as much distance as possible by either running or walking.

TREATMENT OF DATA   1. Distance covered should be rounded off to the nearest 1/8 mile.
2. Consult Table 4-5. Locate the distance covered for either men or women under the appropriate age classification, and determine the level of fitness.

Sample Worksheet for Cooper's 12-Minute Walking/Running Test	
	Example
1. Measure distance covered, and round off to nearest ⅛ mile _____	1. 1.50
2. Locate this distance in appropriate "Age" column _____	2. Age 20
3. Determine fitness level _____	3. Good

Continued

TABLE 4-5

12-Minute Walking/Running Test Distance [Miles] Covered in 12 Minutes

Fitness Category		Age (Years)					
		13-19	20-29	30-39	40-49	50-59	60+
I. Very poor	(men)	<1.30*	<1.22	<1.18	<1.14	<1.03	<.87
	(women)	<1.0	<.96	<.94	<.88	<.84	<.78
II. Poor	(men)	1.30-1.37	1.22-1.31	1.18-1.30	1.14-1.24	1.03-1.16	.87-1.02
	(women)	1.00-1.18	.96-1.11	.95-1.05	.88-.98	0.84-.93	.78-.86
III. Fair	(men)	1.38-1.56	1.32-1.49	1.31-1.45	1.25-1.39	1.17-1.30	1.03-1.20
	(women)	1.19-1.29	1.12-1.22	1.06-1.18	.99-1.11	.94-1.05	.87-.98
IV. Good	(men)	1.57-1.72	1.50-1.64	1.46-1.56	1.40-1.53	1.31-1.44	1.21-1.32
	(women)	1.30-1.43	1.23-1.34	1.19-1.29	1.12-1.24	1.06-1.18	.99-1.09
V. Excellent	(men)	1.73-1.86	1.65-1.76	1.57-1.69	1.54-1.65	1.45-1.58	1.33-1.55
	(women)	1.44-1.51	1.35-1.45	1.30-1.39	1.25-1.34	1.19-1.30	1.10-1.18
VI. Superior	(men)	>1.87	>1.77	>1.70	>1.66	>1.59	>1.56
	(women)	>1.52	>1.46	>1.40	>1.35	>1.31	>1.19

Monitoring heart rate is an indirect method of estimating oxygen consumption. In general, heart rate and oxygen consumption have a direct relationship; the longer the intensity of the exercise, the higher the heart rate. Because of these existing relationships, it should become apparent that the rate of oxygen consumption can be estimated by taking the heart rate.

From Cooper KH: The aerobics program for total wellbeing, New York, 1982, Bantam Books. Reprinted with permission of the publisher, Bantam Books, New York.
*< Means "less than"; > means "more than."

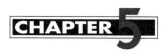

IMPROVING MUSCULAR STRENGTH, ENDURANCE AND POWER

OBJECTIVES

After completing this chapter, you should be able to do the following:

- Define strength, endurance, and power and indicate their relevance to health and skill of performance.
- Describe specific methods for improving muscular strength.
- Discuss differences between males and females in terms of strength development.
- Demonstrate proper techniques for using weights to develop strength and muscular endurance in specific muscle groups.
- Demonstrate various calisthenic exercises that can be used for increasing muscular strength and endurance.

Key Terms

muscular strength
muscular endurance
power
concentric contraction
eccentric contraction
hypertrophy
atrophy
motor unit
myofilaments
isometric exercise
progressive resistance exercise
isokinetic exercise
circuit training
plyometric training
calisthenic exercises

WHY IS MUSCULAR STRENGTH IMPORTANT FOR EVERYONE?

The development of **muscular strength** is an essential component of fitness for anyone involved in a physical activity program. By definition, strength is the ability of a muscle to generate maximum force against some heavy resistance. The development of muscular strength may be considered as both a

muscular strength: the ability of a muscle to generate force against some resistance

health-related and a skill-related component of physical fitness. Maintenance of at least a normal level of strength in a given muscle or muscle group is important for normal healthy living. Muscle weakness or imbalance can result in abnormal movement or gait and can impair normal functional movement. Muscle weakness can also produce poor posture, which can affect appearance. One of the most common health ailments in the United States is lower back pain. In most cases lower back pain is related to lack of muscular fitness, especially lack of muscular strength in the abdominals and loss of flexibility of the hamstrings. Thus strength training may play a critical role not only in fitness programs but also in injury prevention and rehabilitation.

HOW ARE STRENGTH AND MUSCULAR ENDURANCE RELATED?

Muscular strength is closely associated with **muscular endurance**. Muscular endurance is the ability to perform repetitive muscular contractions against some resistance for an extended period of time. As we will see later, as muscular strength increases, there tends to be a corresponding increase in endurance. For example, a person can lift a weight 25 times. If muscular strength is increased by 10 percent through weight training, it is very likely that the maximal number of repetitions would be increased because it is easier for the person to lift the weight. For most people, developing muscular endurance is more important than developing muscular strength, since muscular endurance is probably more critical in carrying out the everyday activities of living. It is important for anyone beginning a physical activity program to understand the need to develop muscular endurance prior to engaging in an aggressive fitness program. This becomes increasingly true with age. However, muscular strength is necessary for anyone involved in certain types of competition.

WHY IS MUSCULAR POWER IMPORTANT IN SPORT ACTIVITIES?

Most movements in sports are explosive and must include elements of both strength and speed if they are to be effective. If a large amount of force is generated quickly, the movement can be referred to as a **power** movement. Without the ability to generate power, your performance capabilities will be limited. It is difficult to hit a softball, drive a golf ball, or kick a soccer ball without generating power.

TYPES OF SKELETAL MUSCLE CONTRACTION

Skeletal muscle is capable of three different types of contraction: (1) an isometric contraction, (2) a **concentric**, or positive, **contraction**, and (3) an **eccentric**, or negative, **contraction**. An isometric contraction occurs when the muscle contracts to produce tension but there is no change in length of the muscle (Figure 5-1). Considerable force can be generated against some immovable resistance, even though no movement occurs. In a concentric contraction, the muscle shortens in length while tension is

muscular endurance: the ability to perform repetitive muscular contractions against some resistance for an extended period of time

power: a large amount of force is generated quickly

concentric contraction: a contraction where the muscle shortens when contracting

eccentric contraction: a contraction where the muscle lengthens when contracting

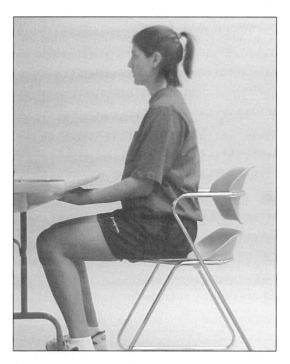

Figure 5-1. Isometric Exercise.

developed to overcome or move some resistance. In an eccentric contraction, the resistance is greater than the muscular force being produced, and the muscle lengthens while producing tension. For example, when lifting a bookbag in your hand, the biceps muscle in the upper arm is shortening as it contracts, which is a concentric contraction. As you lower the bookbag, the biceps muscle is still contracting but now it is lengthening. This is an eccentric contraction. Concentric and eccentric contractions must occur to allow most movements.

FAST-TWITCH VERSUS SLOW-TWITCH FIBERS

As mentioned in Chapter 4, all fibers in a particular muscle unit are either slow-twitch or fast-twitch fibers. Each has distinctive contractile as well as metabolic capabilities. Within a particular muscle, both types of fibers

exist, and the ratio in an individual muscle varies with each person. Those muscles that function primarily to maintain posture against the pull of gravity require more endurance and have a higher percentage of slow-twitch fibers. Muscles that produce powerful, explosive, and strength movements tend to have a much greater percentage of fast-twitch fibers.

Because this ratio is genetically determined, it may play a large role in determining ability for a given sport activity. For example, sprinters and weight lifters have a large percentage of fast-twitch fibers in relation to slow-twitch ones. One study has shown that sprinters may have as many as 95 percent fast-twitch fibers in certain muscles. Conversely, marathon runners generally have a higher percentage of slow-twitch fibers. The question of whether fiber types can change as a result of training has not been completely resolved. However, both types of fibers can improve their metabolic capabilities through specific strength and endurance training.

WHAT DETERMINES HOW MUCH STRENGTH YOU HAVE?

Muscular strength is proportional to the size of a muscle as determined by the cross-sectional diameter of the muscle fibers. The greater the cross-sectional diameter or the bigger a particular muscle, the stronger it is, thus the more force it is capable of generating. The size of a muscle tends to increase in cross-sectional diameter with weight training. This increase in muscle size is referred to as **hypertrophy**. Conversely, a decrease in the size of a muscle is referred to as **atrophy**.

hypertrophy: an increase in muscle size in response to training

atrophy: a decrease in muscle size caused by inactivity

Strength is a function of the number and diameter of muscle fibers composing a given muscle. The number of fibers is an inherited characteristic; a person who inherits a large number of muscle fibers has the potential to hypertrophy to a much greater degree than does someone with relatively few fibers. However, anyone can increase strength through exercise.

Strength is also directly related to the efficiency of the neuromuscular system and the function of the **motor unit** in producing muscular force. Initial increases in strength during a weight-training program can be attributed primarily to increased neuromuscular efficiency. For a muscle to contract, an impulse must be transmitted from the nervous system to the muscle. Each muscle fiber is innervated by a specific motor unit. By overloading a particular muscle, as in weight training, the muscle is forced to work efficiently. Efficiency is achieved by getting more motor units to fire, causing a stronger contraction of the muscle.

Strength in a given muscle is determined not only by the physical properties of the muscle but also by biomechanical factors. Bones along with muscles and their tendons form a system of levers and pulleys that collectively generate force that can move an external object. The position of attachment of a particular muscle tendon on the bone will largely determine how much force this muscle is capable of generating.

The ability to generate muscular force is also related to age. Both men and women seem to be able to increase strength throughout puberty and adolescence, reaching a peak around 20 to 25 years of age. After that, this ability begins to level off and in some cases decline. It has been shown that after about age 25

motor unit: a group of muscle fibers innervated by a single motor nerve

a person generally loses an average of 1 percent of his or her maximal remaining strength each year. Thus at age 65 a person would have only about 60% of the strength he or she had at age 25.

This loss in muscle strength is definitely related to individual levels of physical activity. Those people who are more active, or perhaps those who continue to strength train, considerably reduce this tendency toward declining muscle strength. In addition, exercise may have an effect in slowing the decrease in cardiorespiratory endurance and flexibility, as well as in slowing increases in body fat that tend to occur with aging. Therefore strength maintenance is important for all individuals regardless of age or the level of competition if total wellness and health are an ultimate goal.

Overtraining can have a negative effect on the development of muscular strength. The statement "if you abuse it, you will lose it" is applicable here. Overtraining can result in psychological breakdown ("staleness") or physiological breakdown, which may involve musculoskeletal injury, fatigue, or sickness. Engaging in proper and efficient resistance training, eating a proper diet, and getting appropriate rest can all minimize the potential negative effects of overtraining.

Gains in muscular strength resulting from resistance training are reversible. Individuals who interrupt or stop resistance training altogether will see rapid decreases in strength gains. "If you don't use it, you'll lose it."

WHAT PHYSIOLOGICAL CHANGES OCCUR TO CAUSE INCREASED STRENGTH?

There is no question that weight training to improve muscular strength results in an increased size, or hypertrophy, of a muscle. What causes a muscle to hypertrophy? Over the years, several theories have been proposed to explain this increase in muscle size; most of these have been discounted.

The primary explanation for this hypertrophy is best attributed to an increase in the size and number of small contractile protein filaments within the muscle, called **myofilaments**. Increases in both size and number of the myofilaments as a result of strength training cause the individual muscle fibers to increase in cross-sectional diameter. This increase is particularly found in men, although women will also see some increase in muscle size. It is certainly found that more research is needed to further clarify and determine the specific causes of muscle hypertrophy. In addition to muscle hypertrophy, there are a number of other physiological adaptations to resistance training. The Health Link below identifies them.

Health Link

Adaptations to Resistance Training

- The strength of noncontractile structures such as tendons and ligaments is increased.
- The mineral content of bone is increased, making the bone stronger and more resistant to fracture.
- Aerobic capacity may be improved when resistance training is done at a high enough intensity to increase heart rate to the 60 to 85 percent range.
- There are increases in the levels of several enzymes important to aerobic and anaerobic metabolism.

WHAT ARE THE TECHNIQUES OF RESISTANCE TRAINING?

If you were to go into a weight room and ask ten different people what weight-lifting technique they thought was the most effective for improving muscular strength, you would likely get ten different responses. The key for you is to figure out which technique will best allow you to achieve the goals you have established for yourself. There are a number of different techniques of resistance training for strength improvement, including **progressive resistance exercise**, **isokinetic exercise**, **isometric exercise**, **circuit training**, and **plyometric training**.

myofilaments: small protein structures that are the contractile elements in a muscle fiber

isometric exercise: an exercise in which the muscle contracts against resistance but does not change in length

progressive resistance exercise: a technique that gradually strengthens muscles through a muscle contraction that overcomes some fixed resistance

isokinetic exercise: an exercise in which the speed of movement is constant regardless of the strength of a contraction

circuit training: a series of exercise stations that consist of various combinations of weight training, flexibility, calisthenics, and brief aerobic exercises

plyometric training: a technique of exercise that involves a rapid eccentric (lengthening) stretch of a muscle, followed immediately by a rapid concentric contraction of that muscle for the purpose of producing a forceful explosive movement

OVERLOAD

Regardless of which technique is used, one basic principle of training is extremely important. For a muscle to improve in strength, it must be forced to work at a higher level than that to which it is accustomed. In other words, the muscle must be **overloaded.** Without overload the muscle will be able to *maintain* strength as long as training is continued against a level of resistance to which the muscle is accustomed. However, *no additional* strength gains will be realized. This maintenance of existing levels of muscular strength may be more important in weight-training programs that emphasize muscular endurance rather than strength gains. It is certainly true that many individuals can benefit more in terms of overall health by concentrating on improving muscular endurance. However, to most effectively build muscular strength, weight training requires a consistent, increasing effort against progressively increasing resistance. Progressive resistance exercise is based primarily on the principles of overload and progression. The principle of overload applies to isometric, progressive resistance, and

plyometric exercise. All five training techniques produce improvement of muscular strength over a period of time. Table 5-1 summarizes the five different techniques for improving muscular strength.

PROGRESSIVE RESISTANCE EXERCISE

Progressive resistance exercise is perhaps the most commonly used and most popular technique for improving muscular strength. Progressive resistance exercise training uses exercises that strengthen muscles through a contraction that overcomes some fixed resistance, such as with dumbbells, barbells, or various weight machines. Progressive resistance exercise uses isotonic contractions, in which force is generated while the muscle is changing in length.

Isotonic contractions may be either concentric or eccentric. Suppose you are going to perform a biceps curl (see Figure 5-15, page 97). To lift the weight from the starting position, the biceps muscle must contract and shorten in length (concentric or positive contraction). If the biceps muscle does not remain contracted when the weight is being lowered, gravity

TABLE 5-1
Techniques of Improving Muscular Strength

Technique	Action	Equipment/Activity
Isometric exercise	Force develops while muscle length remains constant	Any immovable resistance
Progressive resistive exercise	Force develops while the muscle shortens or lengthens	Free weights, Universal, Nautilus, Eagle, Body Master
Isokinetic training	Force develops while muscle is contracting at a constant velocity	Cybex, Orthotron, Minigym, Kincom, Biodex
Circuit training	Used as a combination of isometric, PRE, or isokinetic exercises organized into a series of stations	May use any of the equipment listed above Calisthenics
Plyometric exercise	Uses a rapid eccentric stretch of the muscle to facilitate an explosive concentric contraction	Hops, bounds, and depth jumping

would cause this weight to simply fall back to the starting position. Thus to control the weight as it is being lowered, the biceps muscle must continue to contract while at the same time gradually lengthening (eccentric or negative contraction).

Various types of exercise equipment can be used with progressive resistive exercise, including free weights (barbells and dumbbells) or exercise machines such as Universal, Nautilus, Eagle, Cybex, and Body Master, to name a few (Figure 5-2, *A*). Dumbbells and barbells require the use of iron plates of varying weights that can be easily changed by adding or subtracting equal amounts of weight to both sides of the bar. The exercise machines have a stack of weights that is lifted through a series of levers or pulleys. The stack of weights slides up and down on a pair of bars that restrict the movement to only one plane (Figure 5-2, *B*). Weight can be increased or decreased simply by changing the position of a weight key.

There are advantages and disadvantages to both the free weights and the machines. The machines are relatively safe to use in comparison with free weights. For example, if you are doing a bench press with free weights, it is essential to have someone "spot" you (help you lift the weights back onto the support racks if

you don't have enough strength to complete the lift). If you don't, you may end up dropping the weight on your chest. A spotter has three functions: to protect the lifter from injury, to make recommendations on proper lifting technique, and to motivate the lifter. See the Safe Tip on page 86 for proper spotting technique.

With the exercise machines, you can easily and safely drop the weight without fear of injury. It is also a simple process to increase or decrease the weight with the exercise machines by moving a single weight key, although

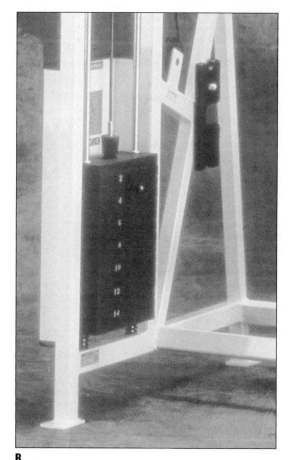

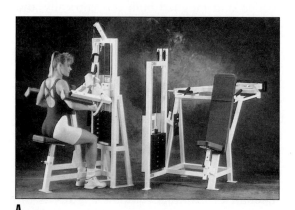

A   **B**

Figure 5-2. Proper Cybex Equipment.
A, This Cybex equipment is isotonic. B, Resistance may be easily altered by changing the key in the stack of weights. (Courtesy CYBEX, Division of LUMEX Inc, New York.)

Safe Tip

Proper spotting techniques

- Make sure the lifter uses the proper grip.
- Check to see that the lifter is in a safe, stable position.
- Make sure the lifter moves through a complete range of motion at the appropriate speed.
- Make sure the lifter inhales and exhales during the lift.
- When spotting dumbbell exercises, spot as close to the dumbbells as possible above the elbow joint.
- Make sure the lifter understands how to get out of the way of missed attempts, particularly with overhead techniques.
- Stand behind the lifter.
- If heavy weights exceed the limits of your ability to control the weight, use a second spotter.
- Communicate with the lifter to know how many reps are to be done, whether a liftoff is needed, and how much help the lifter wants in completing a rep.
- Always be in a position to protect both the lifter and yourself from injury.

changes can generally be made only in increments of 10 or 15 pounds. With free weights, iron plates must be added or removed from each side of the barbell.

Persons who have strength trained using both free weights and the exercise machines realize the difference in the amount of weight that can be lifted. Unlike the machines, free weights have no restricted motion and can thus move in many different directions, depending on the forces applied. Also, with free weights, an element of muscular control on the part of the lifter is required to prevent the weight from moving in any direction other than vertically. This control will usually decrease the amount of weight that can be lifted. Regardless of which type of equipment is used, the same principles of isotonic training may be applied.

In progressive resistance exercise, it is essential to incorporate both concentric and eccentric contractions. It is possible to generate greater amounts of force against resistance with an eccentric contraction than with a con-

centric contraction. Eccentric contractions are less resistant to fatigue than are concentric contractions. The mechanical efficiency of eccentric exercise may be several times higher than that of concentric exercise. Research has clearly demonstrated that the muscle should be overloaded and fatigued both concentrically and eccentrically for the greatest strength improvement to occur.

When training specifically for the development of muscular strength, the concentric or positive portion of the exercise should require 1 to 2 seconds, while the eccentric or negative portion of the lift should require 2 to 4 seconds. The ratio of negative to positive should be approximately one to two. Physiologically, the muscle will fatigue much more rapidly concentrically than eccentrically. Arthur Jones, the inventor of Nautilus equipment, stresses the use of these positive and negative contractions in his training program, although this principle should be applied regardless of which brand of equipment is being used.

It has been argued that a disadvantage of any type of isotonic exercise is that the force required to move the resistance is constantly changing throughout the range of movement. Nautilus (Figure 5-3, *A*) has attempted to alleviate this problem of changing force capabilities by using a cam in its pulley system (Figure 5-3, *B*). The cam has been individually designed for each piece of equipment so that the resistance is variable throughout the movement. This change in resistance at different points in the range has been labeled accommodating resistance or variable resistance. Whether this design does what it claims to do is debatable. It must be remembered that in real-life situations it does not matter whether the resistance is changing. What is important is that you develop enough strength to move objects from one place to another. The amount of strength necessary for each person largely depends on his or her lifestyle and occupation.

▶ Progressive Resistance Exercise Techniques

Perhaps the most confusing aspect of progressive resistance exercise is the terminology used to describe specific programs. The Fit List on page 88, which identifies specific terms with their operational definitions, may provide some clarification.

There are probably as many fallacies and misconceptions associated with resistance training as with any other component of fitness. It seems that everyone has his or her own ideas about the best techniques for increasing muscular strength. A considerable amount of research has been done in the area of resistance training to determine optimal techniques in terms of (1) the intensity or the amount of weight to be used, (2) the number of repetitions, (3) the number of sets, (4) the recovery period, and (5) the frequency of training.

There is no such thing as an optimal strength-training program. Achieving total

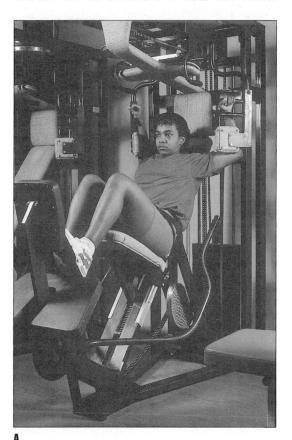

A

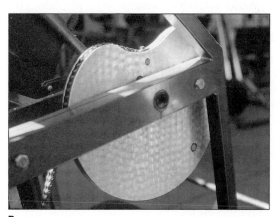

B

Figure 5-3. Nautilus.
*A, Nautilus bench press machine. **B,** The cam on Nautilus is designed to equalize resistance throughout the full range of motion.*

Fit List

Progressive Resistive Exercise Terminology

Repetition	Number of times you repeat a specific movement
Repetition	Maximum number of maximum repetitions at a given weight
Set	A particular number of repetitions
Intensity	The amount of weight or resistance lifted
Recovery	The rest interval between sets
Frequency	The number of times an exercise is done in a week's period

agreement on a program of resistance training that includes specific recommendations relative to repetitions, sets, intensity, and frequency is impossible. However, the following general recommendations will provide you with an effective resistance training program.

For any given exercise, the amount of weight selected should be sufficient to allow six to eight repetitions maximum (RM) in each of the three sets with a recovery period of 60 to 90 seconds between sets. Initial selection of a starting weight may require some trial and error to achieve this six to eight RM range. If at least three sets of six repetitions cannot be completed, the weight is too heavy and should be reduced. If it is possible to do more than three sets of eight repetitions, the weight is too light and should be increased. Progression to heavier weights is determined by the ability to perform at least eight repetitions maximum in each of three sets. When progressing weight, an increase of about 10 percent of the current

weight being lifted should still allow at least six RM in each of three sets.

A particular muscle or muscle group should be exercised consistently every other day. Thus the frequency of weight training should be at least three times per week but no more than four times per week. It is common for serious weight trainers to lift every day; however, they exercise different muscle groups on successive days. For example, Monday, Wednesday, and Friday may be used for upper body muscles, whereas Tuesday, Thursday, and Saturday are used for lower body muscles (Figure 5-4).

It is important to realize that there are many effective techniques and training regimens that weight lifters and body builders can use. One may decide from looking at the size of a muscle or seeing the amount of weight these people are able to lift that they are doing something right even though their training regimens may not always follow the recommendations of researchers.

Regardless of specific techniques used, to improve strength the muscle must be overloaded in a progressive manner. This is the basis of progressive resistance exercise. The amount of weight used and the number of repetitions performed must be sufficient to make the muscle work at a higher intensity than it is used to. This is the single most critical factor in any strength-training program. It is also essential to design the strength-training program to meet the specific needs of a person, whether he or she is a competitive athlete or an individual interested in improving total-body health and fitness.

ISOKINETIC EXERCISE

An isokinetic exercise involves a muscle contraction in which the length of the muscle is changing while the contraction is performed at a constant velocity. In theory, maximal resistance is provided throughout the range of motion by the machine. The resistance provided by the machine will move only at some preset

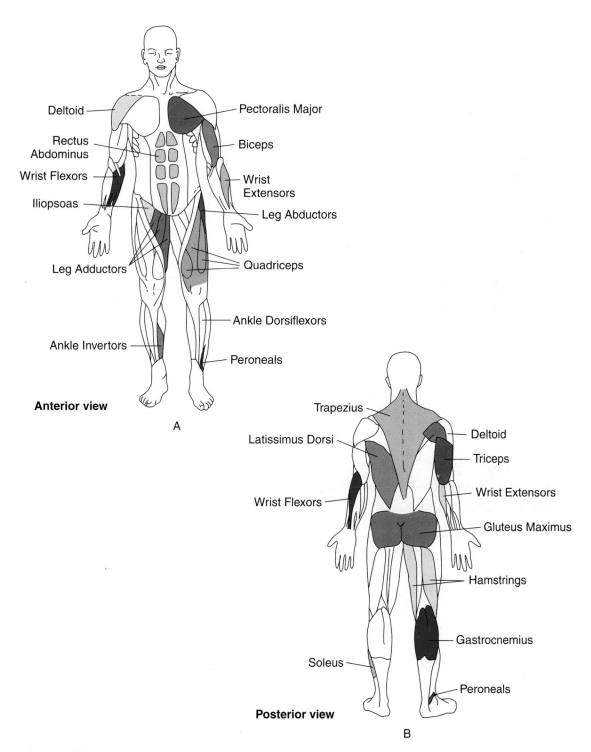

Figure 5-4. Major Muscles of the Body.

speed, regardless of the force applied to it by the individual. Thus the key to isokinetic exercise is not the resistance but the speed at which resistance can be moved.

Several isokinetic devices are available commercially: Cybex, Orthotron, Biodex, Kin-Com, and Mini-gym are among the more common isokinetic devices (Figure 5-5). In general, they rely on hydraulic, pneumatic, and mechanical pressure systems to produce this constant velocity of motion. The majority of the isokinetic devices is capable of resisting both concentric and eccentric contractions at a fixed speed to exercise a muscle.

A major disadvantage of these units is their cost. Many of them come with a computer and printing device and are used primarily as diagnostic and rehabilitative tools in the treatment of various injuries.

Isokinetic devices are designed so that regardless of the amount of force applied against a resistance, it can only be moved at a certain speed. That speed will be the same whether maximal force or only half the maximal force is applied. Consequently, when training isoki-

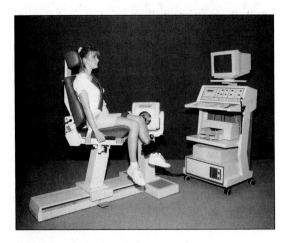

Figure 5-5. Isokinetic Exercise.
Isokinetic exercise works a muscle at a fixed speed of contraction.
Courtesy of CYBEX, Division of LUMEX Inc., 2100 Smithtown Ave, PO Box 9003, Ronkonkoma, Long Island, NY 11779-9003.

netically, it is absolutely necessary to exert as much force against the resistance as possible (maximal effort) for maximal strength gains to occur. This is another one of the major problems with an isokinetic strength-training program. Anyone who has been involved in a weight-training program knows that on some days it is difficult to find the motivation to work out. Because isokinetic training requires a maximal effort, it is very easy to "cheat" and not go through the workout at a high level of intensity. In a progressive resistive exercise program, you know how much weight has to be lifted with how many repetitions. Therefore, isokinetic training is often more effective if a partner system is used primarily as a means of motivation toward a maximal effort.

Assuming that you generate a maximal effort on each repetition, a general recommendation for isokinetic training is to use three sets of 10 to 15 repetitions at whatever speed of movement you select. If you are exerting maximal effort, you should expect that fatigue will usually occur at some point within each set.

It is theoretically possible that maximal strength gains are best achieved through the isokinetic training method, in which the velocity is equal throughout the range of motion, when such training is done properly with a maximal effort. However, there is no conclusive research to support this theory.

ISOMETRIC EXERCISE

An isometric exercise involves a muscle contraction in which the length of the muscle remains constant while tension develops toward a maximal force against an immovable resistance (Figure 5-1, page 81). To develop strength, the muscle should generate a maximal force for 10 seconds at a time, and this contraction should be repeated five to ten times per day.

Isometric exercises are capable of increasing muscular strength; unfortunately, strength gains in a particular muscle will occur only in the position in which resistance is applied. At other positions in the range of motion, the strength curve drops off dramatically because of a lack of motor activity at those angles, and there is no corresponding increase in strength.

Another major disadvantage of these isometric, "sit at your desk" exercises is that they tend to produce a spike in blood pressure that can result in potentially life-threatening cardiovascular accidents. This sharp increase in blood pressure results from holding your breath and increasing pressure within the chest cavity. Consequently, the heart experiences a significant increase in blood pressure. This has been referred to as the *Valsalva effect*. To avoid or minimize this effect, it is recommended that breathing be done during the maximal contraction.

Isometric exercises certainly have a place in a fitness program. There are certain instances in which an isometric contraction can greatly enhance a particular movement. A common use for isometric exercises would be for injury rehabilitation or reconditioning. A number of conditions or ailments resulting either from trauma or from overuse must be treated with strengthening exercises. Unfortunately, these problems may be aggravated with full range-of-motion strengthening exercises. It may be more desirable to make use of isometric exercises until the injury has healed to the point that full-range activities can be performed.

CIRCUIT TRAINING

Circuit training uses a series of exercise stations consisting of various combinations of weight training, flexibility, calisthenics, and brief aerobic exercises. Circuits may be designed to accomplish many different training goals. With circuit training, you move rapidly from one station to the next and perform whatever exercise is to be done at that station within a specified time period. A typical circuit would consist of eight to twelve stations, and the entire circuit would be repeated three times.

Circuit training is definitely an effective technique for improving strength and flexibility. Certainly, if the pace or the time interval be-

▶ Station 1 Push-ups: 30 repetitions
▶ Station 2 Hamstring: low back stretching
▶ Station 3 Bent-knee sit-ups (25 repetitions)
▶ Station 4 Bench press (10 repetitions at 75% maximal weight)
▶ Station 5 Rope skipping (100 repetitions)
▶ Station 6 Knee extensions (15 repetitions at 80% maximal weight)
▶ Station 7 Shoulder adduction (15 repetitions)
▶ Station 8 Knee flexions (15 repetitions at 80% maximal weight)

There would be 60 seconds to complete each station, and the entire circuit would be repeated three times in succession.

Figure 5.6. Example of Circuit Training Setup.

tween stations is rapid and if work load is maintained at a high level of intensity with heart rates at or above target training levels, the cardiorespiratory system may benefit from this circuit. It should be and most often is used as a technique for developing and improving muscular strength and endurance. Figure 5-6 provides an example of a simple circuit training setup that can be easily completed by healthy college students.

PLYOMETRIC EXERCISE

Plyometric exercise is a technique of exercise that involves a rapid eccentric (lengthening) stretch of a muscle, followed immediately by a rapid concentric contraction of that muscle for the purpose of producing a forceful explosive movement over a short period of time. Plyometric exercises involve hops, bounds, and depth jumping for the lower extremity and the use of medicine balls and other types of weighted equipment for the upper extremity.

Depth jumping is an example of a plyometric exercise in which an individual jumps to the ground from a specified height and then quickly jumps again as soon as ground contact is made.

The greater the stretch put on the muscle from its resting length immediately before the concentric contraction, the greater the resistance the muscle can overcome. Plyometrics emphasize the speed of the stretch phase. The rate of stretch is more critical than the magnitude of the stretch. An advantage to using plyometric exercise is that it can help develop eccentric control in dynamic movements. Plyometrics tend to place a great deal of stress on the musculoskeletal system. The learning and perfection of specific jumping skills and other plyometric exercises must be technically correct and specific to one's age, activity, and physical and skill development.

Recommendations for plyometric exercise are variable. However you should once again adhere to the three sets of six to eight repetitions rule as discussed previously.

SHOULD YOU EXERCISE DIFFERENTLY TO IMPROVE MUSCULAR ENDURANCE?

Muscular endurance was defined as the ability to perform repeated muscle contractions against resistance for an extended period of time. Most weight-training experts believe that muscular strength and muscular endurance are closely related. As one improves, there is a tendency for the other to improve also. It is generally accepted that when one is weight training for strength, heavier weights with a lower number of repetitions should be used. Conversely, endurance training uses relatively lighter weights with a greater number of repetitions.

It has been suggested that endurance training should consist of three sets of 10 to 15 repetitions, using the same criteria for weight selection progression and frequency as recommended for progressive resistive exercise. Thus suggested training regimens for both muscular strength and endurance are similar in terms of

sets and numbers of repetitions. Persons who have great strength levels tend to also exhibit greater muscular endurance when asked to perform repeated contractions against resistance.

STRENGTH TRAINING FOR WOMEN

Strength is just as important to women as to men. Unfortunately, a few women are reluctant to engage in a weight-training program because of the fear of developing bulky muscles. This fear is unfounded; the average woman is incapable of building significant muscle bulk through weight training. Significant muscle hypertrophy depends on the presence of an anabolic steroidal hormone called *testosterone.* Testosterone is considered a male hormone, although all women possess some testosterone in their systems. Women with higher testosterone levels tend to have more masculine characteristics, such as increased facial and body hair, a deeper voice, and the potential to develop a little more muscle bulk.

For the average woman, there is no need to worry about developing large bulky muscles with strength training. What does happen is that muscle tone is improved. Muscle tone basically refers to the firmness, or tension, of the muscle during a resting state. For example, doing sit-ups increases the firmness and to some extent the "definition" of the abdominal muscles and makes them more resistant to fatigue. All of us would agree that a person who has a firm, well-toned body is physically attractive.

A woman in weight training will probably see some remarkable gains in strength initially, even though her muscle bulk does not increase. How is this possible? These initial strength gains, which can be attributed to improved neuromuscular system efficiency, tend to plateau, and, in the female, minimal improvement in muscular strength will be realized during a continuing strength-training program. These initial neuromuscular strength gains will also be seen in men, although their strength will continue to increase with appropriate training. It must be repeated that women who do have higher testosterone levels have the potential to further increase their strength because of the development of greater muscle bulk.

Perhaps the most critical difference between men and women regarding physical performance is the ratio of strength to body weight. The reduced strength/body weight ratio in women is the result of their higher percentage of body fat. The strength/body weight ratio may be significantly improved through weight training by decreasing the body fat percentage while increasing lean weight. Strength training programs for women should follow the same guidelines as those for men.

SPECIFIC WEIGHT-TRAINING EXERCISES

To say that a person is strong is probably incorrect. We should instead refer to a specific muscle, muscle group, or movement as being strong because increases in strength occur only in muscles that are regularly subjected to overload. Because muscle contractions result in joint movement, the goal of weight training should be to increase strength in every movement possible about a given joint. Exercises must be designed to place stress on those groups of muscles collectively to produce a specific joint movement.

For this reason our approach to specific strength-training exercises deviates from the traditional approach. The following illustrations are organized to show exercises for all motions about a particular joint rather than for each specific muscle. These exercises are demonstrated using free weights (barbells, dumbbells, weights, and some machine weights). Any of the exercises described may be applied to various commercial weight machines such as Universal or Nautilus. Positions may differ slightly when different pieces of equipment are used. However, the joint motions that affect the various muscles indicated are still the same.

Figures 5-7 to 5-31 describe exercises for strength improvement of shoulder, hip, knee, and ankle joint movements. Complete the worksheets in Table 5-2 to assess your progress in strength increases while doing the following exercises. The Safe Tip on page 105 provides you with guidelines and precautions to be used in resistance training.

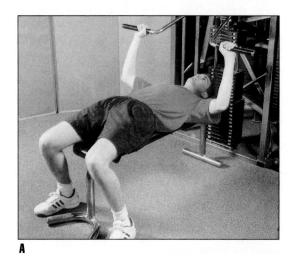

A

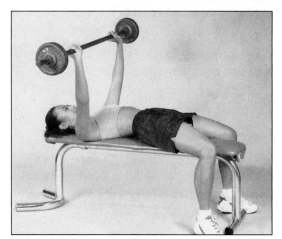

B

Figure 5-7. Bench Press.
A, Machine, B, Free weights.
Joints affected: shoulder, elbow.
Movement: pushing away.
Position: supine, feet flat on bench or floor, back flat on bench.
Primary muscles: pectoralis major, triceps.

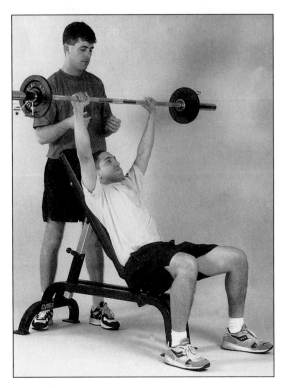

Figure 5-8. Incline Press.
Joints affected: shoulder, elbow.
Movement: pushing upward and away.
Position: supine at an inclined angle, feet flat on floor, back flat against bench.
Primary muscles: pectoralis major, triceps.

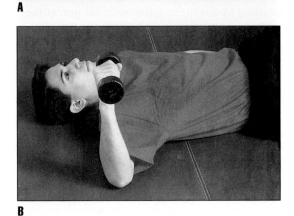

A

B

Figure 5-9. Shoulder Lateral Rotation.
Joints affected: shoulder.
Movement: external rotation.
Position: supine, shoulder at 90-degree angle and elbow flexed at 90-degree angle.
Primary muscles: infraspinatus, teres minor.

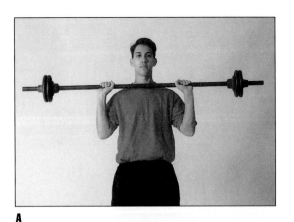

A

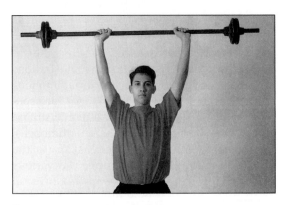

B

Figure 5-10. Military Press.
Joints affected: shoulder, elbow.   Movement: pressing the weight overhead.   Position: standing, back straight.   Primary muscles: deltoid, trapezius, triceps.

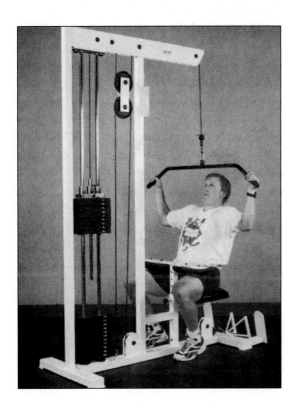

Figure 5-11. Lateral Pull-Downs.
Joints affected: shoulder, elbow.
Movement: pulling the bar down behind the neck.
Position: kneeling, back straight, head up.
Primary muscles: latissimus dorsi, biceps.

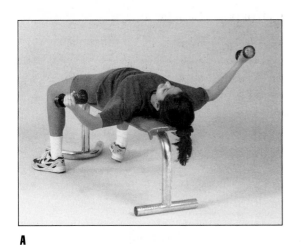

A

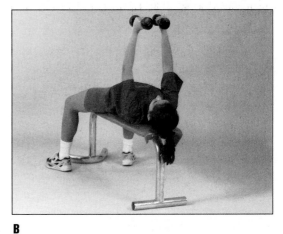

B

Figure 5-12. Flys.
Joint affected: shoulder.
Movement: horizontal flexion. Bring arms together over head.
Position: lying on back, feet flat on floor, back flat on bench.
Primary muscles: deltoid, pectoralis major.

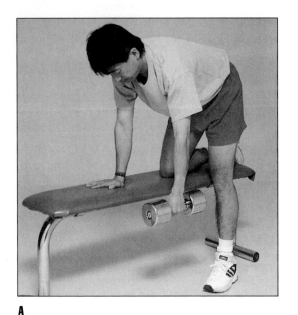
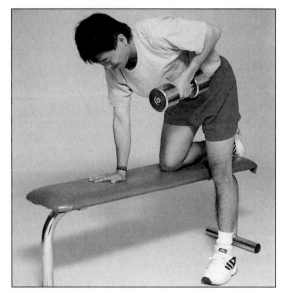

A   B

Figure 5-13. Bent Over Rows.
Joint affected: shoulder.
Movement: adduction of scapula.
Position: standing, bent over at waist.
Primary muscles: trapezius, rhomboids.

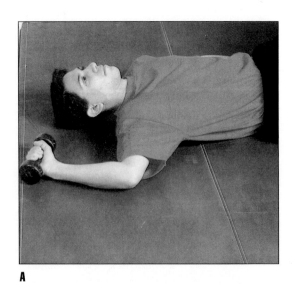
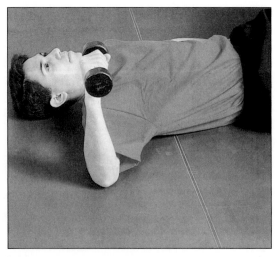

A   B

Figure 5-14. Shoulder Medial Rotation.
Joint affected: shoulder.   Movement: internal rotation.   Lifting weight off the floor.   Position: supine, shoulder abducted and elbow flexed.   Primary muscles: subscapularis.

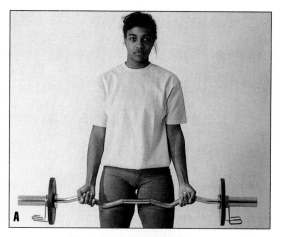
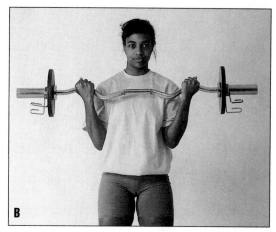

Figure 5-15. Biceps Curls.
Joint affected: elbow.
Movement: elbow flexion. Curling the weight up to the shoulder.   Position: stand-ing feet front and back rather than side to side, back straight, arms extended.
Primary muscles: biceps.

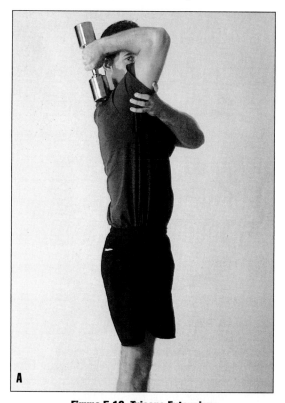
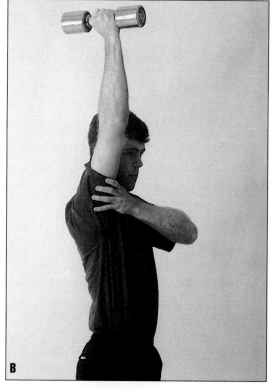

Figure 5-16. Triceps Extensions.
Joint affected: elbow.   Movement: elbow extension. Pressing weight toward ceiling.
Position: standing, elbows pointing directly forward beside ears.
Primary muscles: triceps.

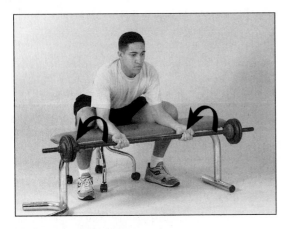

Figure 5-17. Wrist Curls.
Joint affected: wrist.
Movement: wrist flexion. Curling weight upward.
Position: seated, forearms on table, palms up.
Primary muscles: long flexors of forearm.

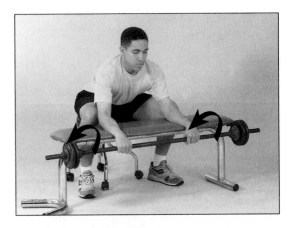

Figure 5-18. Wrist Extensions.
Joint affected: wrist.
Movement: extension. Curling weight upward.
Position: seated, forearms on table, palms down.
Primary muscles: long extensors of forearm.

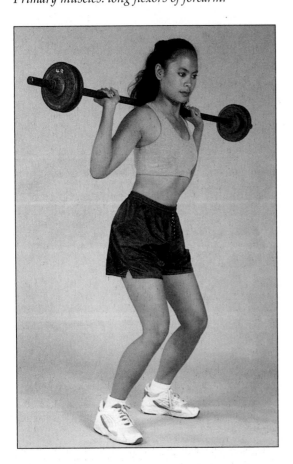

Figure 5-19. Squat.
Joint affected: hips and knees.
Movement: hip flexion and knee extension.
Position: standing, feet shoulder width apart, back straight, barbell resting on shoulders, bend knees to lower to either 3/4 or 1/2 squat position then stand up.
Muscles: hip extensors, quadriceps.

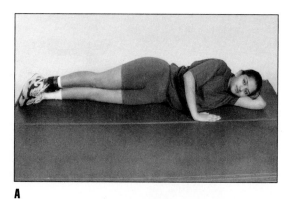

A

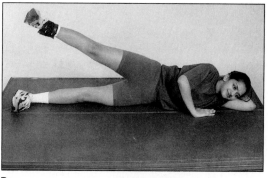

B

Figure 5-20. Leg Raises.
Joint affected: hip.
Movement: hip abduction. Lifting leg up.
Position: sidelying. Weight band strapped around ankle.
Primary muscles: hip abductors.

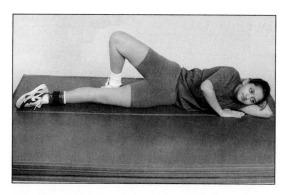

A

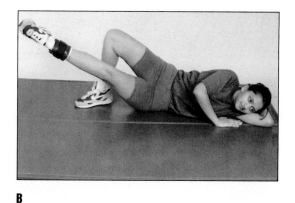

B

Figure 5-21. Leg Lifts.
Joint affected: hip.
Movement: hip adduction, lifting lower leg.
Position: side lying, weight band strapped around bottom ankle.
Primary muscles: hip adductors.

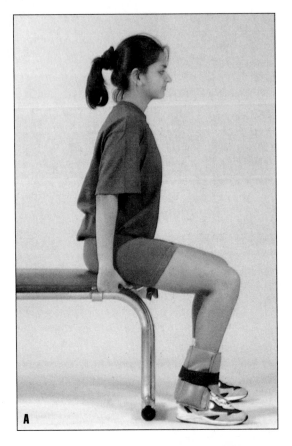
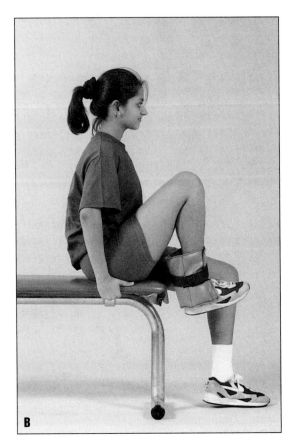

Figure 5-22. Bent-Knee Leg Lifts.
Joint affected: hip.
Movement: hip flexion. Lifting knee up.
Position: sitting, knee flexed, weight around ankle.
Primary muscles: iliopsoas.

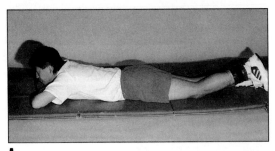
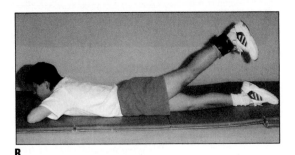
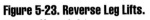

Figure 5-23. Reverse Leg Lifts.
Joint affected: hip.
Movement: hip extension. Lifting leg toward ceiling.
Position: prone, knee extended, weight band around ankle.
Primary muscles: gluteus maximus, hamstrings.

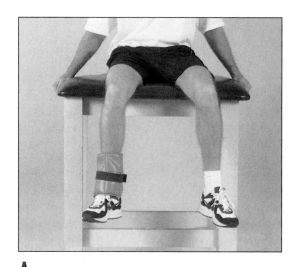

A

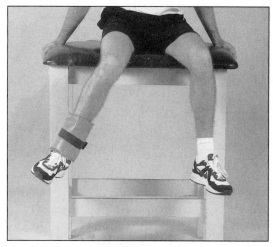

B

Figure 5-24. Hip, Medial Rotation.
Joint affected: hip.
Movement: internal rotation. Rotating lower leg outward.
Position: sitting, knee flexed, weight on ankle.
Primary muscles: medial rotators.

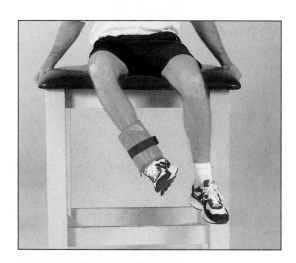

Figure 5-25. Hip, Lateral Rotation.
Joint affected: hip.
Movement: lateral rotation. Rotating lower leg inward.
Position: sitting, knee flexed, weight on ankle.
Primary muscles: lateral rotators.

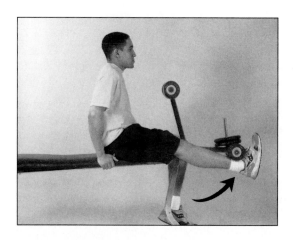

Figure 5-26. Quadriceps Extensions.
Joint affected: knee.
Movement: extension. Straightening knee.
Position: sitting, on knee machine.
Primary muscles: quadriceps group.

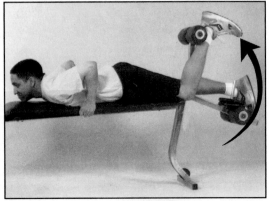

Figure 5-27. Hamstring Curls.
Joint affected: knee.
Movement: flexion. Bending knee and lifting the weight up.
Position: prone, on knee machine.
Primary muscles: hamstring group.

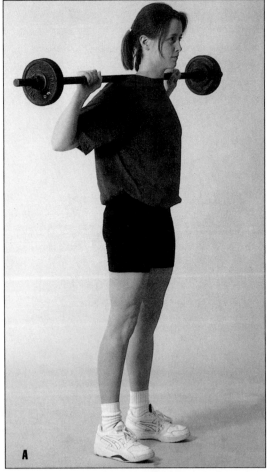

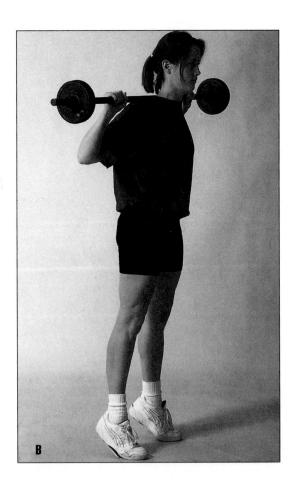

Figure 5-28. Toe Raises.
Joint affected: ankle.
Movement: plantar flexion. Pressing up on toes.   Position: standing and lifting body weight.   Primary muscles: gastrocnemius, soleus.

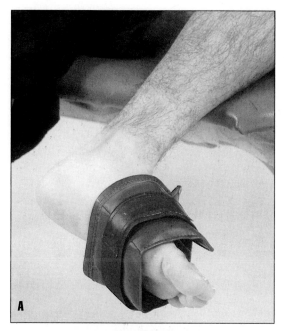

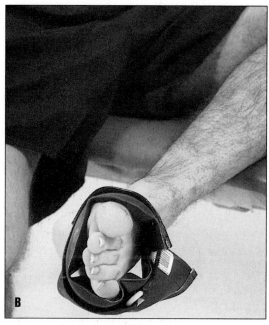

Figure 5-29. Ankle Inversion.

Joint affected: ankle.   Movement: inversion. Lifting the sole of the foot up and in. Position: sitting, knee flexed, instep up, weight on foot.   Primary muscles: anterior tibialis.

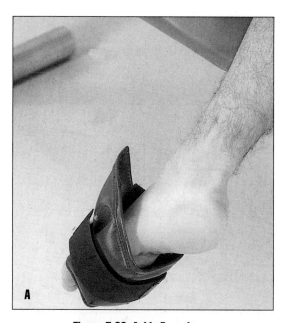

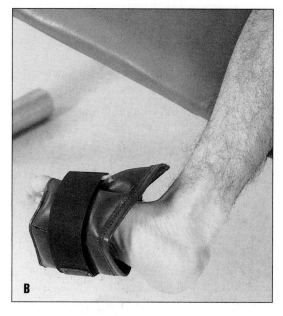

Figure 5-30. Ankle Eversion.

Joint affected: ankle.   Movement: eversion. Lifting the sole of the foot up and out. Position: sitting, knee flexed, instep down, weight on foot.   Primary muscles: peroneals.

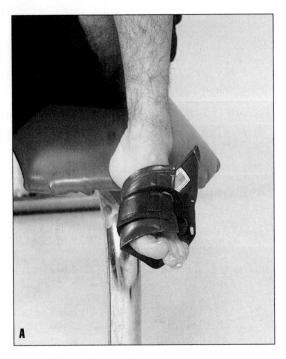
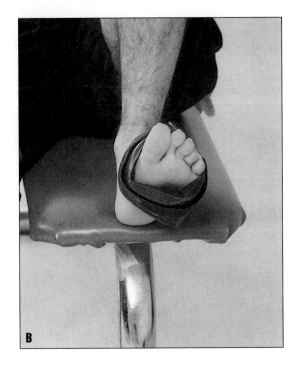

Figure 5-31. Ankle Dorsiflexion.
Joint affected: ankle.
Movement: dorsiflexion. Lifting the toes upward.
Position: sitting, knee flexed, heel on edge of table, weight on foot.
Primary muscles: dorsiflexors in shin.

TABLE 5-2
Strength Training Worksheet I: Upper Body Exercises

Exercise	Reps	Sets		Date and Weight
			Date	
Shoulder lateral rotation	6–8	3	Weight	
Bench press	6–8	3	Weight	
Incline press	6–8	3	Weight	
Military press	6–8	3	Weight	
Lateral pull-downs	6–8	3	Weight	
Flys	6–8	3	Weight	
Reverse flys	6–8	3	Weight	
Shoulder medial rotation	6–8	3	Weight	
Biceps curls	6–8	3	Weight	
Triceps curls	6–8	3	Weight	
Wrist curls	6–8	3	Weight	
Wrist extensions	6–8	3	Weight	

Safe Tip

Guidelines and Precautions in Resistance Training

The following guidelines can improve your effectiveness and your safety during strength training:

- Do appropriate warm-up activities before beginning workout.
- Use proper lifting techniques as recommended on the following pages. Improper lifting techniques can result in injury.
- To ensure balanced development, exercise all muscle groups.
- Avoid doing one-repetition maximum lifts. This can result in muscle strains, especially if you are not properly warmed up.
- Always have a spotter if you are lifting free weights.
- Before using a machine (e.g., Nautilus or Universal) make sure you understand how to use it properly.
- Progress gradually and within your own individual limits.
- Always train throughout a full range of motion.
- Use both concentric and eccentric contractions.
- Try to exercise the larger muscle groups first, and alternate exercises to allow previously exercised muscle groups a chance to recover.
- Do not hold your breath during a lift.
- Do not overtrain. Overtraining may result in injury.
- If you have questions about weight training, seek out an expert who can give you specific, correct advice.
- Do not try to show off; always work within your own limits.

CALISTHENIC STRENGTHENING EXERCISES

Until recently the thought of doing **calisthenic exercise** probably conjured up the image of a hard-nosed Marine drill instructor leading a group of recruits through a boring, regimented exercise session. But add music and bright-colored exercise clothing and change the name to aerobic exercise, aerobic dance, or tae bo and you have a multimillion

> **calisthenic exercises:** exercises done using body weight as resistance

dollar industry that has swept a large segment of the American population into exercise fanaticism. This new fascination with aerobic exercise has shown that calisthenic exercise can be enjoyable without being excessively regimented.

We have already discussed weight training for the development of muscular strength. Calisthenic exercises, if done properly, can improve muscular strength and endurance, flexibility, and cardiorespiratory endurance. However, they are best suited as a supplemental activity to other previously discussed techniques rather than as a substitute for resistance-training exercises.

► Muscle Strength and Endurance

Calisthenics can help to increase muscular strength, tone, and endurance by using the weight of the body and its extremities as resistance. For example, chinning exercises (see Figure 5-40) use the weight of the body to resist the biceps and brachialis muscles in elbow flexion. The primary advantage of calisthenics over training with weights is that you do not need any expensive equipment or machines to provide resistance for you. Most of these exercises can be accomplished without the use of any equipment.

► Flexibility

Calisthenic exercises can also help to improve flexibility as long as each exercise is done through a full range of motion. The weight of a body part can assist in passively stretching a muscle to its greatest length. However, caution must be used when doing calisthenic exercise to improve flexibility. The repetitive, bouncing nature of many of these exercises causes a muscle to be stretched ballistically, which can predispose a muscle to injury, particularly in an untrained person. Through calisthenic exercises, the muscle should be progressively stretched during the set of exercises. Do not neglect a warm-up that includes flexibility exercises before engaging in calisthenics.

► Cardiorespiratory Endurance

There is some question as to whether calisthenic exercises can increase resting heart rate significantly. However, if exercise is of sufficient intensity, frequency, and duration, cardiorespiratory endurance can be improved. Anyone who has gone through a 20- to 30-minute aerobics class will agree that heart rate is elevated to training levels. Calisthenic exercises should be done at a quick pace and without much rest between sets for optimal improvement of cardiorespiratory endurance.

► Specific Exercises

The exercises illustrated in Figures 5-32 to 5-41 are recommended because they work on

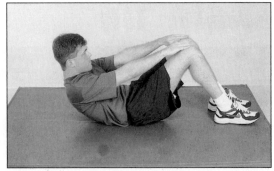

A

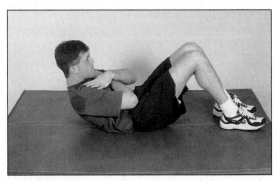

B

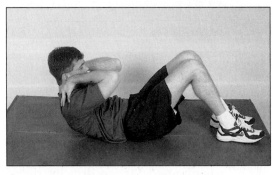

C

Figure 5-32. Sit-Ups.
A, Beginning; B, intermediate; C, advanced.
Joints affected: spinal vertebral joints.
Movement: trunk flexion.
Instructions: lying on back, hands either on chest or behind back, knees flexed to 90-degree angle, feet on floor, curl trunk and head to approximately 45-degree angle.
Primary muscles: rectus abdominis.

specific muscle groups and with a specific purpose. If all exercises are done, most of the major muscle groups in the body will be both stretched and contracted against resistance with the objective of improving strength, flexibility, and endurance. Each exercise can be done at your own pace, although the greater the pace, the greater the stress placed on the cardiorespiratory system. Thus it is recommended that you work quickly and move from one exercise to the next without delay. These exercises can be done to music if you so desire. Most people find it easier to exercise to fast-paced music with a hard, rhythmic beat. However, you should select the type of music most enjoyable to you.

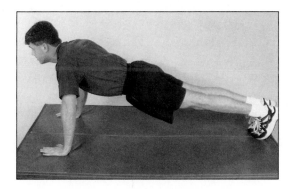 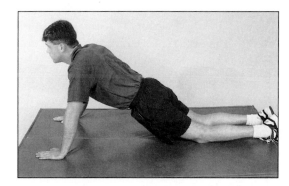

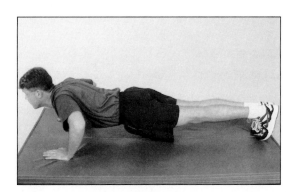 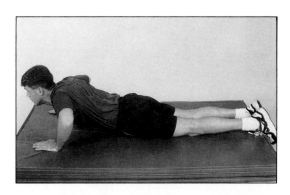

A   **B**

Figure 5-33.
*A, Push-Ups. **B**, Modified Push-Ups.*
Purpose: strengthening.
Muscles: triceps, pectoralis major.
Repetitions: beginner 10; intermediate 20; advanced 30.
Instructions: keep the upper trunk and legs extended in a straight line. Touch floor with chest.
Caution: avoid hyperextending the back, especially in modified push-ups.

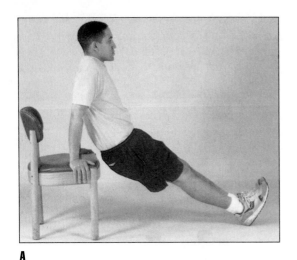
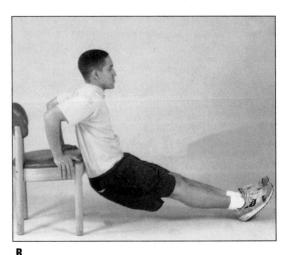

A　　　　**B**

Figure 5-34. Triceps Extensions.
Purpose: strengthening and range of motion at shoulder joint.
Muscles: triceps, trapezius.
Repetitions: beginner 7; intermediate 12; advanced 18.
Instructions: begin with arms extended and body straight. Lower buttocks until they touch the ground, then press back up.

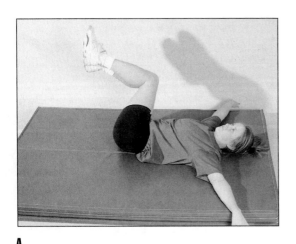
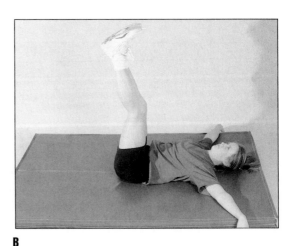

A　　　　**B**

Figure 5-35. Trunk Rotation.
A, Beginner; B, advanced.
Muscles: internal and external obliques.
Repetitions: beginner 10 each direction; intermediate 15 each direction; advanced 20 each direction.
Instructions: rotate trunk from side to side until knees touch the floor, keeping knees slightly bent.
Caution: this exercise should be done only by those who already have strong abdominals.

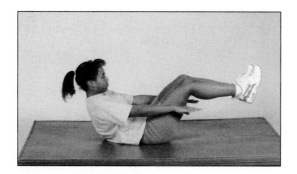

Figure 5-36. Sitting Tucks.
Purpose: strengthen abdominals and stretch low back.   Muscles: rectus abdominis, erector muscles in low back.   Repetitions: beginner 10; intermediate 20; advanced 30.   Instructions: keep legs and upper back off the ground and pull knees to chest. Caution: this exercise should be done only by those who have strong abdominals.

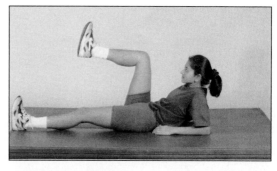

Figure 5-37. Bicycle.
Purpose: strengthen hip flexors and stretch lower back.   Muscles: iliopsoas.
Repetitions: beginner 10 each side; intermediate 20 each side; advanced 30 each side.
Instructions: alternately flex and extend legs as if you were pedaling a bicycle.

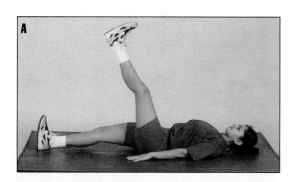

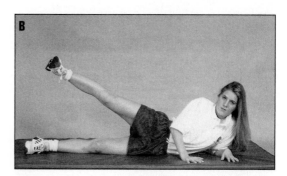

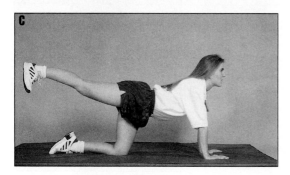

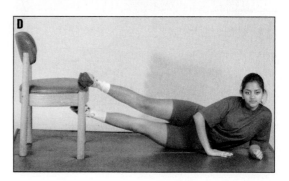

Figure 5-38. Leg Lifts.
A, Front; B, back; C, side (leg up); D, side (leg down).
Purpose: strengthen A, hip flexors; B, hip extensors; C, hip abductors; D, hip adductors.
Muscles: A, iliopsoas; B, gluteus maximus; C, gluteus medius; D, adductor group.
Repetitions: beginner 10 each leg; intermediate 15 each leg; advanced 20 each leg.
Instructions: raise the exercising leg up as far as possible in each position.

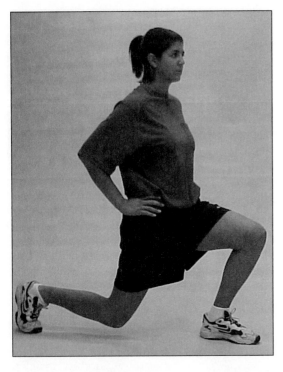

Figure 5-39. Lunges.
Joints affected: hip and knee.
Movement: Forward lunge.
Position: standing, take giant step forward bending knee while holding weights in hands.
Primary muscles: gluteal, hamstrings, quadriceps.

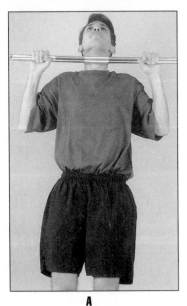

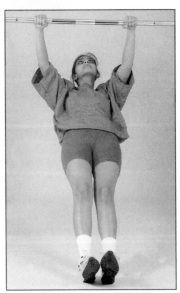

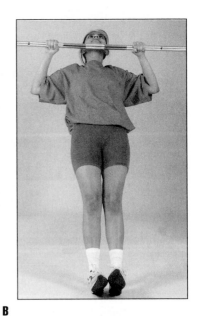

A   **B**

Figure 5-40.
A, Chin-Ups. *B,* Modified Chin-Ups.
Purpose: strengthening and stretch of shoulder joint.   Muscles: biceps, brachialis, and latissimus dorsi.   Repetitions: beginner 7; intermediate 10; advanced 15.
Instructions: pull up until chin touches top of bar.

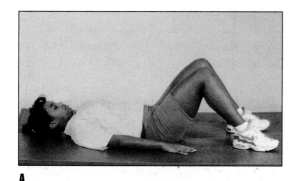

A

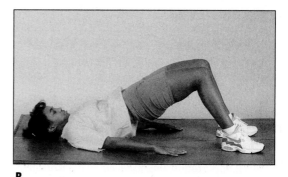

B

Figure 5-41. Buttock Tucks.
Purpose: strengthen muscles of buttocks.
Muscles: gluteus maximus, hamstrings.
Repetitions: beginner 10; intermediate 15; advanced 20.
Instructions: lying flat on back with knees bent, arch back and thrust the pelvis upward.

ASSESSMENT OF MUSCULAR STRENGTH AND ENDURANCE

Lab Activities 5-1 through 5-3 will help you assess your levels of muscular strength, endurance, and power. A worksheet is provided on page 119 on which you can monitor and record your progress on each of the exercises described in this chapter.

SUMMARY

- Muscular strength and endurance are important health-related components of fitness. Power is a skill-related component of fitness.
- The ability to generate force depends on the physical properties of the muscle as well as on the mechanical factors that dictate how much force can be generated through the lever system to an external object.

- Hypertrophy of a muscle is caused by increases in the size of the protein myofilaments, which result in an increased cross-sectional diameter of the muscle.
- The key to improving strength through resistance training is using the principle of overload.
- Five resistance-training techniques can improve muscular strength: progressive resistive exercise, isokinetic exercise, isometric exercise, circuit training, and plyometric training.
- Muscular endurance tends to improve with muscular strength; thus training techniques for these two components are similar.
- Women can significantly increase strength levels but generally will not build large muscle bulk as a result of strength training because of a relative lack of the hormone testosterone.
- If done properly, calisthenic exercises can improve muscular strength and endurance, flexibility, and cardiorespiratory endurance.

SUGGESTED READINGS

Baechle, T.R., and B.R. Groves. 1998. *Weight training: Steps to success,* 2nd edition. Champaign, IL: Human Kinetics.

Bompa, T.O., and L.J. Cornacchia. 1998. *Serious strength training.* Champaign, IL: Human Kinetics.

Chu, D. 1996. *Explosive strength and power.* Champaign, IL: Human Kinetics.

Ebben, W.P., and R.L. Jenson. 1998. Strength training for women: Debunking myths that block opportunity. *Physician and sports medicine* 26(5):86–88, 91–92, 97.

Ebben, W.P., and P.B. Watts. 1998. A review of combined weight training and plyometric training modes: Complex training. *Strength and conditioning* 20(5):18–27.

Field, R.W., and S.O. Roberts. 1999. *Weight training.* Boston: WCB/McGraw-Hill.

Fleck, S., and W. Kramer. 1997. *Designing resistence training programs.* Champaign, IL: Human Kinetics.

Garbutt, G., and N.T. Cable. 1998. Circuit weighttraining. *Sports exercise and injury* 4(2/3):46–49.

Kraemer, W.J., N.D. Duncan, and J.S. Volek. 1998. Resistence training and elite athletes: Adaptations and program considerations. *Journal of Orthopedic and Sports Physical Therapy* 28(2):110–19.

McCartney, N. 1999. Acute responses to resistance training and safety. *Medicine and science in sports and exercise* 31(1):31–37.

Radcliffe, J.C., and R.C. Farentinos. 1999. *Highpowered plyometrics.* Champaign, IL: Human Kinetics.

Roetert, E.P. 1998. Facts and fallacies about strength training for women. *Strength and conditioning* 20(6):172–178.

Stamford, B. 1998. Weight training basics. Part 1: Choosing the best options. *Physician and Sports Medicine* 26(2):115–16.

Stone, M.H., and A.C. Fry. 1998. Increased training volume in strength/power athletes. In Kreider, R.B. et al. (ed). *Overtraining in sport.* Champaign, IL: Human Kinetics.

SUGGESTED WEBSITES

A-Z Fitness
This site presents over 700 excellent links to fitness and bodybuilding. Five certified trainers answer your training questions. Free fitness classifieds, weekly exercise video, new online fitness articles, and more are presented.
http://www.atozfitness.com/

International Sports Sciences Association
ISSA is the fitness certification agency of choice for personal trainers, strength coaches, aerobics instructors, and other exercise enthusiasts. ISSA certified fitness trainers are taught the most current info on strength training, flexibility, bodybuilding, nutrition, fat loss, and lifestyle.
http://www.issaonline.com/certification/index.html

National Council of Strength & Fitness
The NCSF Certification Agency strives to develop the most knowledgeable professional trainers by maintaining the highest standards in the industry.
http://www.ncsf.org/

Plyometrics: Myths and Misconceptions
Visit this site produced by Vern Gambetta.
http://www.gambetta.com/articles/a97008.html

The National Strength and Conditioning Association Home Page
The National Strength and Conditioning Association sponsors this site.
http://www.nsca-lift.org/

WeightsNet - For bodybuilding, fitness, power lifting, sports, and more . . .
WeightsNet is a resource for people who work out with weights for bodybuilding, fitness, power lifting, sports, and more. It's where the 'net pumps up!
http://www.weightsnet.com/

Weight Room Safety
"Weight Room Safety Strategic Planning" by Gary Polson is published as a 6-part article in the National Strength and Conditioning Association's Journal, *Strength and Conditioning.*
http://www.strengthtech.com/weight/safety.htm
http://www.strengthtech.com/weight/weight.htm

Lab Activity 5-1

Push-Ups

Name   Section   Date

PURPOSE   To test muscular endurance.

PROCEDURE
1. *Men:* Begin in the standard push-up position with the weight supported on the hands and toes, with trunk and back straight (Figure 5-42).
   Women: Begin in the push-up position with the weight on the hands and knees (Figure 5-43).
2. Have a partner place his or her fist on the floor directly under your chest.
3. Lower yourself until your chest touches your partner's fist.
4. Count the number of consecutive correctly done push-ups.
5. Consult Table 5-3 to determine your score.

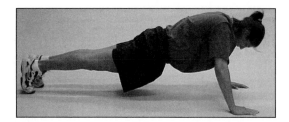

A

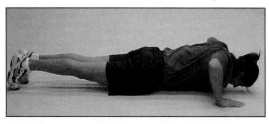

B

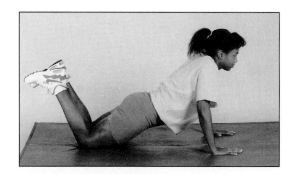

Figure 5-42. Push-Ups

Figure 5-43. Modified Push-Ups.

TABLE 5-3

Push-Up Muscular Endurance Test Standards

	Age (Years)	Fitness Level						
		Superior	Excellent	Very Good	Good	Average	Poor	Very Poor
Males Push-Up	15–29	Above 55	51–54	45–50	35–44	25–34	20–24	15–19
	30–39	Above 45	41–44	35–40	25–34	20–24	15–19	8–14
	40–49	Above 40	35–39	30–34	20–29	14–19	12–13	5–11
	50–59	Above 35	31–34	25–30	15–24	12–14	8–11	3–7
	60–69	Above 30	26–29	20–25	10–19	8–9	5–7	0–4
Females Modified	15–29	Above 49	46–48	34–45	17–33	10–16	6–9	0–5
Push-Ups	30–39	Above 38	34–37	25–33	12–24	8–11	4–7	0–3
	40–49	Above 33	29–32	20–28	8–19	6–7	3–5	0–2
	50–59	Above 26	22–25	15–21	6–14	4–5	2–3	0–1
	60–69	Above 20	16–19	5–15	3–4	2–3	1–2	0

From Pollock ML, Wilmore JH, Fox SM: Health and fitness through physical activity, 1978. All rights reserved. Reprinted by permission of Allyn & Bacon.

Lab Activity 5-2

Bent-Knee Sit-Ups

Name _____   Section _____   Date _____

PURPOSE To measure abdominal muscle endurance.

PROCEDURE 1. Lie flat on your back, and cross your arms across your chest, resting your hands on your shoulders. Knees should be bent to 90 degrees with the feet flat and 18 inches from the buttocks (Figure 5-44).
2. Count the number of sit-ups you are able to complete in 1 minute.
3. Consult Table 5-4 to determine your fitness level.

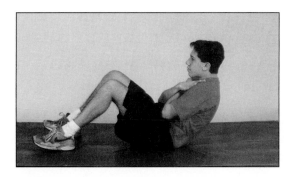

Figure 5-44. Bent-Knee Sit-Ups.

TABLE 5-4

Bent-Knee Sit-Ups Score

	Age (Years)	Fitness Level						
		Very Poor	Poor	Average	Good	Very Good	Excellent	Superior
Males	17–29	0–17	17–35	36–41	42–47	48–50	51–55	55+
	30–39*	0–13	13–26	27–32	33–38	39–43	44–48	48+
	40–49	0–11	11–22	23–27	28–33	34–38	39–43	43+
	50–59	0–8	8–16	17–21	22–28	29–33	34–38	38+
	60–69	0–6	6–12	13–17	18–24	25–30	31–35	35+
Females	17–29	0–14	14–28	29–32	33–35	36–42	43–47	47+
	30–39*	0–11	11–22	23–28	29–34	35–40	41–45	45+
	40–49	0–9	9–18	19–23	24–30	31–34	35–40	40+
	50–59	0–6	6–12	13–17	18–24	25–30	31–35	35+
	60–69	0–5	5–10	11–14	15–20	21–25	26–30	30+

*The value of ages over 30 is estimated.

Lab Activity 5-3

Muscular Endurance Test

Name   Section   Date

PURPOSE   To test general levels of muscular endurance.

EQUIPMENT NEEDED   Chinning bar and a 16-inch bench.

PROCEDURE   1. Perform the following exercises as indicated:

Men: Bent-leg sit-ups, push-ups, static push-ups, pull-ups, bench jumps.

Women: Bent-leg sit-ups, static push-ups, flexed arm hang, modified pull-ups, bench jumps.

Bent-leg sit-ups. Hands on shoulders, knees flexed to 90 degrees. One elbow must touch knee. Fingers must touch the floor between repetitions. Record total number in 1 minute (Figure 5-45).

Push-ups. Standard push-up position. Chest must touch floor during each repetition. Record total number performed consecutively. (Refer to Figure 5-33).

Static push-up. From a standard push-up position, lower the body until the elbow is flexed at 90 degrees or less. Record the number of seconds this position can be maintained without the body touching the floor or losing the proper form (Figure 5-46).

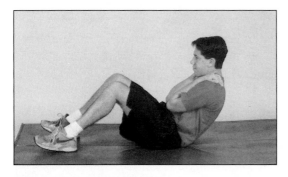

Figure 5-45. Bent-Leg Sit-Ups.

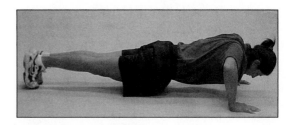

Figure 5-46. Static Push-Up.

Pull-ups. Subject grasps bar with overhand grip. The body is raised until the chin is above the bar and lowered until the arms are fully extended. Record the number of repetitions to failure (Figure 5-47).

Flexed-arm hang. Using an overhand grip, raise the body until the chin is above the bar. Record the number of seconds the chin can be held above the level of the bar (Figure 5-48).

Modified pull-ups. Chinning bar is lowered to the height of the chest. Heels remain in contact with the floor underneath the bar. Arms are fully extended. Then pull up until chin touches bar. Record maximum number of repetitions (Figure 5-49).

Bench jumps. Using a 16-inch bench, record the number of times the subject can either jump or step up onto the bench in a 1-minute period (Figure 5-50).

2. Record the information as indicated on the worksheet.
3. Determine the percentile rank for each exercise by consulting Table 5-5.
4. Determine the overall percentile rank as indicated in the worksheet.

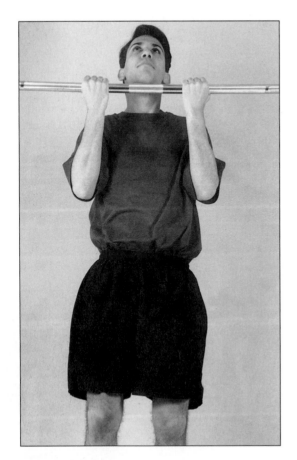

Figure 5-47. Pull-Ups.

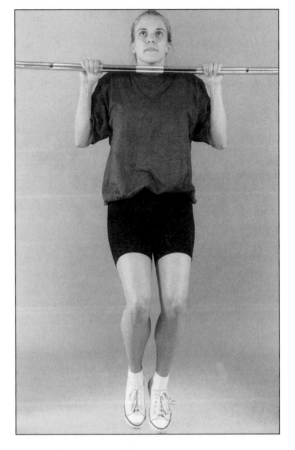

Figure 5-48. Flexed-Arm Hang.

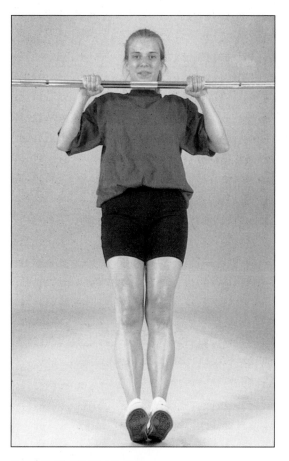

Figure 5-49. Modified Pull-Ups.

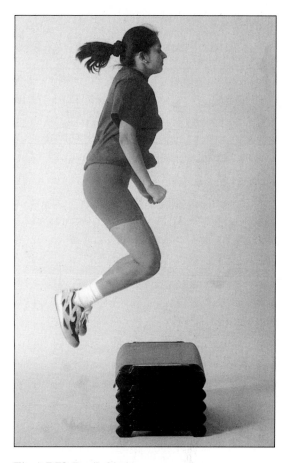

Figure 5-50. Bench Jumps.

Worksheet					
Women				**Men**	
Exercise	*Score*	*Percentile*	*Exercise*	*Score*	*Percentile*
Bent-leg sit-ups	_____	_____	Bent-leg sit-ups	_____	_____
Static push-ups	_____	_____	Push-ups	_____	_____
Flexed-arm hang	_____	_____	Static push-ups	_____	_____
Modified pull-ups	_____	_____	Pull-ups	_____	_____
Bench jumps	_____	_____	Bench jumps	_____	_____
Total of all five percentiles _____			Total of all five percentiles _____	—	
Overall percentile rank _____ (divide by 5)			Overall percentile rank (divide by 5)		

Continued

TABLE 5-5
Muscular Endurance Scoring Table

	Percentile Rank	Bent-Leg Sit-Ups (1 Minute Maximum)	Static Push-Ups (Women); Push-Ups (Men)	Flexed Arm Hang (Women); Static Push-Ups (Men)	Modified Pull-Ups (Women); Pull-Ups (Men)	Bench Jumps
Men	95	50	53	77	14	38
	90	47	49	72	12	36
	80	44	44	67	10	34
	70	41	41	63	9	33
	60	39	38	60	8	31
	50	37	35	57	7	30
	40	35	32	54	6	29
	30	33	29	51	5	27
	20	30	26	47	4	26
	10	27	21	42	2	24
	5	24	17	37	0	22
Women	95	36	38	34	43	28
	90	33	35	28	40	26
	80	30	32	19	36	24
	70	28	30	14	33	22
	60	26	28	10	30	21
	50	24	26	8	28	20
	40	22	24	6	26	19
	30	20	22	4	23	18
	20	18	20	2	20	16
	10	15	17	1	16	14
	5	12	14	0	13	12

CHAPTER 6

INCREASING FLEXIBILITY THROUGH
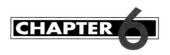
STRETCHING

OBJECTIVES

After completing this chapter, you should be able to do the following:

- Define flexibility and describe its importance as a health-related component of fitness.
- Identify factors that limit flexibility.
- Differentiate between active and passive range of motion.
- Explain the difference between ballistic, static, and PNF stretching.
- Describe stretching exercises that may be used to improve flexibility at specific joints throughout the body.

WHY IS IT IMPORTANT TO HAVE GOOD FLEXIBILITY?

Flexibility may best be defined as the range of motion possible about a given joint or series of joints. Flexibility can be discussed in relation to movement involving only one joint, such as the knee, or movement involving a whole series of joints, such as the spinal vertebral joints, which must all move together to allow smooth bending, or rotation, of the trunk. Flexibility is specific to a given joint or movement. A person may have good range of motion in the ankles, knees, hips, back, and one shoulder joint. However, if the other shoulder joint lacks normal movement, then a problem exists that needs to be corrected before that person can function normally.

Flexibility was identified in Chapter 1 as a health-related as opposed to skill-related

flexibility: the range of motion possible about a given joint or series of joints

121

component of fitness, although for most of us it may be considered important for both. The ability to move a joint or series of joints smoothly and easily throughout a full range of motion is certainly essential to healthy living. The arthritic person who suffers from degeneration in one or more joints loses the capacity of painless, nonrestricted motion and is hampered in the performance of daily acts of healthful living. Lack of flexibility may result in uncoordinated or awkward movements and may predispose a person to muscle strain. Low back pain is frequently associated with tightness of the musculature in the lower spine and also of the hamstring muscles.

If you are physically active, a lack of flexibility will likely impair your performance. For example, if you are a power walker with tight, inelastic hamstring muscles, you may have a problem walking at a fast pace, since tight hamstrings restrict your ability to flex the hip joint, thus shortening your stride length. Most activities you engage in require relatively "normal" amounts of flexibility. However, some activities, such as gymnastics, ballet, diving, karate, tai chi, and yoga, require increased flexibility for superior performance (Figure 6-1). Increased flexibility may increase one's performance through improved balance and reaction time. Experts in the field of training and the de-

velopment of physical fitness generally agree that good flexibility is essential to successful physical performance, although their ideas are based primarily on observation rather than on scientific research.

Most people feel that maintaining good flexibility is important in prevention of injury to muscles and tendons. They will generally insist that stretching exercises be included as part of the warm-up before engaging in strenuous activity. Again, little or no research evidence is available to support this contention.

WHAT STRUCTURES IN THE BODY CAN LIMIT FLEXIBILITY?

A number of different anatomical structures may limit the ability of a joint to move through a full, unrestricted range of motion.

Normal bone structure, fat, and skin or scar tissue may limit the ability to move through a full range of motion. Muscles and their tendons are most often responsible for limiting range of motion. When performing stretching exercises for the purpose of improving a particular joint's flexibility, you are attempting to take advantage of the highly elastic properties of a muscle. Over time, it is possible to increase elasticity, or the length that a given muscle can be stretched. Persons who have a good deal of movement at a particular joint tend to have highly elastic and flexible muscles. Connective tissue surrounding the joint, such as ligaments or the joint capsule, may be subject to contractures. Ligaments and joint capsules do have some elasticity. However, if a joint is immobilized for a period of time, these structures tend to lose some elasticity and actually shorten. This condition is most commonly seen after surgical repair of an unstable joint, but it can also result from long periods of inactivity. Stretching will have a positive effect on muscles, tendons, ligaments, and joint capsules.

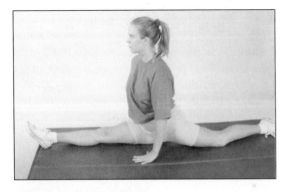

Figure 6-1. Extreme Flexibility.
Certain athletic activities require extreme flexibility for successful performance.

On the other hand, it's also possible for a person to have relatively slack ligaments and joint capsules. These people are generally referred to as being "loose-jointed." Examples of this would be an elbow or knee that hyperextends beyond 180 degrees. Frequently there is instability associated with loose-jointedness that may be as great a problem in movement as a joint that is too tight.

ACTIVE AND PASSIVE RANGE OF MOTION

When a muscle actively contracts, it produces a joint movement through a specific range of motion. However, if passive pressure is applied to an extremity, it is capable of moving farther in the range of motion. **Active range of motion** refers to that portion of the total range of motion through which a joint can be moved by an active muscle contraction. Your ability to move through the active range of motion is not necessarily a good indicator of the stiffness or looseness of a joint because it applies to the ability to move a joint efficiently, with little resistance to motion. **Passive range of motion** refers to the portion of the total range of motion through which a joint may be moved passively. No muscle contraction is needed to move a joint through a passive range of motion. Passive range of motion begins at the end of and continues beyond active range of motion.

It is essential in sport activities that an extremity be capable of moving through a non-restricted range of motion. For example, a hurdler who cannot fully extend the knee joint in a normal stride is at considerable disadvantage because stride length and thus speed will be reduced significantly. Passive range of motion is important for injury prevention. There are many situations in sport in which a muscle is forced to stretch beyond its normal active limits. If the muscle does not have enough elasticity to compensate for this additional stretch, it is likely that the muscle or its tendon will be injured.

AGONIST VERSUS ANTAGONIST MUSCLES

Before discussing the three different stretching techniques, it is essential to define the terms **agonist muscle** and **antagonist muscle**. Most joints in the body are capable of more than one movement. The knee joint, for example, is capable of flexion and extension. Contraction of the quadriceps group of muscles on the front of the thigh causes knee extension, whereas contraction of the hamstring muscles on the back of the thigh produces knee flexion. The muscle that contracts to produce a movement, in this case the quadriceps, is referred to as the agonist muscle. Conversely, the muscle being stretched in response to contraction of the agonist muscle is called the antagonist muscle. In this example of knee extension, the antagonist muscle would be the hamstring group.

Some degree of balance in strength must exist between agonist and antagonist muscle groups. This is necessary for normal, smooth, coordinated movement as well as for reducing the likelihood of muscle strain due to the muscular imbalance. Understanding the relationship between agonist and antagonist muscles is essential for a discussion of the three techniques of stretching.

active range of motion: that portion of the total range of motion through which a joint can be moved by an active muscle contraction

passive range of motion: that portion of the total range of motion through which a joint may be moved passively with no muscle contraction

agonist muscle: the muscle that contracts to produce a movement

antagonist muscle: the muscle being stretched in response to contraction of the agonist muscle

WHAT ARE THE DIFFERENT STRETCHING TECHNIQUES?

Maintaining a full, nonrestricted range of motion has long been recognized as an essential component of physical fitness. Flexibility is important not only for successful physical performance but also in the prevention of injury. The goal of any effective flexibility program should be to improve the range of motion around a given joint by altering the extensibility of the muscles and tendons that produce movement at that joint. It is well documented that exercises that stretch these muscles and tendons over a period of time will increase the range of movement possible about a given joint.

Stretching techniques for improving flexibility have evolved over the years. The oldest technique for stretching is called **ballistic stretching**; it makes use of repetitive bouncing motions. A second technique, known as **static stretching**, involves stretching a muscle to the point of discomfort and then holding it at that point for an extended time. This technique has been used for many years. In recent years, another group of stretching techniques known collectively as **proprioceptive neuromuscular facilitation (PNF)**, involving alternating contractions and stretches, has also been recommended. Researchers have had considerable discussion about which of these techniques is most effective for improving range of motion.

BALLISTIC STRETCHING

If you were to walk out to the track on any spring or fall afternoon and watch people who are warming up to run by doing their stretching exercises, you would probably see them using bouncing movements to stretch a particular muscle. This bouncing technique is more appropriately known as ballistic stretching. Repetitive contractions of the agonist muscle are used to produce quick stretches of the antagonist muscle. The ballistic stretching technique, although apparently effective in improving range

of motion, has been virtually abandoned by most experts because increased range of motion is achieved through a series of jerks or pulls on the resistant muscle tissue. If the forces generated by the jerks are greater than the tissues' extensibility, muscle injury may result.

Successive forceful contractions of the agonist that result in stretching of the antagonist may cause muscle soreness in individuals who are not physically active. For example, forcefully kicking a soccer ball 50 times may result in muscular soreness of the hamstrings (antagonist muscle) as a result of eccentric contraction of the hamstrings to control the dynamic movement of the quadriceps (agonist muscle). Ballistic stretching that is controlled usually does not cause muscle soreness.

STATIC STRETCHING

The static stretching technique is an extremely effective and popular technique of stretching. This technique involves contracting the agonist muscle to passively stretch a given antagonist muscle by placing it in a maximal position of stretch and holding it there for an extended time. Recommendations for the optimal time

> **ballistic stretching:** technique involving repetitive contractions of the agonist muscle that are used to produce quick stretches of the antagonist muscle
>
> **static stretching:** technique involving passively stretching a given antagonist muscle by placing it in a maximal position of stretch and holding it there for an extended time
>
> **proprioceptive neuromuscular facilitation (PNF):** a group of stretching techniques including slow-reversal-hold-relax, contract-relax, and hold-relax techniques, all of which involve some combination of alternating contraction and relaxation of both agonist and antagonist muscles

for holding this stretched position vary, ranging from as short as 3 seconds to as long as 60 seconds. Data are inconclusive at present; however, it appears that 30 seconds may be a good time. The static stretch of each muscle should be repeated three or four times. Much research has been done comparing ballistic and static stretching techniques for the improvement of flexibility. Both static and ballistic stretching are effective in increasing flexibility, and there is no significant difference between the two. However, with static stretching there is less danger of exceeding the extensibility limits of the involved joints because the stretch is more controlled. Ballistic stretching may cause muscular soreness if performed too aggressively, whereas static stretching generally does not and is commonly used in injury rehabilitation of sore or strained muscles.

Static stretching is certainly a much safer stretching technique, especially for sedentary or untrained individuals. However, many physical activities involve dynamic movement. Thus in physically active individuals who routinely engage in dynamic activities, stretching as a warm-up should begin with static stretching and may be safely followed by ballistic stretching, which more closely resembles the dynamic activity.

PROPRIOCEPTIVE NEUROMUSCULAR FACILITATION (PNF) TECHNIQUES

PNF techniques were first used by physical therapists for treating patients who had various types of neuromuscular paralysis. Only recently have PNF stretching exercises been used as a stretching technique for increasing flexibility. A number of different PNF techniques are currently being used for stretching, including slow-reversal-hold-relax, contract-relax, and hold-relax techniques. All involve some combination of alternating contraction and relaxation of both agonist and antagonist muscles (a 10-second pushing phase followed by a 10-second relaxing phase).

Using a hamstring stretching technique as an example (Figure 6-2), the slow-reversal-hold-

relax technique would be done as follows. Lying on your back with the knee extended and the ankle flexed to 90 degrees, a partner passively flexes your leg at the hip joint to the point at which you feel slight discomfort in the muscle. At this point you begin pushing against your partner's resistance by contracting the hamstring muscle. After pushing for 10 seconds, the hamstring muscles are relaxed and the agonist quadriceps muscle is contracted while your partner applies passive pressure to further stretch the antagonist hamstrings. This should move the leg so that there is increased hip joint flexion. The relaxing phase lasts for 10 seconds, at which time you again push against your partner's resistance, beginning at this new joint angle. The push-relax sequence is repeated at least three times.

The contract-relax and hold-relax techniques are variations on the slow-reversal-hold-relax method. In the contract-relax method, the hamstrings are isotonically contracted so that the leg actually moves toward the floor during the push phase. The hold-relax method involves an isometric hamstring contraction against immovable resistance during the push phase. During the relax phase, both techniques involve relaxation of hamstrings and quadriceps while the hamstrings are passively stretched. This same basic PNF technique can be used to stretch any muscle in the body. PNF stretching techniques are perhaps best

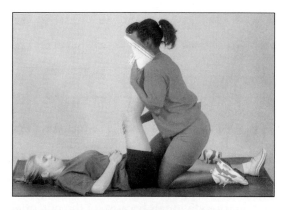

Figure 6-2. Slow-Reversal-Hold-Relax Technique.
This technique stretches hamstring muscles.

Safe Tip

Guidelines and Precautions for Stretching

The following guidelines and precautions should be incorporated into a sound stretching program:

- Warm up using a slow jog or fast walk before stretching vigorously.
- To increase flexibility, overload or stretch the muscle beyond its normal range but not to the point of pain.
- Stretch only to the point where you feel tightness or resistance to stretch or perhaps some discomfort. Stretching should not be painful.
- Increases in range of motion will be specific to whatever joint is being stretched.
- Exercise caution when stretching muscles that surround painful joints. Pain is an indication that something is wrong and should not be ignored.
- Avoid overstretching the ligaments and capsules that surround joints.
- Exercise caution when stretching the low back and neck. Exercises that compress the vertebrae and their discs may cause damage.
- Stretching from a seated position rather than a standing position takes stress off the lower back and decreases the chance of back injury.
- Stretch those muscles that are tight and inflexible.
- Strengthen those muscles that are weak and loose.
- Always stretch slowly and with control.
- Be sure to continue normal breathing during a stretch. Do not hold your breath.
- Static and PNF techniques are most often recommended for individuals who want to improve their range of motion.
- Ballistic stretching should be done only by those who are already flexible and/or are accustomed to stretching and done only after static stretching.
- Stretching should be done at least three times per week to see minimal improvement. It is recommended that you stretch between five and six times per week to see maximum results.

performed with a partner, although they may also be done using a wall as resistance.

PRACTICAL APPLICATION

Although all three stretching techniques have been demonstrated to effectively improve flexibility, there is still considerable debate as to which technique produces the greatest increases in range of movement. The ballistic technique is seldom recommended in sedentary individuals because of the potential for causing muscle soreness. However, it must be added that most sport activities are ballistic in nature (i.e., kicking, running). In highly trained individuals, it is unlikely that ballistic stretching will result in muscle soreness. Static stretching is perhaps the most widely used technique. It is a simple technique and does not require a partner. A full nonrestricted range of motion can be attained through static stretching over time.

PNF stretching techniques are capable of producing dramatic increases in range of motion during one stretching session. Studies comparing static and PNF stretching suggest that PNF stretching is capable of producing greater improvement in flexibility over an extended training period. The major disadvantage of PNF stretching is that a partner is required to help you stretch, although stretching with a partner may have some motivational advantages. More and more athletic teams seem to be adopting the PNF technique as the method of choice for improving flexibility. The *Safe Tip* at left provides some guidelines and precautions for stretching.

▶ Alternative Stretching Techniques

Three exercise techniques, yoga, tai chi, and pilates exercises, integrate some elements of stretching and flexibility into their philosophies of mind/body control. You should consult the suggested readings at the end of this chapter for references that discuss these techniques in greater detail.

IS THERE A RELATIONSHIP BETWEEN STRENGTH AND FLEXIBILITY?

We often hear about the negative effects that strength training has on flexibility. For example, someone who develops large bulk through strength training is often referred to as muscle bound. The expression muscle bound has negative connotations in terms of the ability of that person to move. We tend to think of people who have highly developed muscles as having lost much of their ability to move freely through a full range of motion.

Occasionally a person develops so much bulk that the physical size of the muscle prevents a normal range of motion. When strength training is not properly done, movement can be impaired. However, there is no reason to believe that weight training, if done properly through a full range of motion, will impair flexibility. Proper strength training probably improves dynamic flexibility and, if combined with a rigorous stretching program, can greatly enhance powerful and coordinated move-

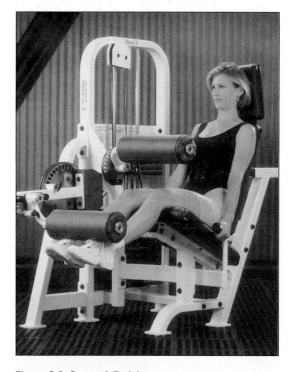

Figure 6-3. Strength Training.
If strength training is combined with flexibility exercise, a full range of motion may be maintained.

ments that are essential for success in many athletic activities. In all cases a heavyweight training program should be accompanied by a strong flexibility program (Figure 6-3).

STRETCHING EXERCISES

Figures 6-4 to 6-16 illustrate stretching exercises that may be used to improve flexibility at specific joints throughout the body. The exercises described may be done statically or with slight modification; they may also be done with a partner using a PNF technique.

There are many possible variations to each of these exercises. The exercises selected are those that seem to be the most effective for stretching of various muscle groups. Table 6-1 is a checklist that can help you monitor your stretching program.

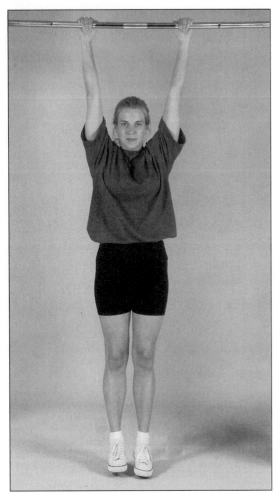

Figure 6-4. Arm Hang Exercise.
Muscles stretched: entire shoulder girdle complex.
Instructions: using a chinning bar, simply hang
with shoulders and arms fully extended for 30 sec-
onds. Repeat five times.

Figure 6-5. Shoulder Towel Stretch Exercise.
Muscles stretched: internal and external rotators.
Instructions: A, Begin by holding towel above
head shoulder-width apart. B, Try to pull towel
down behind back, first with left hand then with
right; you should end up in position C. Reverse
order to get back to position A. Repeat five times
on each side.

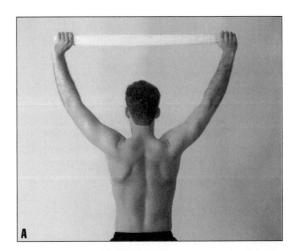

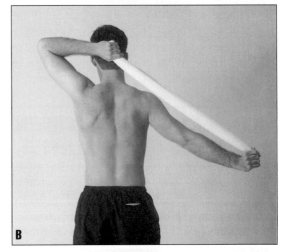

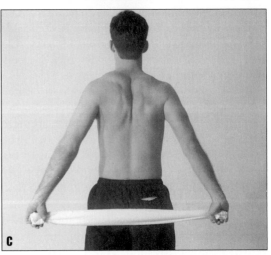

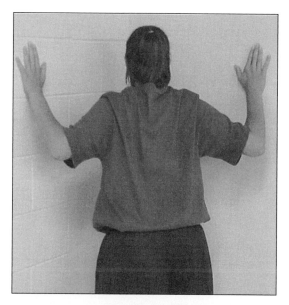

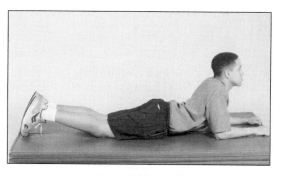

Figure 6-7. Abdominal and Anterior Chest Wall Stretch Exercise.
Muscles stretched: muscles of respiration in thorax, abdominal muscles.
Instructions: extend upper trunk, support weight on elbows, keeping pelvis on the floor. Repeat three times, hold for 30 seconds.
Caution: Do not perform this exercise if you have increased back pain.

Figure 6-6. Chest and Shoulder Stretch Exercise.
Muscles stretched: pectoralis, deltoid.
Instructions: stand in a corner, hands on walls, and lean forward. Repeat three times, hold for 30 seconds.

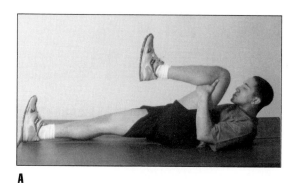

A

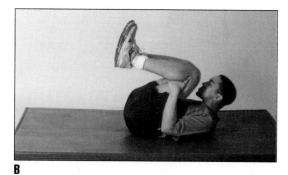

B

Figure 6-8. William's Flexion Exercise.
Muscles stretched: low back and hip extensors.
Instructions:
A, Touch chin to right knee and hold, then to left knee and hold.
B, Touch chin to both knees and hold. Hold each position for 30 seconds.

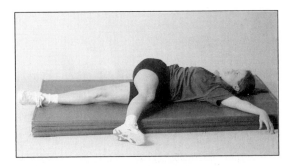

Figure 6-9. Low Back Twister Exercise.
Muscles stretched: rotators of lower back, sacrum, and hip abductors.
Instructions: lie on back on edge of bed or table. Keep shoulders and arms flat on surface. Cross leg farthest from edge over the top and let it hang off the side of bed, keeping knee straight; repeat with other leg. Repeat three times with each leg, hold for 30 seconds.
Caution: if keeping the leg straight produces pain, do this exercise with the leg bent. Be sure to exercise caution in returning the leg to the starting position.

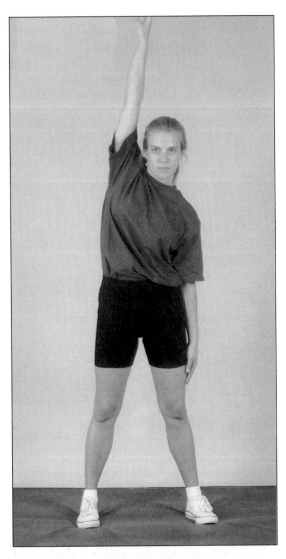

Figure 6-11. Lateral Trunk Stretch Exercise.
Muscles stretched: lateral abdominals, intercostals.
Instructions: standing with feet spread at shoulder width, extend one arm above head and "reach for the sky." Hold for 30 seconds and repeat three times on each side.

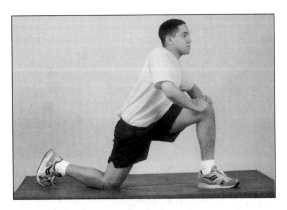

Figure 6-10. Forward Lunge Exercise.
Muscles stretched: hip flexors, quadriceps.
Instructions: Assume a kneeling position with one knee on the ground; thrust pelvis forward. Repeat three times; hold for 30 seconds.

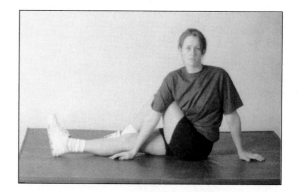

Figure 6-12. Trunk Twister Exercise.
Muscles stretched: trunk and hip rotators.
Instructions: place one foot over opposite knee.
Rotate trunk to bent knee side.

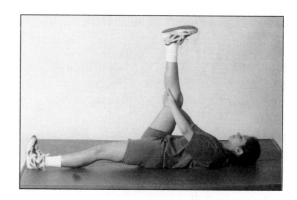

Figure 6-13. Hamstring Stretch Exercise.
Muscles stretched: hip extensors, knee flexors.
Instructions: lie flat on back. Raise one leg straight
up with knee extended and ankle flexed to 90 de-
grees. Grasp leg around calf and pull toward head;
repeat with opposite leg. Repeat three times with
each leg; hold for 30 seconds.

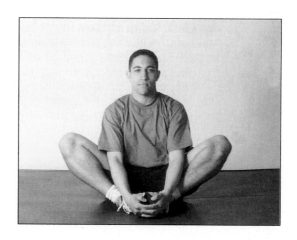

Figure 6-14. Groin Stretch Exercises.
Muscles stretched: hip adductors in groin.
Instructions: sit with knees flexed and soles of feet
together. Try to press knees flat on the floor; if they
are flat to begin with, try to touch face to floor.
Repeat three times; hold for 30 seconds.

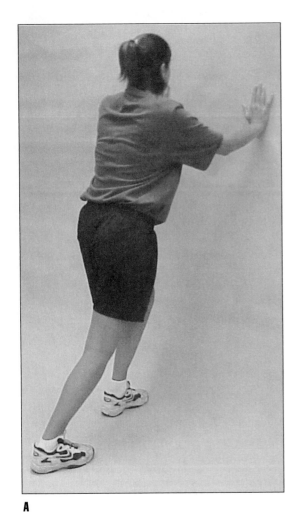

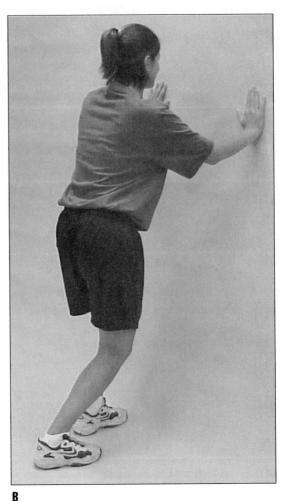

A   B

Figure 6-15. Achilles Heel Cord Stretch Exercise.
*Muscles stretched: foot plantar flexors. **A**, Gastrocnemius; **B**, soleus.*
*Instructions: **A**, Stand facing wall with toes pointing straight ahead and knees straight. Lean forward toward wall, keeping heels flat on floor. You should feel stretching high in calf. **B**, Stand facing wall with toes pointing straight ahead and knees flexed. Lean forward toward wall, keeping heels flat on floor. You should feel stretching low in calf. Repeat each position three times; hold each for 30 seconds.*

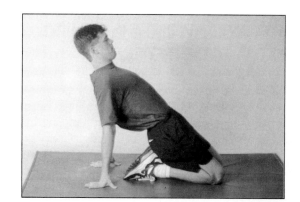

Figure 6-16. Toe Pointer Exercise.
Muscles stretched: foot dorsiflexors.
Instructions: sitting with knees flexed and feet directly under buttocks, lean backward and take weight on hands. Repeat three times; hold for 30 seconds.

TABLE 6-1

Checklist for a Individualized Stretching Program

Exercise	Hold Time (sec)	Repetitions	Day													
			1	2	3	4	5	6	7	8	9	10	11	12	13	14
Arm hang	30	5														
Shoulder towel stretch	10	5														
Abdominal and anterior chest wall stretch	30	3														
Chest and shoulder stretch	30	3														
William's flexion exercise	30*	3														
Low back twister	30	3														
Pelvic thrust	30	3														
Lateral trunk stretch	30	3														
Quadriceps stretch	30	3														
Hamstring stretch	30	3														
Groin stretch	30	3														
Achilles heel cord stretch	30	3*														
Toe pointer	30	3														

*In each position.

HOW DO YOU KNOW IF YOU HAVE GOOD FLEXIBILITY?

Accurate measurement of the range of joint motion is difficult. Various devices have been designed to accommodate variations in the sizes of the joints as well as the complexity of movements in articulations that involve more than one joint. Of these devices, the simplest and most widely used is the goniometer (Figure 6-17).

A goniometer is a large protractor with measurements in degrees. By aligning the two arms parallel to the longitudinal axis of the two segments involved in motion about a specific joint, it is possible to obtain relatively accurate measures of range of movement. The goniometer has its place in a rehabilitation setting, where it is essential to assess improvement in joint flexibility for the purpose of modifying injury rehabilitation programs. Because it is most appropriate to talk about flexibility as being specific to a given joint or movement, there is no doubt that the most accurate method for assessing joint movement is through the use of a goniometer. However, for the average person, it is not practical to assess joint movement using goniometry. Lab Activities 6-1 through 6-3 will help you to assess your existing flexibility.

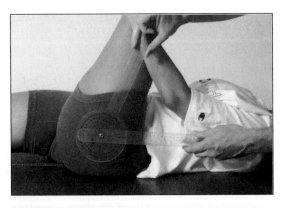

Figure 6-17. Goniometric Measurement of Hip Joint Flexion.

SUMMARY

- Flexibility is the ability to move a joint or a series of joints smoothly through a full range of motion.
- Flexibility may be limited by fat or defects in bone structure, skin, connective tissue, ligaments, or muscles and tendons.
- Passive range of motion refers to the degree to which a joint may be passively moved to the end points in the range of motion, whereas active range of motion refers to movement through a portion of the range of motion resulting from active contraction.
- An agonist muscle is one that contracts to produce joint motion; the antagonist muscle is stretched with contraction of the agonist.
- Ballistic, static, and proprioceptive neuromuscular facilitation (PNF) techniques have all been used as stretching techniques for improving flexibility.
- Strength training, if done correctly through a full range of motion, will probably improve flexibility.
- Measurement of joint flexibility is accomplished through the use of a goniometer.

SUGGESTED READINGS

Alter, M.J. 1998. *Sports stretch,* 2nd edition. Champaign, IL: Human Kinetics.

Anderson, B. 1986. *Stretching.* Bolinas, CA: Shelter Publications.

Bandy, W.D., J.M. Orion, and M. Briggler. 1998. The effect of static stretch and dynamic range of motion training on the flexibility of the hamstring muscles. *Journal of Orthopedic and Sports Physical Therapy* 27(4):295–300.

Clark, A. 1999. *The complete illustrated guide to tai chi: The practical approach to the ancient Chinese movement for health and well-being.* Rockport, MA:Element.

Kent, H. 1999. *The complete illustrated guide to yoga: A practical approach to achieving optimum health for mind, body and spirit.* Rockport, MA:Element.

Knudson, D. 1998. Stretching: From science to practice. *Journal of Physical Education, Recreation and Dance* 69(3): 38–42.

Kurz, T. 1994. *Stretching scientifically: A guide to flexibility training.* Island Pond, Vermont:Stadion.

LaBrusciano, G., S. Lonergan, and S. Pilates. 1996. A method ahead of its time. *Strength and conditioning* 18(4): 74–75.

McAtee, R.E. 1999. *Facilitated stretching.* Champaign, IL: Human Kinetics.

Ninos, J. 1996. PNF Stretching Techniques. *Strength and Conditioning* 18(5):42.

Norris, C. 1999. *The complete guide to stretching.* London: A. and C. Black Publishers, Ltd.

Surburg, P.R., and J.W. Schrader. 1997. Proprioceptive neuromuscular facilitation techniques in sports medicine: A reassessment. *Journal of Athletic Training* 32(1): 34–39.

Wharton, J., P. Wharton, and B. Browning. 1996. *The Wharton's Stretch Book.* New York: Time Books.

Yeager, D. 1999. PNF: A new way to stretch! *Hughston health alert* 11(1):6–37.

SUGGESTED WEBSITES

Brad Appleton's Stretching and Flexibility FAQ
This site presents frequently asked questions with answers on flexibility and stretching. It tells you everything you ever wanted to know.
http://www.enteract.com/~bradapp/docs/rec/stretching/

Practical Tai Chi Chuan
This is an introduction to tai chi chuan with extensive text on tai chi history and principles.
http://www.taichichuan.co.uk/

References on Stretching
This site presents a list of books and articles on stretching and flexibility.
http://www.fitabc.com/stretch/stretch6.htm

SportStretch
This new stretching aid helps improve flexibility by the practice of Active Isolated Stretching.
http://www.sportstretch.com/

Stretching
This site presents stretching for everyday fitness and for running, tennis, racquetball, cycling, swimming, golf, and other sports.
http://www.shelterpub.com/_fitness/_stretching/stretching.ht...

Stretching and Flexibility
This is an essay on types and uses of stretching.
http://www.bath.ac.uk~masrjb/Stretch/stretching_l.html

The Yoga Site - Website directory
This online yoga resource center features a free teacher directory, posture info, Yoga Therapy Report, style guide, Q and A, retreats, books, links, and more.
http://www.yogasite.com/

Lab Activity 6-1

Trunk Flexion

PURPOSE This test measures the flexibility of the lower back muscles and the hip extensors (that is, the hamstrings and gluteals).

PROCEDURE Sit with the legs together, knees flat on the floor, and feet flat against some vertical surface. Bend forward at the waist and reach as far forward as possible with fingers (Figure 6-18).

Your score is determined by measuring the number of inches you can reach either in front of or beyond the vertical surface.

To determine your classification, see Table 6-2.

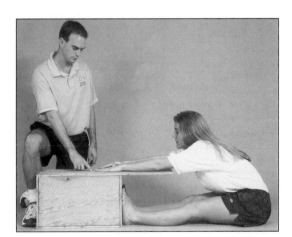

Figure 6-18. Trunk and Hip Flexion Test.
Feet are placed flat against a box with head up.

TABLE 6-2
Flexibility in Trunk and Hip Flexion (Sit and Reach)

Classification	Men	Women
Poor	0 in	0 in
Average	1–3 in	2–4 in
Good	4–6 in	5–7 in
Excellent	7 in	8 in

Lab Activity 6-2

Trunk Extension

Name   Section   Date

PURPOSE   This test measures the flexibility of the abdominal and hip flexor muscles.

PROCEDURE   Lie in a prone position on the floor. Have a partner hold the legs and hips to the ground. Grasp your hands behind the neck, inhale, lift the upper trunk as high off the floor as possible, and hold (Figure 6-19).

Your score is determined by measuring the distance from the chin to the floor. To determine your classification, see Table 6-3.

Caution: If a student has back pain this test should be avoided.

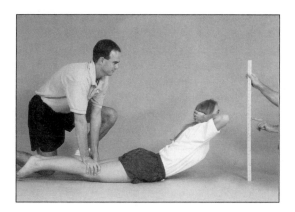

Figure 6-19. Trunk Extension Test.

TABLE 6-3
Flexibility in Trunk and Hip Flexion (Sit and Reach)

Classification	Men	Women
Poor	16 in	17 in
Average	17–18 in	18–19 in
Good	19–21 in	20;23 in
Excellent	22 in	24 in

Lab Activity 6-3

Shoulder Lift Test

Name _____ Section _____ Date _____

PURPOSE   This test measures the flexibility of the shoulder flexors.

PROCEDURE   Lie prone on the floor with arms extended over the head while holding the hands together. Raise hands as high as possible, with the face and chest kept flat on the floor; hold (Figure 6-20).

Your score is determined by measuring the distance from the hands to the ground. To determine your classification, see Table 6-4.

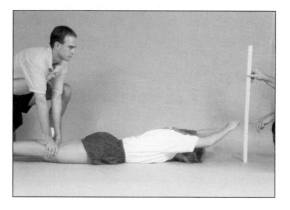

Figure 6-20. Shoulder Lift Test.

TABLE 6-4
Flexibility of the Shoulder Joint

Classification	Men	Women
Poor	0–19 in	0–20 in
Average	20–22 in	21–23 in
Good	23–25 in	24–26 in
Excellent	26 in	27 in

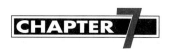

CHAPTER 7

LIMITING YOUR BODY FAT THROUGH
DIET & EXERCISE

OBJECTIVES

After completing this chapter, you should be able to do the following:

- Explain the distinction between body weight and body composition.
- Explain the principle of caloric balance and how imbalances lead to weight gain or loss.
- Identify various methods for weight loss.
- Explain the importance of lifestyle modification in weight loss.
- Develop a program of weight loss or maintenance consistent with your needs.

Key Terms

overweight
obesity
body composition
lean body weight
adipose cell
subcutaneous fat
caloric balance
calorie
kilocalorie
basal metabolic rate
set point theory
spot reducing
bulimia
anorexia nervosa

WHY IS WEIGHT CONTROL IMPORTANT TO YOU?

It seems that every American at one time or another has been concerned about his or her body weight. Very few people seem to be satisfied with it; some would even like to gain weight. Most look in the mirror and study the "roll" of fat that spreads around their midsection or the dimpled fat on their thighs and wonder how to eliminate it. Wearing a bathing suit becomes an act of courage. Our desire to achieve a more ideal appearance makes us easy targets for those interested in profitting from our concern.

The battle against excess body fat has turned into a multi-billion-dollar industry that presents various diet plans, exercise studios, and countless gimmicks and gadgets guaranteed to help you lose those extra pounds and inches. One thing they don't guarantee is that you will be able to maintain the new, reduced weight. Most people who do lose weight eventually regain it and even some extra pounds. So, why bother to lose weight?

Many people decide to lose weight because they are dissatisfied with their appearance. However, there is little question that being overweight can lead to a number of health-related problems. Dr. Herbert deVries has stated, "There are very few, very fat old people around. Your own observations—the national statistics—clearly show that long life does not mean survival of the fattest." If you are overly fat, you run an increased risk of developing heart disease, hypertension, atherosclerosis, stroke, diabetes, infections of the respiratory tract, cancer, and disorders of the kidneys. If you are moderately overweight, you have a 40 percent higher risk of premature death. Individuals who are obese have a death rate 70 percent higher than normal. Obviously, you must be concerned about the amount of body fat you have.

THE AMERICAN LIFESTYLE

There are many reasons why our American lifestyle makes weight control difficult. It is virtually impossible to do anything socially without having something to eat or drink. We associate food with dating, weddings, birthdays, and funerals.

Eating fast food is a way of life in American society. Many people have for the most part grown up as fast-food "junkies." Furthermore budgets and tight schedules often dictate that fast food is a frequent choice. Aside from occasional problems with food flavor, the biggest concern in consuming fast foods is that 40 to 50 percent of the calories consumed are from fats. To compound this problem, these already sizable meals are now being "supersized" at a more affordable price.

Technology has allowed the American lifestyle to become increasingly sedentary as more "labor-saving" devices are invented. The purpose of devices such as garage door openers and remotes for video and audio equipment is to make life and work easier, but there are few associated training effects from pressing a button or moving a joystick.

We do little in our lifestyle that increases physical activity levels. We try to park as close to the entrance as possible so we don't waste time and energy walking back and forth. It is easier to hop on an elevator or escalator than to walk up flights of stairs. Most are not aware of how their behaviors conserve energy rather than burn it.

What is the best way to control your weight? Most people tend to panic when they realize that they have put on a few extra pounds. They either go on starvation diets or become exercise fanatics, neither of which is particularly enjoyable or provides a long-term solution to the problem. The key to being able to maintain your weight is to have the motivation to alter your lifestyle in ways that you can live with. You need to make a commitment to changing your lifestyle so that you burn off extra energy and consume less food. The cumulative effect of these modifications will make weight control an integral part of your lifestyle rather than a behavior you adopt from time to time.

WHAT IS BODY COMPOSITION?

Body composition refers to both the fat and the nonfat components of the body. The portion of total body weight that is composed of fat tissue is referred to as the percentage body fat. The portion of the total body weight that is composed of nonfat or lean tissue, which includes muscles, tendons, bones, connective tissue, and so on, is referred to as **lean body weight**. Assessment of body composition is

> **body composition:** the fat and nonfat components of the body
>
> **lean body weight:** the portion of the total body weight that is composed of nonfat or lean tissue

perhaps a bit more difficult than simply stepping on a scale and measuring actual body weight in pounds. However, body composition measurements are more accurate in attempting to determine precisely how much weight a person may gain or lose.

In the traditional college student age range, the average female has between 18 and 25 percent of her total body weight made up of fat. The average male has between 12 and 18 percent body fat. However, persons who engage in strenuous physical activities on a regular basis tend to have a lower percentage body fat. Male endurance athletes may get their fat percentage as low as 8 to 12 percent, and female endurance athletes may reach 12 to 18 percent body fat. It is recommended that body fat percentage not go below 5 percent in men and 12 percent in women because a certain amount of body fat is necessary for good health. As age increases, average percent body fat for both males and females will also increase. Individuals whose body fat percentage is above these normal ranges are said to be **overfat** while those below the normal ranges are referred to as **underfat**.

HOW IS FAT STORED AND WHERE DO YOU FIND IT?

Fat is found in all of the body's cells. Some **essential fat** is necessary for cushioning organs, regulating temperature, and storing energy for future needs. **Non-essential fat** gradually accumulates when your food intake exceeds your energy demands. A special type of cell, the **adipose cell**, stores fat. The adipose cell stores triglyceride (a liquid form of fat), which moves in and out of the cell according to energy needs. The greater the amount of triglyceride contained in the adipose cells, the greater the amount of total body weight that is composed of fat.

About half of the body's fat is located under the skin (**subcutaneous fat**). The fat distribu-

tion in adults tends to follow particular patterns that are largely inherited. In general, people tend to have large stores of fat in the abdominal area; women tend to store more fat in their hips and thighs than men. Recent evidence indicates that fat deposited in the abdominal area as opposed to the buttocks seems to pose an increased health risk. Risk of developing heart disease and diabetes has been linked to a waist measurement that is greater than hip measurement. (See the Fit List "Simple Tests for Excess Fat" for the waist to hip ratio.)

The term cellulite is often used in magazines and advertisements to identify a type of fat that appears to be dimpled and usually is deposited in the buttocks, upper thighs, and upper arms. Cellulite is a nonmedical term for the ordinary adipose tissue that is found in these sites. Losing weight and exercising will reduce all body fat, including cellulite.

WHAT DETERMINES HOW MUCH FAT YOU HAVE?

Two factors determine the amount of fat found in the body: (1) the number of adipose cells and (2) the size of the adipose cell. The number of adipose cells increases before birth and continues to rise until puberty. Children who become obese at an early age are believed to have too many fat cells (hyperplasia). Adolescents who become overweight seem to develop a greater number of fat cells than those of normal weight. It is thought that by early adulthood the number of fat cells becomes fixed. However, some recent evidence suggests that fat cell number may increase under certain conditions during adulthood.

adipose cell: a type of cell that stores triglyceride, a liquid form of fat

subcutaneous fat: the fat that is found directly under the skin

In addition to cell number, cell size is a factor in obesity. The size of the adipose cell depends on the amount of fat stored within it. Fat cell size increases (hypertrophies) until early adulthood. In the mature adult, fat cell size fluctuates as a function of caloric balance. If more calories are consumed than are needed, the excess is converted to fat and stored in the adipose cells. Under this condition, adipose cells swell with fat. When the energy from fat is needed to fuel activities, the fat cells lose stored fat and shrink in size.

Contrary to popular belief, a fat baby does not necessarily become a fat child or fat young adult. However, after the age of two, a child begins to adopt the eating behaviors and activity patterns of his or her family members. If this child is still too fat by the time he or she starts school, then it is more likely that he or she will become a fat adolescent and adult. In fact the chances of this happening are three times greater in the obese child than in children of normal body weight.

In children who become obese at an early age, weight increases are primarily due to increases in the number of fat cells. In adults, weight loss or gain is primarily a function of the changes in fat cell size, not cell numbers. Thus obese adults tend to exhibit a great deal of adipose cell hypertrophy.

WHAT CAUSES OBESITY?

Some terms used to describe degrees of obesity are useful. Being overweight and being obese are different conditions. Being **overweight** implies having excess body weight relative to bone structure and height. The term overweight is not very precise. On the other hand, **obesity** clearly describes a condition of having an excessive amount of fat. An individual who is 20 percent or more above his or her recommended weight is said to be obese. It has been estimated that in America about 50 million adult men and 60 million adult women are

> **overweight:** having excess body weight relative to bone structure and height
>
> **obesity:** an excessive amount of body fat

too fat and need to do something to lose this excess. The problem of having too much body fat is reaching epidemic proportions in the United States.

The development of obesity has been attributed to several factors, including heredity, social environment, and a lifestyle that includes poor nutritional habits and sedentary behavior. Many people have a tendency to overeat, but most fail to get enough exercise to "burn" up the energy from food. The excess energy is stored as fat for future energy needs. This chapter will briefly examine some of the major factors that contribute to the development of obesity. Emphasis will be given to the impact of a sedentary lifestyle on the development of obesity and how to modify your body fat level safely and for a lifetime.

How do you know if you are overweight? The Fit List at right gives you some simple tests for excess fat. More sophisticated tests will be described later.

HOW DO YOU ACHIEVE CALORIC BALANCE?

It is important to reemphasize that fat in the form of triglyceride moves in and out of the adipose cell according to energy demands. If you have been able to maintain your weight,

---

*A calorie is simply a measure of the energy value of a foodstuff. A calorie by definition is the amount of energy necessary to raise the temperature of 1 gram of water 1°C. However, this unit is too small to be easy to use, so the term **kilocalorie** is more appropriate. A kilocalorie is equal to 1000 calories. Thus subsequent mention to a specific number of calories in this text refers to kilocalories, which will be denoted as kcal or Calories.

Fit List

Simple Tests for Excess Fat

Pinch-an-inch test: Using the thumb and index finger, pinch the skin and fat on the hip directly under the armpit, on the back just under the shoulder blade, on the back of the upper arm over the triceps, and at your waist above the hip bone. If there is more than 1 inch (25 mm) of skin and fat between your fingers, you are probably too fat.

Waist to Hip ratio: Using a tape measure, measure the circumference of your waist at the navel. Then measure hip circumference at the widest point around the hips. Divide the waist measurement by the hip measurement to get a waist-to-hip ratio. If the ratio is greater than 0.95 for males and 0.80 for females, you have too much fat around your belly and you are at risk.

Mirror test: Perhaps the best of the three. Simply look at yourself naked in front of a full length mirror. Now bounce up and down. If parts of your body jiggle that should not, you are overweight.

You must be prepared to honestly answer the question, "Am I too fat?"

---

you are in a state of **caloric balance**. That is, the number of **calories*** that you consume in food equals the number that you use or expend. If you are trying to gain weight, then you need to consume more calories than you expend. The extra calories will be stored, and you will gain weight (*positive caloric balance*). Conversely, if you want to lose weight, you need to expend more energy than you are consuming so that the body has to use its fat stores for energy (negative caloric balance). **Any excess of calories, whether from foods or supplements that contain the basic food-**stuffs (protein, carbohydrates, or fat) can be converted to body fat and stored.** See Chapter 8 for a more detailed discussion of the various foodstuffs.

There are differences in the caloric content of these three foodstuffs.

Carbohydrate = 4 Calories per gram
Protein = 4 Calories per gram
Fat = 9 Calories per gram

It becomes extremely important to consider the implications of caloric values when considering programs for weight loss or gain. The percentage of total body weight that is composed of fat is highly related to the level of physical activity. Persons who have an excess of fat tend to be sedentary and therefore are in a positive calorie situation. In behavioral terms, the number of calories in food ingested and the number of calories expended can be modified. You can eat less and exercise more. However, for many who do not overeat, gradual weight gain often occurs as a result of

caloric balance: the number of calories consumed equals the number of calories expended

calories: a measure of the energy value of a foodstuff

kilocalorie: 1000 calories

aging. The caloric expenditure of physical activities and resting metabolism declines with aging. It will become necessary to decrease caloric intake by about 2.5 percent for every 10 years over the age of 25. Thus, as you age, it becomes increasingly important to either increase exercise levels or decrease caloric intake to avoid gaining body fat.

HOW DO YOU MEASURE BODY COMPOSITION?

There are several methods of assessing body composition:

1. Hydrostatic (underwater) weighing involves placing a subject in a specially designed underwater tank to determine body density.
2. Measurement of electrical impedance predicts the percentage body fat by assessing resistance to the flow of electrical current through the body between selected points.
3. Measurement of skinfold thickness is the simplest and most commonly used method.

The third technique is based on the idea that about 50 percent of the fat in the body is subcutaneous (under the skin). By measuring the thickness of this layer of fat, the total percentage of body fat can be estimated. Skinfolds are measured at various body sites using skinfold calipers. Men and women tend to develop fat deposits in different body areas; skinfold measurements must be taken at these specified places. A number of different methods for calculating body fat percentages using skinfold measurements have been developed. The technique proposed by McArdle and co-workers, which measures the triceps and subscapular skinfold, will be used in Lab Activity 7-1 to determine body fat composition (see Figures 7-2 and 7-3). Although skinfold measurement is a less accurate method than underwater weighing and about the same as electrical impedence, almost everyone can learn to perform this technique. Furthermore, the calipers are less costly and time-consuming to use than the other equipment.

When taking a series of skinfold measurements over time to determine changes, it is important that the same person take the measurements all the time. Due to the potential error that is always possible with caliper measures, having the same person take repeated measurements will minimize errors and give a more accurate indication of absolute changes in body composition.

HOW DO YOU DETERMINE DESIRED BODY WEIGHT?

Once you have calculated the percentage of your total body weight that is made up of fat tissue, you may determine that you have too much fat. It would be helpful to determine how much weight you have to lose to achieve a normal percentage of body fat. Figure 7-1 will help you calculate your desired body weight.

HOW MANY CALORIES DO YOU EXPEND EACH DAY?

Before you can plan your weight modification program, you need to know (1) how much energy you typically use each day (caloric expenditure) and (2) how much energy you consume in your diet each day. Physical activity, whether competitive or recreational, results in an increased need for energy. The goal is to consume enough nutritious foods to meet basic tissue needs plus an additional amount to meet increased energy needs for the activity. Generally, people who participate in physical activity need more energy supplied by the three foodstuffs but not additional vitamins or minerals. As they increase their activity, people usually increase their food intake, which meets nutritional needs. Chapter 8 will explore the topic of nutrition in greater detail.

If a physically active person's daily energy intake does not match the energy expenditure,

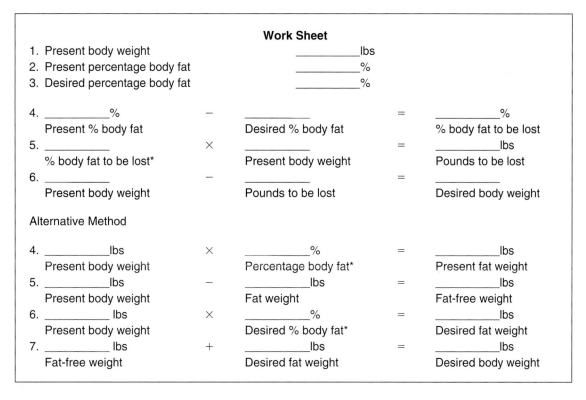

Figure 7-1. A Worksheet for Calculating Desired Body Weight.

body weight loss will occur. For individuals who want to maintain or alter their weight, some estimation of caloric expenditure and intake is necessary.

To estimate caloric expenditure, you must calculate both your **basal metabolic rate** (BMR) and the total energy required for all activities you are involved in throughout the course of a day. It is first necessary to determine the number of calories (energy) needed to support your basal metabolism. This is the minimal level of energy required to sustain the

body's vital functions such as respiration, circulation, and maintenance of body temperature. The BMR is the rate at which calories are spent for these maintenance activities. The Fit List on page 150 describes various factors that influence BMR. Lab Activity 7-2 will help you determine your BMR.

Once BMR has been determined, Lab Activity 7-3 will help you calculate energy requirements of all activities done in a 24-hour period. There is a wide variation in energy output for different types of activity and thus there is some difficulty in achieving accuracy in this exercise. It is determined by the type, intensity, and duration of a physical activity. Body size is also a factor; heavier people expend more energy in an activity than lighter ones. Specific energy expenditures may be determined by consulting charts that predict

basal metabolic rate: the rate at which calories are spent for carrying on the body's vital functions and maintenance activities

Fit List

Factors Influencing BMR

Age: In general, the younger the person, the higher the BMR.

Body surface area: The greater the amount of body surface area, the higher the BMR.

Gender: Men generally have a higher metabolic rate than women.

Diet: There is a dramatic and sustained reduction in BMR that occurs with very-low-calorie dieting.

Exercise: Consistent exercise tends to increase the BMR during the activity and for a period of time after the activity ceases.

energy used in an activity based on (1) the time spent in each activity in minutes and (2) the metabolic costs of each activity in kilocalories per minute per pound (kcal/min/lb) of body weight. If you were to carefully calculate energy costs of all daily activities such as sitting, walking, and studying, you can estimate the amount of energy used in a day. By determining your caloric needs for BMR and daily activities, you can calculate your total daily caloric expenditure.

HOW MANY CALORIES DO YOU EAT EACH DAY?

Once you have some idea of how many calories you expend each day, you need to determine how many calories you are consuming. A physically active person needs a sufficient number of calories from food to maintain body weight and composition. Determining caloric intake requires consulting food composition tables such as the ones in Appendix A. Appendix A indicates the nutritive value of commonly used foods. This chart identifies specific foods and indicates the number of calories per specified serving size. For example, if you consult Appendix A, you will see that 1 ounce of cheddar cheese provides 115 Calories. Maintaining a daily food intake log such as in Lab

Activity 7-4 can determine not only your caloric intake but also your eating patterns and habits. Factors unrelated to nutrition often influence what kinds of foods are selected and how much is eaten. These factors include your mood and social environment at mealtimes. From this table you may calculate your daily caloric intake.

ASSESSING YOUR CALORIC BALANCE

If the daily logs for estimating caloric intake and caloric expenditure have been accurately kept, it will be relatively easy to compare the total caloric values to determine whether you are in caloric balance. It is not easy to maintain caloric balance on a daily basis. One reason is that schedules never seem to be the same from one day to the next. Eating meals may be inconsistent, as are times spent engaged in physical activity. Estimations of caloric intake range from between 1000 to 5000 Calories per day. Estimations of caloric expenditure range from between 2200 and 4400 Calories per day. Energy demands will be higher for those who are physically active and considerably higher for endurance-type athletes, who may require 7000 Calories or more per day. If you desire to lose weight, you must modify your behaviors so that you are burning more calories for energy than you are taking in. If you want to gain weight, you must consume more calories than you expend. The Worksheet for Estimating Caloric Balance (page 177) will determine whether you are in a state of positive or negative caloric balance based on your estimation of caloric intake and expenditure.

SET POINT THEORY OF WEIGHT CONTROL

If you completed the Lab Activities and kept track of your weight, you may have noticed that although your caloric balance fluctuated from day to day, your weight did not go up or down. The **set point theory** provides an explanation of why it is so difficult to lose or gain weight. The body tends to maintain a certain level of body fat. This theory maintains that the body has a "set point" or some mechanism for maintaining a specific body weight. It operates like a thermostat that is set to control a house's temperature. When the temperature in the house drops below the set point, the furnace turns on. When the temperature warms to the setting, the furnace shuts off. For people, it may be that the body's fat level is set at a particular point, and attempts to reduce this level are met with resistance by the body.

It is unclear how this set point is controlled. It may be that the fat cells tend to maintain a certain degree of fat stored within them and resist efforts to reduce their size. Exercise in combination with caloric restriction appears to be the only way to reduce the set point. In any case, the set point theory is just that, a theory that may explain why so many people are unsuccessful at keeping off the fat lost through dieting.

> **set point theory:** a mechanism for maintaining body weight at a specific level

WHAT CAN YOU DO TO LOSE WEIGHT?

There are many weight reduction techniques available; some are based on sound scientific and nutritional principles, and others are dangerous or a waste of money. Losing weight boils down to creating a situation of negative caloric balance. First, food intake may be decreased by dieting. Second, caloric expenditure may be increased by increasing the amount of physical activity. Finally, a combination of approaches can be attempted.

LOSING WEIGHT BY DIETING

Weight loss through dieting alone is difficult. Much of what we choose to eat is influenced not by hunger but by other factors such as customs, advertising, our moods, and the attractiveness and availability of the food supply. Pizza can be delivered to your door with a phone call. Food has meaning to us; we associate sweet, "rich" desserts with rewards for good performances or just to make us feel better. Furthermore, dieting is viewed as the deprivation and punishment one must endure for overindulgence. Every so often, we literally starve ourselves, lose a few pounds, and then promptly return to our old eating habits and regain the lost weight. The behavior is repeated without achieving lasting weight control. Thus periodic dieting is ineffective. At best, long-term weight control by dieting alone is successful only 20 percent of the time.

Obviously, in any weight-loss program the goal is to lose fat, not lean tissue. Unfortunately, many popular diets, the so-called starvation diets, recommend reduction of caloric intake to dangerous levels. It is recommended that the minimum caloric intake for a female not go below 1000 to 1200 Calories per day and for a male not below 1200 to 1400 Calories per day. A minimum level of 1200 Calories may be needed to avoid entering a starvation metabolism. It should also be added that it is difficult to maintain adequate nutrition when caloric intake is at this level for long periods of time. Low calorie eating plans require careful planning to avoid nutritional deficits.

Starvation diets that restrict caloric intake below these recommended levels may actually reduce metabolic rate, thus making weight loss more difficult. The body's metabolic rate goes into "low gear" and conserves calories. The ideal situation is to keep the metabolic rate at normal or raise it to burn more calories. The initial weight loss that occurs with severe caloric restriction for the first few days of the diet may be encouraging. However, the majority of this weight loss is not due to the loss of much fat but results from loss of water weight (dehydration). More moderate reductions of total Calories are recommended to lose body fat.

LOSING WEIGHT BY EXERCISING

Clearly, dieting alone is not the answer to long-term loose weight control. However, the weight lost through exercise involves primarily loss of fat tissue (estimates are as high as 90 percent) and almost no loss of lean tissue. Establishing new behaviors that include daily physical activity takes a great deal of motivation. For most of us, exercise habits were established early in life. Physical activity in adolescence can prevent the formation of excess adipose tissue and results in an increase in lean body weight. At any age, physical activity, when combined with caloric reduction, can lead to substantial losses of body fat while preserving lean tissue. Keep in mind that physical activity in the sedentary college student may result in increases in muscle tissue, which is more dense and has greater weight than fat tissue. Thus, for anyone, initial attempts at weight loss through increased activity levels may be frustrating. You weigh yourself and see no change or even an increase in weight. Instead of relying on scales, which provide no in-

formation about changes in body composition, every few weeks you should measure skinfold thickness.

Many try techniques for **spot reducing**. Trying to reduce the level of body fat at specific sites such as the waist or thighs is useless. During exercise, the energy is supplied from fat stores throughout the body, not just the muscles being moved. However, actively exercising a specific area may increase muscle tone and possibly muscle strength, although the fat in that area will not be reduced. You lose inches off your body, which makes clothing fit more comfortably. Nevertheless, the benefits of aerobic exercise on the entire body are important to overall health.

Weight loss through exercise alone is almost as difficult as losing weight through dieting. People trying to exercise solely for the purpose of losing weight are not likely to stick with an exercise program for a long time. However, it is essential to realize that physical exercise not only will result in weight reduction but also may enhance cardiorespiratory endurance, improve strength, and increase flexibility. For this reason, exercise has some distinct advantages over dieting in any weight-loss program.

LOSING WEIGHT BY DIETING AND EXERCISING

Undoubtedly the most efficient method of decreasing the percentage of body fat is through some combination of diet and exercise. A moderate caloric restriction combined with a moderate increase in caloric expenditure will result in a negative caloric balance. This method is relatively fast and easy compared with either of the others, especially if it

spot reducing: a useless attempt to reduce fat stored in a specific area

focuses on changing eating habits and activity levels. You don't have to starve and run 6 miles a day. If caloric intake is reduced by 200 to 300 Calories per day and if caloric expenditure is increased by 200 to 300 Calories per day, over a 7-day period this will result in a loss of approximately 3500 Calories, or 1 pound of body fat.

In any weight-loss program, the maximum weight loss should be 1 to 2 pounds per week. The rate of weight loss depends on how much body fat the person has at the start of the period of caloric restriction. In general, the greater the amount of body fat, the more rapidly one loses while on a calorie-reduced diet. This explains why some people lose 4 pounds or more the first week on a low-calorie diet. They had maintained their excess weight on relatively high calorie levels, and the reduction creates a major need for energy from fat stores.

A slower rate of weight loss indicates that the person is making minor lifestyle changes, particularly in regard to eating and physical activity behaviors, that they can maintain over time. The adoption of new behaviors and attitudes takes time. The Fit List below lists suggestions for weight-loss strategies to help keep one motivated in weight control efforts.

Fit List

Weight Loss Strategies

A number of strategies may be involved in a behavior modification approach to weight loss. Some of these approaches include the following:

- Keeping a log of the times, settings, reasons, and feelings associated with your eating
- Controlling negative emotions such as boredom, loneliness, anger, and frustration while eating.
- Setting realistic, long-term goals (for example, loss of a pound per week instead of 5 pounds per week)
- Avoiding the total deprivation of enjoyable foods (occasionally reward yourself with a small treat)
- Eating slowly and realizing that the sacrifices you are making are what *you* feel are important for *your* health and happiness
- Putting more physical activity into your daily routine (taking stairs instead of elevators, or parking in the distant part of a parking lot, for example)
- Rewarding yourself when you reach your goals (with new clothes, sporting equipment, a vacation trip)
- Sharing your commitment to weight loss with your family and friends (then they can support your efforts)
- Keeping careful records of daily food consumption and weight change
- Being prepared to deal with occasional plateaus and setbacks in your quest for weight loss

From Payne W, Hahn D: Understanding your health, St Louis, 1998, WCB/McGraw-Hill.

EMPHASIZING THE LONG-HAUL APPROACH TO WEIGHT LOSS

In any weight-loss program, the "long haul" must be emphasized. It generally took a long time to accumulate that extra weight, and it will take time to lose it safely. This fact is frustrating to the impatient individual who wants results fast. Many of these people starve themselves to lose weight, shed some pounds, then return to their former eating habits and experience weight gain, the so-called "yo-yo" effect. This behavior makes subsequent weight-loss efforts even more difficult, since the body tends to protect its existing fat stores.

WEIGHT-LOSS GIMMICKS AND FADS

Even educated people will resort to almost anything in a desperate effort to lose weight. Each year (especially before the summer months), Americans spend billions of dollars trying to find any method that promises they will lose weight quickly and without much effort. People are willing to spend money and time on diet programs, pills, creams, gadgets, books, and equipment that claim to "melt pounds fast." Claims are made for rubberized suits that are supposed to "sweat" off pounds, mechanical devices to shake, vibrate, or roll off the fat; and pills, creams, and powders to remove "cellulite." Advertisements display physically attractive people who are reported to have lost dozens of pounds while using a device or diet plan. Most weight-loss gimmicks are based on unsound nutritional information and have no basis in scientific fact. Although people may lose weight at first, they become bored with the technique and lose interest. Any weight that was lost is regained.

What about the numerous diet plans? It seems that a new diet plan appears in a book that makes the best-seller list monthly. It is not easy to determine whether or not a diet plan is reliable and safe to follow. Table 7-1 reviews some of the more popular weight-loss plans.

You will continue to see or hear about unreliable methods as long as people are unable to make the lifestyle changes needed to maintain control over their body weight.

SETTING REALISTIC GOALS FOR WEIGHT LOSS

Once you have decided to change your lifestyle to decrease your percentage of body fat, you must set some weight-loss goals. First, determine a desirable weight that is realistic in terms of your age, height, and bone structure. Goals must be reasonable and attainable. If you set too high a goal, you may become dissatisfied with any degree of weight loss that does not meet the goal. Ultimately, your goal should be to reach the standards for at least achieving the "good" body fat percentages for your age group as shown in Table 7-2 (page 158). The second important goal is to determine a reasonable and safe rate of weight loss; it may be as low as ½ pound per week or as high as 2 pounds, depending on how much weight you have to lose. You may lose weight faster at first, but the rate slows and eventually averages out to become close to the goal rate within a few weeks.

WHAT IF YOU WANT TO GAIN WEIGHT?

As a society we seem to be preoccupied with losing weight. However, there are people who would like to gain weight. The aim of a weight-gaining program should be to increase lean body mass, that is, muscle, as opposed to body fat. Muscle mass should be increased only by muscle work combined with an increase in food consumption. It cannot be increased by the intake of any special food or vitamin. Unfortunately, as will be indicated in Chapter 8, muscle mass and weight may also be increased in an unsafe manner through the use of steroids or growth hormones.

TABLE 7-1
Overview of Diet Plans

Type of Diet	Advantages	Disadvantages	Examples
High-Protein, Low-Carbohydrate Diets Usually include all the meat, fish, poultry, and eggs you can eat Occasionally permit milk and cheese in limited amounts Prohibits fruits, vegetables, and any bread or cereal products	Rapid initial weight loss because of diuretic effect Very little hunger	Too low in carbohydrates Deficient in many nutrients—vitamin C, vitamin A (unless eggs are included), calcium, and several trace elements High in saturated fat, cholesterol, and total fat Will result in ketosis because the major energy sources are protein and fat—both dietary and body. Extreme diets of this type could cause death Impossible to adhere to these diets long enough to lose any appreciable amount of weight Dangerous for people with kidney disease Weight loss, which is largely water, is rapidly regained Diet does not develop a new and useful set of eating habits Expensive Unpalatable after first few days Difficult for dieter to eat out	Dr. Stillman's Quick Weight Loss Diet Calories Don't Count by Dr. Taller Dr. Atkin's Diet Revolution Scarsdale Diet Air Force Diet Mastering the Zone Diet Carbohydrate Addict's Lifespan Program
Low-Calorie, High-Protein Supplement Diets Usually a premeasured powder to be reconstituted with water or a prepared liquid formula	Rapid initial weight loss Easy to prepare—already measured Palatable for first few days Usually fortified to provide recommended amounts of micronutrients Must be labeled if >50% protein	Usually prescribed at dangerously low kilocalorie intake of 300 to 500 kcal Will result in ketosis Do not retrain dieters in acceptable eating habits Overpriced; initially, users are often urged to buy several large cans of different flavors of the diet food (which is usually non-fat dried milk) Low in fiber and bulk—constipating in short amount of time Frequently cause loss of potassium with resultant weakness and heart arrhythmias Often contain poor quality protein	Metracal Diet Cambridge Diet Liquid Protein Diet Last Chance Diet Oxford Diet

From Guthrie HA: Introductory nutrition, St. Louis, 1989, Mosby.   *Continued*

TABLE 7-1

Overview of Diet Plans—cont'd

Type of Diet	Advantages	Disadvantages	Examples
Restricted-Calorie, Balanced Food Plans			
	Sufficiently low in kilo-calories to permit steady weight loss	Do not appeal to people who want a "unique" diet	Weight Watchers Diet
	Nutritionally balanced	Do not produce immediate and large weight losses	Prudent Diet (American Heart Association)
	Palatable		The I Love New York
	Include readily available foods		UCLA Diet
	Reasonable in cost		Time-calorie Displacement (TCD)
	Can be adapted from family meals		Overeaters Anonymous
	Permit eating out and social eating		The Beyond Diet
	Promote a new set of eating habits		Take Off Pounds Sensibly (TOPS)
			Fit or Fat Target Diet
Fasting/Starvation Diet			
	Rapid initial loss	Nutrient deficient	ZIP Diet
		Danger of ketosis	5-day Miracle Diet
		>60% loss is muscle	
		<40% loss is fat	
		Low long-term success rates	
High-Carbohydrate Diet			
	Emphasizes grains, fruits, vegetables	Limits milk, meat	Beverly Hills Diet
	High in bulk	Nutritionally very inadequate for calcium, iron, and protein	Quick Weight Loss Diet
	Low in cholesterol		Pritikin Diet
			Carbohydrate Cravers
			Hilton Head Metabolism Diet

TABLE 7-1
Overview of Diet Plans—cont'd

Type of Diet	Advantages	Disadvantages	Examples
High-Fiber, Low-Kilocalorie Diets	High satiety value Provide bulk	Irritating to the lower colon Decrease absorption of trace elements, especially iron Nutritionally deficient Low in protein	Pritikin Diet F Diet Zen Macrobiotic Diet Rice Diet Eat More, Weigh Less
Protein-Sparing Modified Fats <50% protein: 400 kcal	Safe under supervision High-quality protein Minimize loss of lean body mass	Decreases BMR Monotonous Expensive	Optifast Medifast Cambridge Diet Last Chance Diet Slimfast Ultrafast
Premeasured Food Plans	Provides the prescribed portion sizes—little chance of too small or too large a portion Total food programs Some provide adequate kilocalories (1200) Nutritionally balanced or supplemented	Expensive Do not retrain dieters in acceptable eating habits Precludes eating out or social eating Often low in bulk Monotonous Low long-term success rates	Nutri-System Carnation Plan Jenny Craig Herbalife Genesis
Limited Food Choice Diets	Reduce the number of food choices made by the users Limited opportunity to make mistakes Almost certainly low in calories after the first few days	Deficient in many nutrients, depending on the foods allowed Monotonous—difficult to adhere to Eating out and eating socially are difficult Do not retrain dieters in acceptable eating habits Low long-term success rates No scientific basis for these diets	Banana and milk diet Grapefruit and cottage cheese diet Kempner rice diet Lecithin, vinegar, kelp, vitamin B_6 diet Beverly Hills Diet Fit for Life

TABLE 7-2

Percentage Fat Based on Skinfolds

	9%–17% Men			
Rating	Ages 20–29	Ages 30–39	Ages 40–49	Ages 50+
Dangerously Low	<5	<5	<5	<5
Excellent	5–8.9	5–10.9	5–11.9	5–12.9
GOOD	**9–12.9**	**11–13.9**	**12–15.9**	**13–16.9**
Fair	13–16.9	14–17.9	16–20.9	17–21.9
Poor	17–19.9	18–22.9	21–25.9	22–27.9
Very Poor	>19.9	>22.9	>25.9	>27.9

	17%–25% Women			
Rating	Ages 20–29	Ages 30–39	Ages 40–49	Ages 50+
Dangerously Low	<12	<12	<12	<12
Excellent	12–16.9	12–17.9	12–19.9	12–20.9
GOOD	**17–20.9**	**18–21.9**	**20–23.9**	**21–24.9**
Fair	21–23.9	22–24.9	24–27.9	25–30.9
Poor	24–27.9	25–29.9	28–31.9	31–35.9
Very Poor	>27.9	>29.9	>31.9	>35.9

The recommended rate of weight gain is a maximum of 1 to 2 pounds per week. This can be achieved through positive caloric balance. One pound of fat represents the equivalent of 3500 Calories. Lean body tissue, which contains less fat, more protein, and more water than fat tissue, represents approximately 2500 Calories. Therefore to gain 1 pound of muscle, a weekly excess of approximately 2500 Calories is needed. Adding 500 to 1000 Calories daily to the usual diet will provide the energy needs of gaining 1 to 2 pounds per week and fuel the increased energy expenditure of the muscle training program. Weight training must be part of the program; otherwise, the excess energy intake will be converted to fat. The Safe Tip on page 159 offers suggestions for an individual concerned about a safe weight-gaining program. For recommendations regarding weight training, refer to Chapter 5.

Athletes in training for competition require very high-calorie diets. They often believe that more protein is needed to build bigger muscles. Actually, a relatively small amount of additional protein is needed for the muscles developed in a training program. Most Americans consume about twice the amount of protein needed; therefore protein is obtained by eating natural food sources rather than by consuming protein supplements. Furthermore, protein supplements may have undesirable effects on the body.

One should monitor body weight weekly to ensure a gradual weight gain. Having the same person measuring skinfold thickness regularly will detect any increases in body fat. An increase in the skinfold thickness indicates a need for a reduction in caloric intake or an increase in training, or both, until it is demonstrated that the percentage of body fat is not increasing.

WHAT ARE EATING DISORDERS?

Unfortunately for many people in our society, weight loss has become an obsession that poses a threat to health and well-being. The media bombard the public with an ideal body image that is fashion-model thin. This creates social and internal pressures, especially for young women, to become overly concerned with the relationship of body image to self-image. Pursuing an ideal body image, even one that is unrealistic and unhealthy, becomes an attainable goal. When one believes that a

Safe Tip

Guidelines for Gaining Weight

- Set a reasonable goal. An exercise program should begin in advance of the competing season. Rapid weight gain indicates increase in fat, not muscle.
- Follow an exercise program prescribed by a fitness professional and designed to develop the desired muscles (see Chapter 3).
- Determine the usual caloric intake, then estimate the additional calories needed daily to gain lean weight.
- For a young individual, an additional 500 to 1000 Calories per day may be needed to gain lean weight. Therefore it is important to plan both the composition and the timing of meals and snacks. The diet should be based on the food groups (see Chapter 8), with additional calories obtained from larger portions of foods rich in complex carbohydrates. It is recommended that the diet contain less than 25% of calories from fat. The fat component of the diet should be low in saturated fats and cholesterol.

thinner body is the key to becoming more satisfied with one's self, the individual is susceptible to adopting bizarre behaviors in an attempt to find happiness. In some cases, dieting behavior is so extreme that people literally starve themselves to death. Descriptions of some of the more common eating disorders associated with self-image problems follow. Also, the Fit List on page 160 provides some clues to identifying those with dangerous weight-control behaviors.

BULIMIA

Bulimia, believed to be one of the more common eating disorders, involves recurrent episodes of binge-type eating ("pigging out") followed by purging (vomiting and laxative

bulimia: an eating disorder involving recurrent episodes of binge-type eating followed by purging

abuse). Usually the binge consists of foods high in calories from fat or sugar, such as bags of cookies, doughnuts, and chips. A typical binge involves the consumption of 1000 Calories or more during a 1- to 2-hour time period. These binges may occur once a month or, in severe cases, several times a day. To avoid gaining weight from the positive caloric situation, the person follows the binge with purging through vomiting, laxatives, or fasting. People who engage in such behavior tend to binge and purge in secret; in particular, the purging behavior is hidden from friends and family members.

Persons with bulimia are generally college-aged women who are about average or not excessively overfat. Reports of bulimic behavior in young men involve the consumption of large quantities of beer and foods such as pizza followed by vomiting.

Although bulimics are often extroverts and socially active, they tend to have problems with interpersonal relationships. They suffer from low self-esteem and feel isolated because

Fit List

Identifying Behaviors Associated with Eating Disorders

Reports or observation of the following signs or behaviors should arouse concern:
- Repeated expression of concerns about being or feeling fat even when weight is below average.
- Expressions of fear about being or becoming obese that do not diminish as weight loss continues.
- Refusal to maintain even a minimal normal weight consistent with the individual's sport, age, and height.
- Consumption of huge amounts of food not consistent with the person's weight.
- A pattern of eating substantial amounts of food, followed promptly by trips to the bathroom and resumption of eating shortly thereafter.
- Periods of severe calorie restriction or repeated days of fasting.
- Evidence of purposeless, excessive physical activity.
- Depressed mood and expression of self-deprecating thoughts after eating.
- Apparent preoccupation with the eating behavior of other people, such as friends, relatives, or teammates.
- Known or reported family history of eating disorders or family dysfunction.

of their behavior. Bulimics believe that this behavior is disgusting and beyond their control. They become depressed and anxious, which in turn leads to more binging and purging episodes. In severe cases, bulimics become so obsessed with obtaining enough food and laxatives that they have little money for other needs. Sometimes they are arrested in the act of shoplifting these items from stores.

If untreated, the purging episodes can damage the body. The depressed bulimic may decide that suicide is the only solution to this abnormal behavior. If you know someone who seems to be able to eat huge amounts of food, is not physically active, yet is not gaining weight, you may suspect this disorder. It often helps to discuss the possibility of bulimia with them and to encourage them to obtain counseling. Treatment should focus on the causes of the behavior, including reasons for the low self-esteem and how to build supportive relation-

ships. Individuals benefit from counseling that teaches how to cope with stress in a more constructive manner than binging and purging. Success is often measured in reducing the behavior rather than totally eliminating it. Thus it is essential to be realistic about changing bulimic behaviors; habits take time to change.

ANOREXIA NERVOSA

Anorexia nervosa is a psychological disease in which a person develops an aversion to food and a distorted body image. Over a period of time, the person loses a considerable amount of body weight so that health and life are threatened. Recently, anorexia nervosa has become a more widespread problem, although not as widespread as bulimia. About 90 percent of the cases involve females, and the disorder usually begins around puberty. It is very obvious that these individuals are anorexic. They are so thin that they appear to have a terminal disease such as cancer. The subcutaneous fat layer is nearly absent, so veins can be seen on arms and legs. The typical feminine shape that is due to body fat deposits is absent. Extreme physical activity behaviors are also characteristic of the illness; the anorexic may jog or work out tirelessly. The normal female hormonal cycle depends on a certain minimal level of body fat; most of these women fail to menstruate.

In certain sports, anorexic behaviors may be apparent, particularly for those athletes who think a thin appearance is important. These sports include gymnastics, wrestling, dancing, cheerleading, track, and, to some degree, tennis. This has been called *anorexia athletica.* These athletes seem to associate a slender appearance with the ability to perform successfully and appear more attractive.

In many instances the condition begins as an attempt to reduce body fat through caloric reduction and increased exercise. Instead of being satisfied with reaching a healthy goal weight, these individuals become obsessed with the ability to control body weight and continue the effort. They may fast, but often they eat small, precisely measured quantities of food that do not supply enough calories to fuel the high energy demands of their physical activity and maintain a reasonable amount of body fat. Reports of a combination of anorexia nervosa and bulimic behaviors are not uncommon. This is often called *bulimia nervosa.* An estimated 20 percent of those affected with this psychological disease die from the effects of severe malnutrition or the chemical imbalances created by purging.

Individuals with anorexia nervosa cannot be convinced that they are "too thin." Their body image is so distorted that even while looking at themselves in a mirror, they think they could

> **anorexia nervosa:** a psychological disease in which a person develops an aversion to food and a distorted body image

lose some more weight. Therefore treating the condition is beyond the abilities of a health or physical educator. Simply referring the person to a health clinic is not effective unless specialists are on staff who are qualified to deal with these cases. Anorexics should be referred to a licensed psychologist or a medical doctor who specializes in treating such cases. In severe cases, long-term hospitalization is necessary. The key to treatment is getting patients to realize that they can gain control over their lives in ways that do not involve dieting. Unfortunately, many of those who do survive do not fully recover but remain underweight and fearful of any future weight gain.

SUMMARY

- Body composition analysis indicates the percentage of total body weight composed of fat tissue versus the percentage composed of lean tissue.
- The size and number of adipose cells determine percentage body fat, which can be measured by measuring the thickness of the subcutaneous fat with a skinfold caliper at specific areas.
- Changes in body weight are caused almost entirely by a change in caloric balance, which is a function of the number of calories taken in and the number of calories expended.
- Caloric expenditure may be calculated by maintaining accurate records of the number of calories expended for metabolic needs and in activities performed during the course of a day. Caloric intake measurement requires recording the number of Calories consumed.
- Weight can be lost either by increasing caloric expenditure through exercise or by decreasing caloric intake through reducing food intake. Most effective is a combination of moderate caloric restriction and a moderate increase in physical exercise during the course of each day.
- Weight loss should be accomplished gradually over a long period.

- Weight gain should be accomplished by increasing caloric intake and engaging in a weight-training program.
- Bulimia is an eating disorder that involves periodic binging and subsequent purging.
- Anorexia nervosa is a form of mental illness in which a person reduces food intake and increases energy expenditure to the extent that the loss of body fat threatens health and life.

SUGGESTED READINGS

Andersen, R.E. 1995. Is exercise or increased activity necessary for weight loss and weight management? *Medicine, exercise, nutrition and health* 4(2):57–59.

Anderson, A. 1999. *The 1999 Multi-diet: Taming the beast!* Jeffersonville, IN: Hamilton/Wolcott Publishing.

Brownell, K., and C. Fairburn. 1999. *Eating disorders and obesity: A comprehensive handbook.* New York, NY: Guilford Press.

Clarkson, P. et al. 1998. Methods and strategies for weight loss in athletics. *Sports science exchange-roundtable* 9(1):1–5.

Claude-Pierre, P. 1999. *The secret language of eating disorders.* New York, NY: Vintage Books.

DeLorenzo, A. et al. 1998. Comparison of different techniques to measure body composition in moderately active adolescents. *British Journal of Sports Medicine* 32(3):215–19.

Grilo, C.M. 1995. The role of physical activity in weight loss and weight loss management. *Medicine, exercise, nutrition and health.* 4(2):60–76.

Marks, B.L., and J.M. Rippe. 1996. The importance of fat free mass maintenance in weight loss programmes. *Sports medicine* 22(5):273–81.

McArdle, W., F. Katch, and V. Katch. 1996. *Exercise physiology, energy, nutrition and human performance.* Philadelphia: Lea and Febiger.

McQuillan, S., E. Khosrova, and E. Saltzman. 1998. *The complete idiot's guide to losing weight.* Indianapolis, IN: MacMillan.

Parr, R.B. 1998. Weight loss: What works and what doesn't. *American College of Sports Medicine's Health and Fitness Journal* 2(2):12–17.

Rhea, D.J., E.A. Jambor, and K. Wiginton. 1996. Preventing eating disorders in female athletes. *Journal of Physical Education, Recreation and Dance* 67(4):66–68.

Ross, R. 1997. Effects of diet- and exercise-induced weight loss on visceral adipose tissue in men and women. *Sports medicine* 24(1):55–64.

Sinning, W.E. 1996. Body composition in athletes. In Roche, A.F. et al. (ed). *Human body composition.* Champaign, IL: Human Kinetics.

Wallberg-Rankin, J. 1998. Guiding athletes in weight loss. *Sport health* 16(2):38–40.

Waltine, R.S. 1997. Starvation diets revisited. *Strength and conditioning* 19(4):70–71.

SUGGESTED WEBSITES

National Association of Anorexia Nervosa and Associated Disorders (ANAD)
This is the oldest non-profit organization helping victims of eating disorders and their families. [For information assembled by ANAD, see Healthtouch Online.]
http://members.aol.com/anad20/index.html

National Eating Disorders Organization
Get answers to any questions about eating disorders and their prevention. If you have (or know someone who has) an eating disorder, NEDO has information that may help.
http://www.laureate.com/nedointro.html

iVillage.com's Better Health's Diet & Nutrition Center
Get the latest dieting news & research, expert advice, interactive health assessment tools, scheduled chats, message boards and more.
http://www.betterhealth.com/diet/

The Weight Directory—
This is a directory of weight-loss resources, products, and services.
http://www.weightdirectory.com/

Weightloss2000
This site provides news about obesity and weight control, as well as an online support group for people dealing with weight issues.
http://www.weightloss2000.com/

Weight Loss Support Groups
This is a comprehensive directory and list of weight support groups that can help you lose weight.
http://www.weightdirectory.com/support.htm

Weight Loss Tips
This site presents tips from *Prevention Magazine*.
http://www.healthyideas.com/report/980610/

Lab Activity 7-1

Name   Section   Date

PURPOSE   To calculate percentage body fat using skinfold measures.

PROCEDURE
1. The triceps skinfold is measured over the right arm triceps muscle (back of the upper arm) halfway between the elbow and the tip of the shoulder (Figure 7-2).
   a. Instruct the subject to let the arm hang limply at the side. Grasp the skinfold parallel to the vertical axis of the arm. Lift the skinfold away from the arm, and make sure that no muscle tissue is caught in the fold.
   b. Place the contact surfaces of the calipers ½ inch (12 mm) above the fingers. Release the lever arm on the caliper, and allow pressure from the instrument to bring the two sides together. The caliper pointer then indicates the skinfold thickness in millimeters (mm). Repeat and record the measurement two or three times; then record the average of these measurements on the worksheet provided.

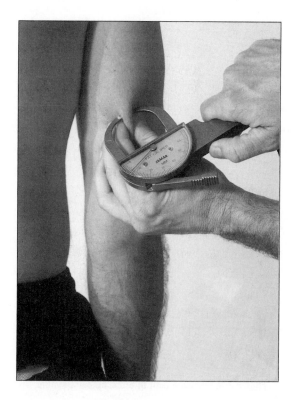

Figure 7-2. Measurement of Triceps Skinfold.

2. The subscapular (below the shoulder blade) measurement site is approximately ½ inch below the inferior angle of the scapula in line with the natural cleavage lines of the skin (Figure 7-3).

   a. Have the subject stand erect with shoulders thrust backward, arm at side. The point of the scapula (shoulder blade) located toward the spine should be obvious. Mark this point, then measure ½ inch below it and place a mark that will be the measurement site.

   b. Standing behind the subject, use the thumb and index fingers and grasp the skinfold in the natural cleavage line (along an imaginary line from elbow to neck). Lift the skinfold away from the scapula, and shake it to make sure no muscle tissue is caught in the fold. Use the caliper to measure as described previously, and record your average on the worksheet.

3. Now that the measurements for the triceps and the subscapular skinfolds are known, percentage body fat can be easily calculated using the following equations.

$$\text{Women: Percentage body fat} = 0.55(A) + 0.31(B) + 6.13$$
$$\text{Where } A = \text{Triceps skinfold (mm)}$$
$$B = \text{Subscapular skinfold (mm)}$$
$$\text{Men: Percentage body fat} = 0.43(A) + 0.58(B) + 1.47$$
$$\text{Where } A = \text{Triceps skinfold (mm)}$$
$$B = \text{Subscapular skinfold (mm)}$$

4. Consult Table 7-2 to determine the classification of your total percentage body fat.

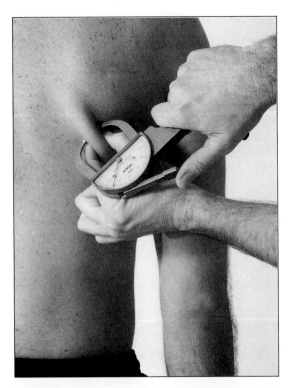

Figure 7-3. Measurement of Subscapular Skinfold.

INTERPRETATION   Ideal body composition consists of low fat and high muscle mass. Height-weight tables only assess one's weight in relation to insurance risk; they do not accurately reflect ideal body composition.

Your percentage body fat can be estimated from skinfold measures. It is recommended that women stay within 17 to 25 percent fat and men within 9 to 17 percent fat.

Too little body fat may be just as detrimental to your health as too much fat. The critical level for women is no less than 12 percent and for men is no less than 5 percent.

Worksheet for Calculating Percentage of Body Fat

1. Triceps skinfold thickness _____ mm
2. Subscapular skinfold thickness _____ mm

Calculation of Body Fat Percentage
1. Use the following formulas to determine percentage of body fat.

   Men
   $(0.43 \times$ _____ mm$) + (0.58 \times$ _____ mm$) + 1.47 =$ _____ %
         triceps   subscapular   body fat
         skinfold   skinfold

   Woman
   $(0.55 \times$ _____ mm$) + (0.31 \times$ _____ mm$) + 6.13 =$ _____ %
         triceps   subscapular   body fat
         skinfold   skinfold

2. Using Table 7-2, find your gender and age range category. Take the percentage determined above, and determine which health rating you are in. For example, if your percentage is 23 and you are a 22-year-old woman, your health rating is fair.

Lab Activity 7-2

Determining Your Basal Metabolic Rate (BMR)

Name _____ Section _____ Date _____

PURPOSE To determine your basal metabolic rate.

PROCEDURE 1. Use Figure 7-4 to determine your body surface area. Using a ruler, draw a straight line from your height to your weight. The point at which that line crosses the

Scale I Height		Scale III Surface area	Scale II Weight	
in	cm	m²	lb	kg
8"		2.9	340	160
6'6"	200	2.8	320	150
4"		2.7	300	140
2"	190	2.6	280	130
6'0"		2.5	260	120
10"	180	2.4		
		2.3	240	110
8"		2.2		105
5'6"	170	2.1	220	100
	165	2.0	200	95
4"	160	1.9	190	90
2"	155	1.8	180	85
5'0"	150	1.7	170	80
10"	145	1.6	160	75
8"		1.5	150	70
	140		140	65
4'6"	135	1.4	130	60
4"	130	1.3	120	55
2"	125	1.2	110	50
4'0"	120	1.1	100	45
10"	115	1.0	90	40
8"	110	0.9	80	35
3'6"	105		70	30
4"	100	0.8	60	25
2"	95	0.7	50	20
3'0"	90		40	
	85	0.6 0.58		15

Figure 7-4. Estimating Total Body Surface Area.
Locate your height on Scale 1 and then your weight on Scale 2. Using a straight edge, connect the two points with a line. The intersection of the line on Scale 3 is your body surface area.

middle column shows your surface area in square meters (m²). Record this number beside "Estimated Body Surface Area" on the worksheet. For example, for a 20-year-old man whose height is 6 feet (180 cm) and weight is 170 pounds (77.3 kg), his body surface area on the nomogram would be 1.99 square meters.

2. Next use Table 7-3 find the factor for your sex and age, and multiply your surface area by this factor. Record this number for "BMR factor" on the worksheet below. For example, for a 20-year-old man, the factor is 39.9 kcal per square meter per hour (kcal/m²/h).

TABLE 7-3
Basal Metabolic Rate According to Age and Sex

Age	BMR (kcal/m²/h) Men	BMR (kcal/m²/h) Women	Age	BMR (kcal/m²/h) Men	BMR (kcal/m²/h) Women
10	47.7	44.9	29	37.7	35.0
11	46.5	43.5	30	37.6	35.0
12	45.3	42.0	31	37.4	35.0
13	44.5	40.5	32	37.2	34.9
14	43.8	39.2	33	37.1	34.9
15	42.9	38.3	34	37.0	34.9
16	42.0	37.2	35	36.9	34.8
17	41.5	36.4	36	36.8	34.7
18	40.8	35.8	37	36.7	34.6
19	40.5	35.4	38	36.7	34.5
20	39.9	35.3	39	36.6	34.4
21	39.5	35.2	40–44	36.4	34.1
22	39.2	35.2	45–49	36.2	33.8
23	39.0	35.2	50–54	35.8	33.1
24	38.7	35.1	55–59	35.1	32.8
25	38.4	35.1	60–64	34.5	32.0
26	38.2	35.0	65–69	33.5	31.6
27	38.0	35.0	70–74	32.7	31.1
28	37.8	35.0	75+	31.8	

3. Next, multiply "Estimated body surface" by the "BMR factor" and record on the worksheet.

Worksheet for Calculating Basal Metabolic Rate (BMR)

1. Estimated body surface area (see Figure 7-4) = _____
2. BMR factor (see Table 7-3) = _____
3. _____ × _____ = _____
    Estimated body surface area   BMR factor   BMR
4. _____ = _____ × 24 hours
    Basal metabolic needs for 1 day   BMR

---

4. Finally, multiply this product by 24 hours per day to find your BMR needs per day.

Lab Activity 7-3

Calculating Caloric Expenditure

Name _____   Section _____   Date _____

PURPOSE   To keep a 24-hour log of all activities done during the day: everything from eating breakfast to biking to school or work, recreational activities, and so forth.

PROCEDURE
1. Consult Table 7-5 (page 172), Energy Expenditure During Physical Activity. Use the guidelines in Table 7-4 below for activities not included in Table 7-5.
2. Record your activities on the worksheet provided, listing the following:
   a. Clock time—Specify the time of day.
   b. Activity—The type of activity you were involved in.
   c. Total number of minutes spent in the activity.
   d. kcal/min/lb—Locate your nearest body weight in pounds, and use the appropriate column.
   e. Total Calories expended—Multiply total number of minutes by kcal/min/lb.
3. To calculate expenditure during sleep, multiply the number of hours you slept by the BMR calculated in Lab Activity 7-2.
4. Total the Calories expended during activities on the worksheet.
5. Add in the Calories expended in basal metabolism during a 24-hour period as calculated in Lab Activity 7-2.

*Every minute of the day should be accounted for.

TABLE 7-4
General Guidelines for Energy Expenditure

Activity	kcal/min/lb
Very light (such as typing, driving)	0.010
Light (such as shopping)	0.021
Moderate (such as dancing, bowling)	0.032
Heavy (such as football, running)	0.062

TABLE 7-5

Energy Expenditure During Physical Activity

To determine the number of calories expended during an activity, multiply the number of calories per minute per pound by your body weight in pounds. Then multiply this figure by the number of minutes you were involved in the activity.

Activity	Cal/min/lb	Activity	Cal/min/lb
Archery	.030	Fishing	.028
Badminton	.044	Football	.060
Baseball	.031	Gardening	
Basketball	.063	Digging	.057
Billiards	.018	Mowing	.051
Boxing (sparring)	.062	Raking	.025
Canoeing		Golf	.039
Leisure	.020	Gymnastics	.030
Racing	.047	Handball	.063
Circuit training		Hiking	.042
Hydra-Fitness	.060	Horseback riding	
Universal	.053	Galloping	.062
Nautilus	.042	Trotting	.050
Free weights	.039	Walking	.019
Climbing hills	.055	Ice hockey	.095
Croquet	.027	Jogging	.069
Cycling		Judo	.089
5.5 mph	.029	Jumping rope	
9.4 mph	.045	70 per min	.074
Racing	.079	80 per min	.075
Dancing		125 per min	.080
Aerobic, medium	.047	145 per min	.089
Aerobic, intense	.061	Lacrosse	.095
Ballroom	.023	Lying at ease	.010
Eating (sitting)	.010	Painting (outside)	.035
Field hockey	.061	Racquetball	.081

Data from Bannier EW, Brown SR: The relative energy requirements of physical activity. In Falls HB, editor: Exercise physiology, New York, 1968, Academic Press; Howley ET, Glover ME: The caloric costs of running and walking one mile for men and women, Med Sci Sports 6:235, 1974; Passmore R, Durnin JVGA: Human energy expenditure, Physiol Rev 25:801, 1955.

TABLE 7-5
Energy Expenditure During Physical Activity—cont'd

Activity	Cal/min/lb	Activity	Cal/min/lb
Running		Squash	.096
11.5 min per mile	.061	Swimming	
9 min per mile	.088	Backstroke	.077
8 min per mile	.095	Breast stroke	.074
7 min per mile	.104	Butterfly	.078
6 min per mile	.115	Crawl, slow	.070
5.5 min per mile	.131	Crawl, fast	.071
Cross-country	.074	Side stroke	.055
Sailing	.002	Treading, fast	.077
Sitting quietly	.009	Treading, normal	.028
Skiing		Table tennis	.031
Cross-country	.074	Tennis	.050
Downhill	.064	Volleyball	.023
Water	.052	Walking (normal pace)	.036
Skindiving		Weight training	.032
Considerable motion	.125	Wrestling	.085
Moderate motion	.094	Writing (sitting)	.013
Soccer	.059		

Name _____   Date _____

Worksheet for Calculating Daily Energy Expenditure
(Daily Activities Log)

Clock Time	Activity	Total Minutes Spent in Activity	kcal/min/lb	Total Calories Expended

Total Calories expended during activities   _____

Add Calories expended in basal metabolism during sleeping only   _____

Total Calories expended   _____

Lab Activity 7-4

Calculating Caloric Intake

Name   Section   Date

PURPOSE   To determine your daily caloric intake.

PROCEDURE   1. A daily food intake log such as the one in the worksheet on page 176 can be kept over a period of several days to let you know about how many Calories are being consumed on the average each day. College students are notorious for skipping meals and eating multiple snacks. Thus, it is important to record everything you consume during the entire 24-hour period. Don't neglect to record extras such as mustard and pickles that you include on a hamburger. Those columns that deal with hunger level and mood may help you to determine what causes you to eat when you do.
2. As with caloric expenditure, adding up the caloric values of all foods consumed during a 24-hour period can give you a reasonably accurate estimate of daily caloric intake.

Name _____ **Date** _____

Worksheet for Calculating Calorie Intake
(Daily Food Intake Log)

Time	Food Eaten	Amount	Number of Calories	How Cooked	Meal or Snack	Hunger Level* (0–3)	Activity and Location when Eating	Mood† (1–3)

Total number of Calories consumed =

*Hunger rating: 0, not hungry; 3, very hungry
†Mood: 1, good, happy; 2, fair, "OK"; 3, upset.

Worksheet for Estimating Caloric Balance

_____   _____   _____
Name   Section   Date

PURPOSE   To help you estimate whether you are in caloric balance, based on your assessment of a day's caloric intake and expenditure.

PROCEDURE   1. Consult Lab Activity 7-2 for estimated BMR caloric needs. Fill in below. Consult Lab Activity 7-3 for your estimation of activity caloric needs. Fill in below. Add the two numbers together.

_____ + _____ = _____ Calories
BMR Calories   Activity Calories

2. Multiply the sum from step 1 by 0.1 to estimate the number of Calories that are needed for the thermic effect of food (10% of BMR + Activity Calories).

_____ × 0.1 = _____ Calories

3. Add the sum of Calories from step 1 with the number obtained in step 2 to obtain an estimate of a day's caloric needs.

_____ + _____ = _____ Total Calories
Step 1 Calories   Step 2 Calories

4. Consult Lab Activity 7-4 for an estimation of your caloric intake. Record the number below.

_____ Calories

5. Compare the total number of energy expenditure Calories obtained in step 3 with the total for intake in step 4.
   Check which situation applies:
   a. Caloric intake is greater than expenditure   _____
   b. Caloric expenditure is greater than intake   _____
   c. Caloric expenditure equals intake   _____

Is this day's energy situation in balance, in negative balance, or in positive balance? _____

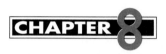
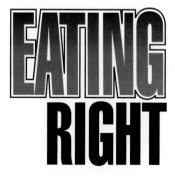

CHAPTER 8

EATING RIGHT

OBJECTIVES

After completing this chapter, you should be able to do the following:

- Identify the six classes of nutrients.
- Describe the major function of the nutrients.
- Analyze your diet for nutritional quality.
- Identify common nutrition myths that relate to fitness.
- Explain the relationship of nutrition to physical performance.

WHY DO YOU NEED TO KNOW ABOUT NUTRITION?

"Sports drinks," "anabolic amino acids," "antioxidants," "fat burners"—it seems that every day you read or hear about the health benefits of some nutrition-related product or service. Nutrition "experts" promote their latest books on radio talk shows, salespeople in health food stores praise the virtues of nutrient supplements, and friends give advice about diets that guarantee to melt pounds fast. Nutrition appears to be the key that unlocks the door

Key Terms
nutrition
diet
nutrients
deficiencies
overnutrition
diuretics
nutrient dense
requirements
recommendations

to a healthy, more attractive body. How true are all of the nutrition claims about foods, nutrients, or diet plans? What role does nutrition play in maximizing fitness? Lab Activity 8-1 will help you determine how much you know about nutrition. By understanding the basics of nutrition, you will be more likely to recognize the many forms of nutritional misinformation.

nutrition: the science of certain food substances

And, armed with some basic nutrition information, you will be able to identify "weak" areas of your diet and work to strengthen them. Are you eating a nutritious diet now? Lab Activity 8-2 will help you assess your eating patterns and find out whether or not you are currently eating a nutritious diet.

BASIC PRINCIPLES OF NUTRITION

What do you think of when you hear the word diet? Although many people think of losing weight, diet actually refers to your usual food selections. Everyone is on a diet! When a person eats less food in an effort to lose weight, he or she is on a weight reduction diet. Nutrition is the science of certain food substances, nutrients, and what they do in your body. Nutrients perform three major roles:

1. Growth, repair, and maintenance of all body cells
2. Regulation of body processes
3. Supply of energy for cells

The Fit List below, summarizes the various nutrients, which are categorized into six major classes: carbohydrates, fats (often called lipids), proteins, vitamins, minerals, and water. Most foods are actually mixtures of these nutrients. Although we think of bread as being a carbohydrate food, it supplies fats, proteins, and other nutrients too. Some nutrients can be made by the body; an essential nutrient must be supplied by the diet. Not all substances in foods are considered nutrients. For example, caffeine is found in some foods and beverages. Caffeine has definite effects on the body, but we can live without it. Furthermore, there is no such thing as a perfect food; that is, no single natural food contains all of the nutrients needed for health.

Without an adequate supply of nutrients, cells soon lose their ability to perform their jobs. Eventually the rest of the body is affected, and various health disorders called nutritional deficiencies develop. Thanks to our varied food supply, cases of people suffering from nutritional deficiencies are uncommon in the United States. Nevertheless, some Americans consume diets that are borderline deficient in certain nutrients. Occasionally, days with hectic schedules often result in careless eating or skipped meals. If your usual diet is good, it is unlikely that a few "off days" will lead to the development of a nutritional deficiency disease. However, if your diet is consistently of low quality, you run the risk of not being able to function at your peak level. Also, you could develop a deficiency disorder.

Fit List

Essential Nutrients

- Carbohydrates
- Fat
- Protein
- Vitamins
- Minerals
- Water

diet: refers to the types of food substances consumed

nutrients: perform three major roles including growth, repair, and maintenance of all body cells, regulation of body processes, and supplying energy for cells

deficiencies: consuming an inadequate supply of nutrients eventually affects the cells' ability to function and disease results

Just as low levels of nutrients can lead to health problems, nutrient excesses create trouble for your body. **Overnutrition**, eating too much food or specific nutrients, is common in the United States. Eating more food than needed can lead to obesity, which was discussed in Chapter 7. Many nutrients are toxic (poisonous) when taken in large doses. However, it is difficult to obtain toxic levels of nutrients by consuming a varied diet. Most cases of nutrient overdoses are the result of overzealous self-treatment with vitamin/mineral supplements. People think that nutrient supplements are foods and therefore perfectly safe to consume in large quantities.

> **overnutrition:** eating too much food or taking too many supplements can have negative effects on your body

However, the body is designed to obtain its nutrients from foods, not supplement pills or powders.

Running your body requires energy. This energy is supplied by the carbohydrates, fats, and proteins found in foods. Alcohol also provides energy, but it is not a nutrient. The energy value of food is measured by calories. Fats are the most concentrated source of calories in our diet. A gram of fat (there are about 28 grams in an ounce) supplies 9 Calories. Carbohydrates and proteins each contribute 4 Calories per gram. Alcohol, the nonnutrient, supplies 7 Calories per gram. Water, vitamins, and minerals do not supply any calories and therefore no energy. Most Americans eat too much fat and too little carbohydrate. Scientists recommend that we alter the proportions of fat and carbohydrate in diets (Figure 8-1). Later in this chapter, we'll focus on energy use during physical activity.

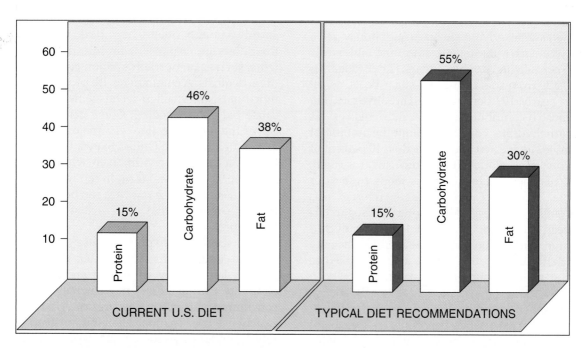

Figure 8-1. Comparison of Calories from Carbohydrates, Fats, and Proteins.

THE NUTRIENTS

▶ Carbohydrates (CHO)

The major role of carbohydrates is to provide energy for the body. Although muscles run on fats and carbohydrates, nerve tissue, especially brain cells, prefer to burn carbohydrates for energy. People should consume at least 55 percent of their total caloric needs from carbohydrates. Carbohydrates are classified as simple (sugars) or complex (starch, glycogen, and most forms of fiber). Let's take a closer look at some of the more important carbohydrates.

Sugars. Sugars are simple carbohydrates that occur as single-sugar or double-sugar chemical units. Glucose (blood sugar) is needed for fueling all cells. It is crucial for the body to maintain normal blood sugar levels. Food sources of glucose include fruits, syrups, and honey. Fructose (fruit sugar) occurs naturally in honey and is added to processed foods. Honey is often promoted as a substitute for sugar. However, honey supplies the same simple carbohydrates as table sugar, so there is no nutritional advantage in using honey as a sweetener. Milk sugar (lactose) and table sugar (sucrose) are double sugars. Table sugar is made from sugar cane and sugar beets, and it is nearly 100 percent pure carbohydrate. Because it contributes no other nutrients besides carbohydrate, you should limit the amount of table sugar eaten to no more than 10 percent of your total calories. If too much sugar is eaten, it displaces more nutritious foods from your diet. That's why sugary foods are referred to as "empty calories." Although table sugar has been blamed for causing hyperactivity in children, criminal behavior, and allergies, the only health problem that can be actually linked to sugar consumption is dental decay.

Sugars are often referred to as "quick" energy. However, you really don't obtain energy the instant you eat a candy bar. While it's true that it takes more time to break down starches, table sugar still has to be broken down and have its single-sugar units absorbed by the digestive tract before it can supply cells with energy.

Starches. Starches are called complex carbohydrates because they consist of long chains of glucose units. Plants make starches, such as those found in cereal grains, potatoes, and beans. During digestion, the long starch chains are broken down, releasing individual glucose units that are absorbed. Individual glucose units combine to form glycogen which is stored in muscle and the liver. When cells need energy, glycogen is broken down to release glucose.

Fiber. Your grandparents knew the importance of eating plenty of roughage to stay "regular" (avoid constipation). We now call roughage fiber. There are many different types of fiber, but they share the common characteristic of being from plant foods. Although most forms are complex carbohydrates, fiber cannot be digested in the small intestine, so it moves through the digestive tract relatively unchanged. Rich sources of fiber include fruits, vegetables, whole grain breads and cereals, nuts, beans, and peas.

Researchers believe that our diet does not supply enough fiber. They think that low-fiber diets are responsible for intestinal problems, such as hemorrhoids, colon cancer, and diverticulosis. A common health problem, hemorrhoids are swollen rectal veins that can cause pain and bleeding. Colon cancer (cancer of the large intestine) is a major cause of cancer deaths in the United States. Diverticulosis is a common condition in which small "blowouts" (pouches) form in the wall of the large intestine. These pouches can become infected (diverticulitis) and cause serious health problems.

Fiber seems to help prevent these conditions because certain forms attract water. This helps to form large, bulky stools that are easier to eliminate during bowel movements. People consuming diets rich in fiber are not as likely to experience constipation. Therefore, instead of relying on laxatives for simple cases of constipation, just eat more fiber-rich foods!

Besides helping to prevent constipation, certain forms of fiber may help to lower blood cholesterol levels. High blood cholesterol levels are a major risk factor for cardiovascular diseases. The fiber from oats, fruits, and vegetables is recommended for its cholesterol-lowering ability. These forms of fiber seem to interfere with cholesterol absorption from the intestinal tract. The less cholesterol absorbed means less enters the bloodstream and causes trouble in your arteries.

Try to obtain about 25 grams of fiber daily. (Nutrition labels often include information about fiber content.) One way to eat more fiber is to choose fruit for snacks or desserts. Increase your fiber intake by making sandwiches from whole-grain breads rather than from the low-fiber white breads. Interest in the healthful benefits of fiber has led to a flood of new whole grain cereal products. Try some of those containing nuts and dried fruits, and your fiber intake will reach more optimal levels. Keep in mind that eating more fiber-rich foods requires extra water, so you'll need to drink plenty of fluids.

▶ Fats

Recently, fat has received a lot of negative publicity for a nutrient that has many important jobs. Extra calories supplied by dietary carbohydrates, proteins, and fats may all be converted to triglyceride and stored in adipose cells as body fat for future energy needs. These body fat deposits cushion organs and give the body rounded contours (especially in women). Fat supplies a major portion of the energy used by muscles. Furthermore, certain types of fat cannot be formed by the body and are essential for health. We like to include fat in our meals because it makes eating more enjoyable by contributing flavor and texture. However, most Americans eat too much fat, a major factor in the development of obesity and cardiovascular diseases.

Depending on their chemical nature, fats may be either saturated or unsaturated. In general, unsaturated fat is from plants and is liquid at room temperature. Canola, peanut, olive oil, and vegetable oils from corn, cottonseed, sunflower, and soybean sources are rich in unsaturated fat. Saturated fats are derived mainly from animal sources. These include the fat in meats, such as beef, pork, and lamb, as well as much of the fat in eggs and dairy products—cream, butter, milk, and cheese. Coconut and palm oils, unlike most plant oils, are highly saturated.

Saturated fat and cholesterol are believed to be responsible for creating blocked arteries that lead to cardiovascular diseases. Cholesterol is a fat-related substance that is only found in animal foods. People think that cholesterol is "bad," but actually it is very important. Even if you avoid all foods that contain cholesterol, your body would make what it needs. The body makes vitamin D and its own steroid hormones from cholesterol. However, when a form of blood cholesterol becomes too high, the risk of developing cardiovascular diseases also increases.

Many studies show that eating saturated fat and cholesterol seems to increase blood cholesterol levels. Beef, milk, butter, and cheese are rich sources of saturated fat. Also, foods from animal sources, including dairy products, egg yolks, liver, and meats, contribute lots of cholesterol. Margarine made from plant fats (oils) is a good substitute for butter because all plant oils are cholesterol-free. Unsaturated fats do not raise blood cholesterol levels like saturated fats. Since certain kinds of saturated fats contribute to the development of high blood cholesterol levels, it is wise to reduce your consumption of these foods made with tropical oils.

Most experts believe it is more important to cut back on your total fat intake than worry about eating specific types of fats. The typical American eats about 40 percent of his or her total calories from fat. Experts think that this is too much and recommend levels of about 25 to 30 percent. These experts also suggest that cholesterol intake be limited to around 300 milligrams a day. Considering that one egg yolk has about 250 milligrams of cholesterol, this recommendation may be tough to meet if you like to eat eggs or products made from eggs every day. The American Heart Association recommends that you eat no more than four eggs a week. The good news is that food consumption surveys show that we have cut back on our saturated fat and cholesterol consumption. This appears to be helping to reduce the number of cardiovascular deaths, especially in younger people. Although not all of this decline is due to eating fewer eggs and drinking more skim milk, reducing overall fat consumption is believed to be partially responsible.

▶ **Protein**

Protein is needed for growth, repair, and maintenance of all cells. Major body structures, such as bone, muscles, and organs, are made of protein. Your skin, hair, and nails are made up of protein. Proteins are needed to make the enzymes that speed up chemical reactions, certain hormones, and components of the immune system. A small amount of protein can be used for energy, too. However, the body prefers to use carbohydrate and fat for energy, conserving protein for its other important functions.

Your body's need for protein increases during periods of growth. For example, protein needs are very high in infancy, during childhood and adolescent growth spurts, and during pregnancy. Breast-feeding women need more protein to supply their nursing infant's needs. During active body-building, athletes have a greater need. However, the typical American diet contains plenty of protein to meet an athlete's needs.

The recommended amount of protein is based on body weight; the typical adult recommendation is 0.8 gram of protein per kilogram of body weight. To determine how many grams of protein are recommended for your weight, take your weight in pounds and divide by 2.2 to obtain your weight in kilograms. Multiply that number times 0.8 to obtain the grams of protein that meet recommended levels of intake. Dietary surveys show that Americans eat more protein than needed, well over 100 grams per day. Much of that protein is from fatty animal sources. Your diet should contain about 12 to 15 percent of its calories from protein.

Proteins are made up of smaller units called amino acids. There are about 20 amino acids in the body. Nine essential amino acids must be supplied by the diet; the remainder can be made by the body. In order to grow, you need to have all of the essential amino acids available. If the diet is protein-deficient, growth slows or stops. During digestion, food proteins are broken down and amino acids are released and absorbed. Most animal proteins, such as those found in meat, fish, poultry, and eggs, contain ample amounts of the essential amino acids and are called complete or high-quality proteins.

Plant proteins, such as those found in beans, peas, nuts, seeds, and cereals, also contribute protein to the diet. For example, a slice of bread supplies 2 grams of protein. Plant food proteins are incomplete, that is, they are not good sources of the essential amino acids. However, the quality improves when they are mixed with proteins from animal sources of food. Many of our favorite food combinations, such as cereal and milk, macaroni and cheese, chili con carne, and tuna or chicken noodle casserole, combine small amounts of high-quality animal proteins with larger amounts of plant proteins. You do not have to eat large portions of animal foods to obtain enough protein.

Vegetarianism is an alternative to the usual American diet that is rich in animal sources of food. All vegetarians use plant foods to form the foundation of their diets; animal foods are either excluded or included to varying degrees. Vegetarian diets are usually lower in fat and higher in fiber and antioxidant nutrients than typical American food selections. However, you run the risk of nutritional deficiencies if you don't consider which nutrients are low in a totally plant-based diet. People who eat only plant foods (total vegetarians) must carefully plan their menus to make certain that they obtain adequate amounts of the essential amino acids and the other nutrients that are found primarily in animal foods.

▶ Water

Water is the most essential nutrient. You can live for weeks, months, even years without the other nutrients, but you will perish after a few days without water. About 60 percent of the adult's body weight is water. Many materials used in the body are water soluble, that is, dissolved in water. Although water does not supply any calories, an adequate supply of water is needed for energy production. Water also takes part in digestion and maintaining the proper environment inside and outside of cells. When your body burns fuels for energy, it produces a great deal of heat energy. Sweating is how your body uses water to keep itself from overheating.

The average adult requires a minimum of 2.5 liters of water or about 10 glasses of water a day. Because it is so vital, the healthy body carefully manages its internal water levels. When body water weight drops by 1 to 2 percent, you begin to feel thirsty. By drinking water, you help your internal water levels return to normal. If you ignore thirst signals and body water continues to decrease, dehydration results. People who are dehydrated cannot generate energy and feel weak. Other symptoms include nausea, vomiting, and fainting. If water losses become too great, the individual dies.

Dehydration is more likely to occur when you are outdoors and heavily sweating while engaging in some strenuous activity. To prevent dehydration, make sure you replace the lost water by drinking plenty of fluids. Don't rely on thirst as a signal that it's time to have a drink. Many people ignore their thirst, or, if

they do heed it, they don't drink enough. Avoid replacing water with caffeinated beverages and alcohol; these fluids act as **diuretics**, pulling more vital water out of your body.

Most adults can benefit from drinking more water. You don't need to buy canned or bottled waters. Drinking tap water may not impress people but it will quench your thirst for a lot less money.

Do you need to drink special sports beverages? These sport drinks are very popular and are widely marketed to the American public.

During physical activity it is essential to replace fluids lost through sweating. Replacing lost fluids with a sport drink is more effective than using water alone. Research has shown that because of the flavor you are likely to drink more sport drinks than water. Sport drinks quickly replace both fluids and electrolytes that are lost in sweat and also provide energy to the working muscles. Water is a good "thirst quencher," but it is not a good "rehydrator" because water "turns off" your thirst before you're completely rehydrated. Water also "turns on" the kidneys prematurely so you lose fluid in the form of urine much more quickly than when drinking a sport drink. A small amount of sodium allows your body to hold onto the fluid you consume rather than losing it through urine.

Not all sport drinks are the same. How a sports drink is formulated dictates how well it works in providing rapid rehydration and energy. The optimal level of carbohydrate is 14 gms per 8 oz of water for quickest absorption and energy. It has been shown that a sport drink can be effective in improving performance during both endurance activities as well as short-term high-intensity activities such as soccer, basketball, and tennis that last from 30 minutes to an hour.

diuretics: foods or chemicals that eliminate natural fluids from your body

▶ Vitamins

Like carbohydrates, proteins, and fats, vitamins are organic compounds that are essential for health. Although required in very small amounts, vitamins perform many roles, primarily as regulators of body processes. Humans need thirteen vitamins for health. You are probably familiar with their letter names, such as vitamins A, B_1, and C. Today, many are referred to by their chemical names. For example, if you see the word thiamin on a label, it's the chemical name for vitamin B_1. During the past 50 years, no new vitamins have been discovered, but scientists are still learning about their many roles.

People mistakenly think that vitamins provide energy. In fact, the body cannot break them down to release energy. However, many of the B-vitamins participate in the various chemical steps that release energy from carbohydrate, fat, and protein. Table 8-1 provides information about vitamins, including rich food sources, deficiency symptoms, and toxicity potential from high doses.

Vitamin deficiencies are uncommon in the United States. A few groups of people, such as the elderly, alcoholics, and those who severely restrict their food intake, are at risk of developing vitamin deficiency diseases. However, nutrition experts are concerned that many people are nutritionally on the "borderline," that is, close to being deficient. We may be too busy to plan nutritious meals, and we rely too much on vending machines or fast food restaurants. Furthermore, many young people are smoking cigarettes and drinking alcoholic beverages, behaviors that increase vitamin and other nutrient needs.

Fat-soluble Vitamins. Vitamins are grouped according to the ability to dissolve in water or fat. Vitamins A, E, D, and K dissolve in fat rather than water. Extra amounts of the fat-soluble vitamins are not easy to eliminate from the body in urine, which is mostly water. Instead they are stored in the liver or body fat until needed. This feature makes them potentially toxic, so be careful if you choose to take supplements of these vitamins. See Table 8-1 for information about the fat-soluble vitamins, including their toxicity potential.

Water-soluble Vitamins. The water-soluble vitamins, B-complex and C, dissolve in water. This feature makes it easier for the body to eliminate excesses in urine. Many of the B-vitamins help produce energy from carbohydrates, proteins, and fats. When these vitamins are unavailable, every cell cannot generate energy to perform its numerous jobs. The result is feeling tired. Don't think that by taking extra amounts of the B-vitamins that you'll have more energy. Once your cells have enough of the B-vitamins, any additional doses will not make cells generate extra amounts of energy. Although excesses of most water-soluble vitamins are excreted in urine, high doses of certain water-soluble vitamins have been linked to toxic effects. See Table 8-1 for information about the water-soluble vitamins, including their toxicity potential.

Antioxidant Nutrients. Nutrition experts are generating excitement and controversy over reports that certain nutrients, called antioxidants, may prevent premature aging, certain cancers, heart disease, and other health problems. An antioxidant protects vital cell components from the destructive effects of certain agents, including oxygen. Vitamin C, vitamin E, and beta carotene are antioxidants. Beta carotene is a plant pigment that is found in dark green, deep yellow, or orange fruits and vegetables. The body can convert beta carotene to vitamin A. In the early 1980s, researchers reported that smokers who ate large quantities of beta carotene-rich fruits and vegetables were less likely to develop lung cancer than other smokers. Since that time, more evidence is accumulated about the benefits of a diet rich in the antioxidant nutrients. The Fit List on page 188 lists foods rich in the antioxidant nutrients.

Some experts believe people should increase their intake of antioxidants, even if it means taking supplements. Others are more

TABLE 8-1
Vitamins

Vitamin	Major Function	Most Reliable Sources	Deficiency	Excess (Toxicity)
A	Maintains skin and other cells that line the inside of the body; bone and tooth development; growth; vision in dim light	Liver, milk, egg yolk, deep green and yellow fruits and vegetables	Night blindness; dry skin; growth failure	Headaches, nausea, loss of hair, dry skin, diarrhea
D	Normal bone growth and development	Exposure to sunlight; fortified dairy products; eggs and fish liver oils	"Rickets" in children—defective bone formation leading to deformed bones	Appetite loss, weight loss, failure to grow
E	Prevents destruction of polyunsaturated fats caused by exposure to oxidizing agents; protects cell membranes from destruction	Vegetable oils, some in fruits and vegetables, whole grains	Breakage of red blood cells leading to anemia	Nausea and diarrhea; interferes with vitamin K if vitamin D is also deficient. Not as toxic as other fat-soluble vitamins
K	Production of blood-clotting substances	Green leafy vegetables; normal bacteria that live in intestines produce K that is absorbed	Increased bleeding time	
Thiamin	Needed for release of energy from carbohydrates, fats, and proteins	Cereal products, pork, peas, and dried beans	Lack of energy, nerve problems	
Riboflavin	Energy from carbohydrates, fats, and proteins	Milk, liver, fruits and vegetables, enriched breads and cereals	Dry skin, cracked lips	
Niacin	Energy from carbohydrates, fats, and proteins	Liver, meat, poultry, peanut butter, legumes, enriched breads and cereals	Skin problems, diarrhea, mental depression, and eventually, death (rarely occurs in US)	Skin flushing, intestinal upset, nervousness, intestinal ulcers
B_6	Metabolism of protein; production of hemoglobin	White meats, whole grains, liver, egg yolk, bananas	Poor growth, anemia	Severe loss of coordination from nerve damage
B_{12}	Production of genetic material; maintains central nervous system	Foods of animal origin	Neurological problems, anemia	

Continued

TABLE 8-1
Vitamins—cont'd

Vitamin	Major Function	Most Reliable Sources	Deficiency	Excess (Toxicity)
Folate (Folic acid)	Production of genetic material	Wheat germ, liver, yeast, mushrooms, green leafy vegetables, fruits	Anemia	
C (Ascorbic acid)	Formation and maintenance of connective tissue; tooth and bone formation; immune function	Fruits and vegetables	"Scurvy" (rare); swollen joints, bleeding gums, fatigue, bruising	Kidney stones, diarrhea
Pantothenic acid	Energy from carbohydrates, fats, proteins	Widely found in foods	Not observed in humans under normal conditions	
Biotin	Use of fats	Widely found in foods	Rare under normal conditions	

Fit List

Foods Rich in Antioxidants

Beta Carotene Foods

- Sweet potatoes
- Pumpkin
- Squash
- Carrots
- Red bell peppers
- Dark green vegetables
- Apricots
- Mango
- Cantaloupe

Vitamin C Foods

- Kiwifruit
- Citrus fruits
- Berries
- Cantaloupe
- Honeydew
- Bell peppers
- Tomatoes
- Cabbage
- Broccoli

Vitamin E Foods

- Vegetable oils
- Nuts
- Seeds
- Margarine
- Wheat germ
- Olives
- Leafy greens
- Asparagus

cautious. Excess beta carotene pigments circulate throughout the body and may turn your skin yellow. However the pigment is not believed to be toxic like its nutrient cousin, vitamin A. On the other hand, increasing your intake of vitamins C and E is not without some risk. Excesses of vitamin C are not well absorbed; the excess is irritating to the intestines and causes diarrhea. Although less toxic than vitamins A or D, too much vitamin E causes health problems, as indicated in Table 8-1.

▶ Minerals

Over 20 mineral elements need to be supplied by the diet. These include the minerals listed in Table 8-2. Other mineral elements are found in the body. The role of minerals is unclear. Minerals are needed for a variety of jobs, such as forming strong bones and teeth, helping to generate energy, activating enzymes, and maintaining water balance. Most minerals are stored in the body, especially in the bones and liver. Vitamins are stored in the liver, too. That explains why liver usually leads the list of most nutritious foods. Vitamins and minerals interact with one another—if you don't get enough of one, the other may not work the way it is supposed to.

Calcium. You are probably aware that calcium is needed for building strong bones and teeth, but it is also needed for nerve and muscle function. Milk products are rich in calcium, but many people do not like to drink milk. For young women, poor food choices and efforts to lose weight are believed to be responsible for low intakes of calcium. Over a lifetime, this may lead to osteoporosis, a condition in which the

TABLE 8-2
Minerals of Major Concern

Mineral	Major Role	Most Reliable Sources	Deficiency	Excess
Calcium	Bone and tooth formation; blood clotting; muscle contraction; nerve function	Dairy products	May lead to osteoporosis	Calcium deposits in soft tissues
Phosphorus	Skeletal development; tooth formation	Meats, dairy products, and other protein-rich foods	Rarely seen	May contribute to the development of hypertension
Sodium	Maintenance of fluid balance	Salt (sodium chloride) added to foods and sodium-containing preservatives	Iron-deficiency anemia	Can cause death in children from supplement overdose
Iron	Formation of hemoglobin; energy from carbohydrates, fats, and proteins	Liver and red meats, enriched breads and cereals	Anemia	Nausea and vomiting
Copper	Formation of hemoglobin	Liver, nuts, shellfish, cherries, mushrooms, whole grain breads and cereals	Skin problems, delayed development, growth problems	Interferes with copper use; may decrease HDL levels
Zinc	Normal growth and development	Seafood and meats	Mental and growth retardation; lack of energy	
Iodine	Production of the hormone thyroxin	Iodized salt, seafood		
Fluorine	Strengthens bones and teeth	Fluoridated water	Teeth are less resistant to decay	Damage to tooth enamel

bones become less dense and break easily. Osteoporosis leads to loss of height, a humped-shaped upper back, and hip fractures that can result in disabling injuries and even death. Most affected bones are those in the wrist, hip, and spine. Factors contributing to osteoporosis include heredity, cigarette smoking, menopause, lack of physical activity, and a lifetime of poor calcium intake.

The calcium in milk products is well absorbed by the body. To increase your dietary calcium intake without eating too much fat, choose low-fat cheeses, milks (skim or 1 percent), or yogurt products. Although cottage cheese is made from milk, it is not a good source of calcium because the mineral is lost from the milk during processing.

Iron. Iron is needed to form the oxygen-carrying pigment in red blood cells called hemoglobin. When hemoglobin picks up oxygen in the lungs, it turns the blood bright red. In cases of iron-deficiency anemia, red blood cells are smaller and do not contain enough hemoglobin. The cells cannot get the oxygen needed to make energy. As a result, one feels tired and looks pale. Iron-deficiency anemia is a fairly common disorder, especially for young women who experience menstrual blood losses and who avoid eating meat. This deficiency can be due to a lack of iron in the diet or excessive blood losses. Donating blood is a worthwhile activity, but it increases the need for iron as the body replaces red blood cells. Among the best food sources of iron are red meats, which contain a type of iron that is well absorbed. However, some people need to take iron pills to treat the anemia. Furthermore, some people absorb too much iron, which causes health problems. Keep in mind that there are many possible causes of anemia; iron-deficiency anemia is just one type of the disorder.

Others. The other minerals are just as important, but there are so many minerals needed by the body, it is beyond the scope of this text to delve further. Review Table 8-2 to learn more about calcium, iron, and several other minerals known to play important roles in the body.

PRODUCTION OF ENERGY

Energy is produced when cells break down the chemical units of glucose, fats, or amino acids to release energy stored in these compounds. Glycogen is not used directly for energy; it must first be broken down to release its supply of glucose units. This process is often referred to as "burning" the energy-supplying nutrients for energy. It is similar to burning a log, except your cells are the "fireplaces." Cellular combustion releases heat energy that maintains your body temperature and generates a form of energy that allows your cells to do work. For example, muscle cells need energy to keep moving, brain cells for thinking, and bone cells for building bone.

Logs cannot burn without oxygen; cells cannot produce much energy without oxygen, too. In Chapter 4, we discussed how anaerobic and aerobic conditions influence the amount of energy that can be generated. Recall that under aerobic conditions, muscle can generate more energy, especially from fat. Figure 8-2 shows the relative proportions of carbohydrate, fat, and protein fuels used for different kinds of physical activity. As shown in the graph, the proportions of nutrient fuels that are burned at any time depend on the type, duration, and intensity of the activity. These factors influence the amount of oxygen that cells need to generate energy.

When sitting around watching TV or reading, oxygen needs are low, and the body runs mostly on fat. As you can see in Figure 8-2, carbohydrates provide the major proportion of energy for short-term, high-intensity muscular contractions. As the duration and the intensity of the activity increase, breathing also increases, supplying more oxygen for the cells and maximizing energy production. When the activity is prolonged, such as in an endurance

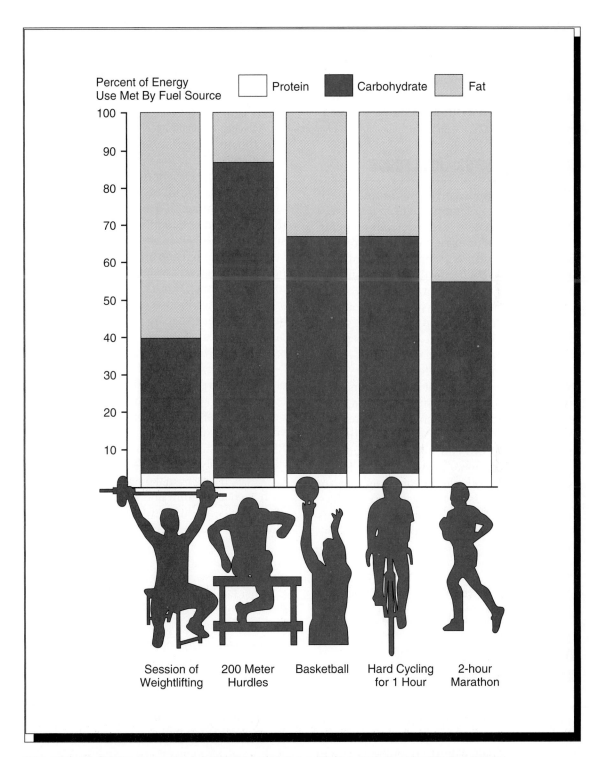

Figure 8-2. The Relative Proportions of Carbohydrates, Fat and Protein Fuels Used for Physical Activity.

type of sport, the percentage of fat and carbohydrate used for fuel is similar. Under usual conditions, proteins supply less than about 5 percent of energy. However, when you are engaged in an endurance type of activity, protein supplies as much as 10 to 15 percent of your energy needs.

NUTRIENT-DENSE VS. JUNK FOODS

Foods that contain considerable amounts of vitamins, minerals, and proteins in relation to their caloric content are referred to being nutrient dense. For example, a cup of orange juice is a more nutrient-dense source of vitamin C, folate (a B-vitamin), and potassium (a mineral) than a cup of orange drink made from only 10 percent fruit juices. Although it has added vitamin C, the additional water and sugar make the orange drink a less nutritious choice. Candy, chips, doughnuts, cakes, and cookies are often referred to as "junk foods." These foods are not nutrient dense because they provide too many calories from fats and sugars in relation to vitamins and minerals. If your overall diet is nutritious, and you can "afford" the extra calories, it's alright to eat occasional fatty or sugary foods. However, many people live on diets that are rich in these kinds of foods, which displace more nutritious food items in their diets. This is not a healthy behavior to practice in the long run.

HOW DO YOU KNOW IF YOU'RE EATING A NUTRITIOUS DIET?

NUTRIENT REQUIREMENTS AND RECOMMENDATIONS

A nutrient requirement is that amount of the nutrient that is needed to prevent the nutrient's deficiency disease. Nutrient needs vary among individuals within a population. A rec-

ommendation for a nutrient is different than the requirement. Scientists establish recommendations for nutrients and calories based on extensive scientific research and assessment of present dietary intakes.

The *U.S. Recommended Daily Allowances* (US RDA) were designed to help consumers compare the nutritional value of many food products (Table 8-3A). Currently the RDAs are being changed to *Dietary Reference Intakes* (DRI). The term RDA is still being used as the actual amount recommended and for some nutrients these recommendations have not changed since 1989. However several old RDAs have been downgraded and are now called *Adequate Intakes* (AI) because of insufficient knowledge to establish new DRIs. (Table 8-3B)

You may want to estimate the nutritional quality of your diet by using the RDA as a guide. It takes a lot of work, but you need to record everything you eat and drink over a 3-day period. Then use the computerized dietary analysis program or the food composition tables in the appendices to analyze the nutritional value of your food intake. In general, if you are consuming at least two-thirds of the RDA for most nutrients on a daily basis, your diet is probably adequate (see Lab Activity 8-2). However, trying to make sense out of the RDA, with their milligram and microgram amounts of nutrients, is difficult for many consumers. How can these nutrient recommendations

nutrient dense: foods that contain considerable amounts of vitamins, minerals, and proteins in relation to their caloric content

requirements: the amount of a nutrient needed to prevent that nutrient's deficiency disease

recommendations: the requirement plus an extra amount referred to as a "margin of safety"

TABLE 8-3A

Recommended Dietary Allowances,[a] Revised 1989 (Abridged) from the Food and Nutrition Board, National Academy of Sciences—National Research Council

Designed for the maintenance of good nutrition of practically all healthy people in the United States

Category	Age (year) or Condition	Weight[b] (kg)	Weight[b] (lb)	Height[b] (cm)	Height[b] (in)	Protein (g)	Vitamin A (μg RE)[c]	Vitamin E (mg α-TE)[d]	Vitamin K (μg)	Vitamin C (μg)	Iron (mg)	Zinc (mg)	Iodine (μg)	Selenium (μg)
Males	15–18	66	145	176	69	59	1,000	10	65	60	12	15	150	50
	19–24	72	160	177	70	58	1,000	10	70	60	10	15	150	70
	25–50	79	174	176	70	63	1,000	10	80	60	10	15	150	70
	51+	77	170	173	68	63	1,000	10	80	60	10	15	150	70
Females	15–18	55	120	163	64	44	800	8	55	60	15	12	150	50
	19–24	58	128	164	65	46	800	8	60	60	15	12	150	55
	25–50	63	138	163	64	50	800	8	65	60	15	12	150	55
	51+	65	143	160	63	50	800	8	65	60	10	12	150	55
Pregnant						60	800	10	65	70	30	15	175	65
Lactating	1st 6 months					65	1,300	12	65	95	15	19	200	75
	2nd 6 months					62	1,200	11	65	90	15	16	200	75

[a]The allowances, expressed as average daily intakes over time, are intended to provide for individual variations among most normal persons as they live in the United States under usual environmental stresses. Diets should be based on a variety of common foods in order to provide other nutrients for which human requirements have been less well defined.

[b]Weights and heights of Reference Adults are actual medians for the U.S. population of the designated age. The use of these figures does not imply that the height-to-weight ratios are ideal.

[c]Retinol equivalents. 1 retinol equivalent = 1μg retinol or 6 μg β-carotene.

[d]α-tocopherol equivalents. 1 mg d-α tocopherol = 1 α-TE.

TABLE 8-3B
Dietary Reference Intakes: Recommended Levels for Individual Intake from the Food and Nutrition Board, Institute of Medicine—National Academy of Sciences

Life-Stage Group		Calcium (mg/d)	Phosphorus (mg/d)	Magnesium (mg/d)	(μg/d)[a,b]	Fluoride (mg/d)	Thiamin (mg/d)	Riboflavin (mg/d)	Niacin (mg/d)[c]	B$_6$ (mg/d)	Folate (μg/d)[d]	B$_{12}$ (μg/d)	Pantothenic Acid (mg/d)	Biotin (μg/d)	Choline[e] (mg/d)
Males	14–18 yr	1,300*	1,250*	410	5*	3*	1.2	1.3	16	1.3	400	2.4	5*	25*	550*
	19–30 yr	1,000*	700	400	5*	4*	1.2	1.3	16	1.3	400	2.4	5*	25*	550*
	31–50 yr	1,000*	700	420	5*	4*	1.2	1.3	16	1.3	400	2.4	5*	30*	550*
	51–70 yr	1,200*	700	420	10*	4*	1.2	1.3	16	1.7	400	2.4[f]	5*	30*	550*
	>70 yr	1,200*	700	420	15*	4*	1.2	1.3	16	1.7	400	2.4[f]	5*	30*	550*
Females	14–18 yr	1,300*	1,250*	360	5*	3*	1.0	1.0	14	1.2	400[g]	2.4	5*	25*	400*
	19–30 yr	1,000*	700	310	5*	3*	1.1	1.1	14	1.3	400[g]	2.4	5*	30*	425*
	31–50 yr	1,000*	700	320	5*	3*	1.1	1.1	14	1.3	400[g]	2.4	5*	30*	425*
	51–70 yr	1,200*	700	320	10*	3*	1.1	1.1	14	1.5	400[g]	2.4[f]	5*	30*	425*
	>70 yr	1,200*	700	320	15*	3*	1.1	1.1	14	1.5	400	2.4[f]	5*	30*	425*
Pregnancy	≤18 yr	1,300*	1,250*	400	5*	3*	1.4	1.4	18	1.9	600[h]	2.6	6*	30*	450*
	19–30 yr	1,000*	700	350	5*	3*	1.4	1.4	18	1.9	600[h]	2.6	6*	30*	450*
	31–50 yr	1,000*	700	360	5*	3*	1.4	1.4	18	1.9	600[h]	2.6	6*	30*	450*
Lactation	≤18 yr	1,300*	1,250*	360	5*	3*	1.5	1.6	17	2.0	500	2.8	7*	35*	550*
	19–30 yr	1,000*	700	310	5*	3*	1.5	1.6	17	2.0	500	2.8	7*	35*	550*
	31–50 yr	1,000*	700	320	5*	3*	1.5	1.6	17	2.0	500	2.8	7*	35*	550*

NOTE: This table presents Recommended Dietary Allowances (RDAs) in bold type and Adequate Intakes (AIs) in ordinary type followed by an asterisk (*). RDAs and AIs may both be used as goals for individual intake. RDAs are set to meet the needs of almost all (97 to 98 percent) individuals in a group. For healthy breastfed infants, the AI is the mean intake. The AI for other life-stage groups is believed to cover their needs, but lack of data or uncertainty in the data prevent clear specification of this coverage.

[a] As cholecalciferol. 1 μg cholecalciferol = 40 IU vitamin D.
[b] In the absence of adequate exposure to sunlight.
[c] As niacin equivalents. 1 mg of niacin = 60 mg of tryptohan.
[d] As dietary folate equivalents (DFE). 1 DFE = 1 μg food folate = 0.6 μg of folic acid (from fortified food or supplement) consumed with food = 0.5 μg of synthetic (supplemental) folic acid taken on an empty stomach.
[e] Although AIs have been set for chlorine, there are few data to assess whether a dietary supply of choline is needed at all stages of the life cycle, and it may be that the choline requirement can be met by endogenous synthesis at some of these stages.
[f] Since 10 to 30 percent of older people may malabsorb food-bound B$_{12}$, it is advisable for those older than 50 years to meet their RDA mainly by consuming foods fortified with B$_{12}$ or a B$_{12}$-containing supplement.
[g] In view of evidence linking folate intake with neural tube defects in the fetus, it is recommended that all women capable of becoming pregnant consume 400 μg of synthetic folic acid from fortified foods and/or supplements in addition to intake of food folate from a varied diet.
[h] It is assumed that women will continue consuming 400 μg of folic acid until their pregnancy is confirmed and they enter prenatal care, which ordinarily occurs after the end of the periconceptional period—the critical time for formation of the neural tube.

translate into amounts of foods? How do you know if your diet supplies enough nutrients and is healthy?

FOOD PYRAMID

The answer is to use food guides as a practical way to analyze your diet. You may recall learning about the "Basic Four" food groups, which divided foods into four categories and included recommended numbers of servings. More recently, concern over the role of diet and health led nutritionists to redesign this educational tool to address current health issues. The latest food guide, the Food Pyramid (Figure 8-3), incorporates generally accepted health-related recommendations concerning fat, sugar, and complex carbohydrate intake within its design. At the base of the pyramid, breads and cereal products form the founda-

tion of the diet, supplying complex carbohydrates and dietary fiber. As you move up to the next tier, you'll see separate groups for the fruits and vegetables. These two groups also provide complex carbohydrates, fiber, vitamins, and minerals. The third tier has groups for meat and meat alternates (dried beans, peas, nuts, and eggs) and milk foods. These foods are important sources of vitamins, minerals, and protein. Foods that are not nutrient dense, sweets, and fatty foods, occupy the top of the pyramid. The idea is to go easy on the amounts of fatty or sugary foods in your diet.

Using the Food Pyramid can make planning nutritious meals simple, that is, if you eat plain foods that are easy to classify into specific food groups. Ethnic dishes and casseroles can make analyzing your diet more difficult. For example, how do you classify an

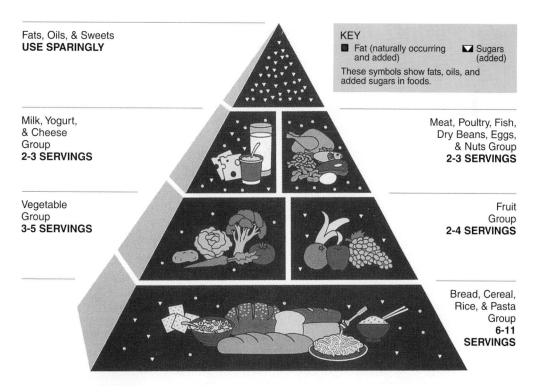

Figure 8-3. Food Pyramid.

enchilada or pizza? Not everyone will find the Food Pyramid helpful. For these people, more general dietary recommendations make sense. These are referred to as the U.S. Dietary Guidelines.

It is important to emphasize that you do not have to eat foods from each of the food groups every day. Also, it is alright to eat "junk" foods on occasion. However, over several days it is important for you to try to eat a well-balanced and nutritious diet. Lab Activity 8-3 will help you to determine your eating habits during a 7-day period.

U.S. DIETARY GUIDELINES

In 1990, experts presented the latest version of the U.S. Dietary Guidelines. The Health Link below recommends food choices to help you meet the U.S. Dietary Guidelines. Note that the key words are variety and moderation. For example, if you eat pears three times a day, you may be missing out on some nutrients that other fruits, such as peaches and strawberries, contribute to the diet. Furthermore it's alright to eat a doughnut or a few cookies, but don't expect to maximize your nutrient intake or maintain a healthy weight if these replace

Health Link

Food Choices for a Healthy Body

- Eat less fat and cholesterol. Eat more lean meats, fish, and poultry. Eat less fried foods, chips, and fatty spreads, such as margarine and butter.
- When ordering a salad, ask for the dressing "on the side" so that you can control the amount.
- Achieve and maintain a desirable body weight. Chapter 7 addressed this in detail. Eat less fatty foods and exercise more.
- Choose foods that are high in fiber and complex carbohydrates; whole grain breads and cereals; rice, tortillas, potatoes, and pasta.
- Eat less sugary foods. Drink less sugar-sweetened soft drinks.
- Reduce sodium intake by cutting back on salty foods and foods with sodium-containing additives. Read labels for sodium content; don't add salt to foods while cooking; taste foods before adding salt; avoid salty snacks, processed luncheon meats, ham, and pickled foods.
- Use alcohol in moderation, if you choose to drink. Moderation means a limit of two drinks per day. Don't drink and drive or operate other machines. Don't drink if you are trying to become or if you are pregnant.
- Drink fluoridated water. Check with your local water authority to see if fluorine is added to your community's water supply.
- Increase calcium intake by drinking more milk (low-fat) or eating more low-fat yogurt and cheeses.
- Eat more iron-rich foods. Eat food containing vitamin C with vegetable sources of iron to improve the mineral's absorption. Enriched breads and cereals are good sources.

meals. By keeping these basic guidelines in mind as you shop for food or select fast food items, you can feel more assured that your diet is healthful.

READING LABELS

Over the past 20 years, food labels have provided helpful nutritional information for consumers. In 1994, a new nutritional labeling format changed the look and importance of food product packaging. It was changed because people were becoming concerned over the amount of fat, cholesterol, sodium, and fiber in the typical American diet, thus producing the drive for a more health-conscious label. Health educators believe that the new format has made it easier for consumers to make more informed, healthful food selections.

Examine the sample label shown in Figure 8-4. The manufacturer must list the total number of Calories per serving, a popular feature of the former label. The new label includes information about the number of total Calories contributed by fat. Unfortunately, you have to do some math to figure out what percentage of total Calories is fat Calories. This is crucial if you are trying to limit the total amount of fat in your diet to about 25 to 30 percent of total Calories. Furthermore the new format presents the information in the form of percentages that are based on "percent daily values" and a standard 2000 Calories. For example, the label shown in Figure 8-4 indicates that the ½-cup-sized serving contributes 15 percent of the percent daily value of calcium. If you are to meet 100 percent of the value for this mineral, the other foods in your daily diet should supply the remaining 85 percent of the value for calcium. Although there are a few exceptions, most packaged supermarket foods must include nutritional labels. Not everyone is satisfied with the new format; consumers will ultimately decide its usefulness.

Nutrition Facts	
Serving Size ½ cup (114g)	
Servings Per Container 4	
Amount Per Serving	
Calories 260	Calories from Fat 120
	% Daily Value*
Total Fat 13g	20%
Saturated Fat 5g	25%
Cholesterol 30mg	10%
Sodium 660mg	28%
Total Carbohydrate 31g	11%
Dietary Fiber 0g	0%
Sugars 5g	
Protein 5g	
Vitamin A 4%	Vitamin C 2%
Calcium 15%	Iron 4%

*Percent Daily Values are based on a 2000 Calorie diet. Your daily values may be higher or lower depending on your calorie needs.

	Calories:	2000	2500
Total Fat	Less than	65g	80g
Sat. Fat	Less than	20g	25g
Cholesterol	Less than	300mg	300mg
Sodium	Less than	2,400mg	2,400mg
Total Carbohydrate		300g	375g
Dietary Fiber		25g	30g

Calories per gram
Fat 9 · Carbohydrate 4 · Protein 4

Figure 8-4. New Label Indicating Nutrition Information per Serving.

WHAT IS THE ROLE OF NUTRITION IN PHYSICAL ACTIVITY?

Interest in the value of nutrition to fitness is very high. Physically active people often believe that certain nutrients can help them achieve their fitness goals or a competitive edge. Depending on personal experiences and beliefs, certain foods may be valued or avoided by athletes. Let's explore some of the more common beliefs and examine what the experts have determined about the role of nutrients and foods in physical performance.

NUTRITIONAL SUPPLEMENTS

You may know people who take vitamin, mineral, and protein supplements. Every year, Americans spend millions of dollars on nutrient supplements. These products often contain amounts of nutrients that are well beyond the minimum needed and the levels recommended. Although claims about the value of supplements abound, there is no scientific evidence that vitamin, mineral, or protein supplements enhance physical performance or boost energy.

▶ Protein Supplements

The experts do not agree on how much additional protein is needed during bodybuilding. For most, it appears that any increase in protein needs for conditioning, bodybuilding, and weight training is easily met by your usual diet. As mentioned earlier, the typical American eats over 100 grams of protein a day, so even those trying to "bulk up" are probably consuming plenty of protein. There seems to be no advantage to consuming greater amounts of protein, especially from protein supplements. Extra proteins or amino acids are not anabolic, that is, they do not stimulate the growth of muscle cells. In fact, using amino acids supplements can be harmful. The body is designed to digest and absorb proteins from foods, not synthetic mixtures of amino acids. These protein supplements can create amino acid imbalances, can cause dehydration (loss of body water), and may increase losses of calcium.

Physical activity increases the need for energy, not protein. If the body is not supplied with enough energy, the valuable amino acids can be used for energy. Therefore, make certain that you are eating enough carbohydrates (preferably starches) to meet your body's energy needs and spare amino acids for other uses. The excess amino acids from foods or supplements can be converted to fat and stored for future energy needs.

▶ Vitamin and Mineral Supplements

There are people, such as the elderly or ill, who have difficulty obtaining all of the vitamins and minerals they need through the diet. These individuals often benefit from supplementation. Even for healthy people, obtaining adequate levels of antioxidant nutrients as well as calcium and iron requires careful dietary planning. The Fit List on page 188 lists foods rich in antioxidants. Although there is disagreement, some experts believe that selecting antioxidant-rich foods is not enough and taking supplements of these specific nutrients is warranted. Furthermore, supplements of the following minerals may be necessary for some people.

Calicum. Some physical activity helps to strengthen bone. However, for very active women, too much physical activity disrupts their normal hormonal levels, leading to premature osteoporosis. Extra calcium may help, but the hormonal problem needs to return to normal if bones are to be protected. These women should check with their doctors before taking calcium supplements.

Iron. There have been reports of a type of anemia, sports or runner's anemia, that often occurs in those involved in training and long-distance running. It is not clear whether or not this is a true anemia. If the person is mildly anemic and experiences a reduction in performance, he or she should try to increase the amounts of iron-rich foods in the diet. If the anemia is serious, a physician should be consulted for advice regarding iron supplements.

▶ Creatine Supplements

Creatine is a naturally occurring organic compound made by the kidneys, liver, and pancreas. Creatine can also be obtained from the ingestion of meat and fish. It also seems that oral supplementation with creatine may enhance muscular performance during high-intensity resistance exercise. Creatine has an integral role in energy metabolism.

There are two main types of creatine, free creatine and phosphocreatine. Phosphocreatine is stored in skeletal muscle and is used during anaerobic activity to produce energy. With creatine supplementation, phosphocreatine depletion is delayed, and performance may be enhanced through the maintenance of the normal metabolic pathways.

The positive physiological effects of creatine include allowing for increased intensity in a workout; prolonging maximal effort and improving exercise recovery time during maximal intensity activities; stimulating protein synthesis; decreasing total cholesterol; decreasing total triglycerides; and, increasing fat free mass. Side effects of creatine supplementation include weight gain and occasional muscle cramping. However, there are apparently no other known long-term side effects.

▶ A Final Word About Supplements

If you choose to take a supplement, do not use it as a food, use it with food. Read the label; avoid supplements that contain more than 150 percent of the recommended levels for each of the nutrients. Do not be misled into thinking that you need to take vitamins with the words organic or natural on the label. Your body does not care if the vitamin C came from a potato, a rose "hip," or a laboratory. If it is called vitamin C

(ascorbic acid), it has a specific chemical structure that cells use. Furthermore, all vitamins are organic, that is, their chemical structures include carbon atoms attached to hydrogen atoms. These terms are meant to impress average consumers and entice them into spending more for their supplements. Select the plain label or generic vitamin/mineral supplements, which are just as effective as the highly advertised brand name ones.

Keep in mind that taking nutrient supplements is no substitute for eating food and that many nutrients are toxic in large amounts. Unlike supplements, foods usually contain nutrients in the proper forms and proportions. Therefore, take the time to analyze the nutritional quality of your diet.

SUGAR

It was proposed that eating large quantities of simple carbohydrates, such as those supplied by candy bars, honey, or pure sugar, immediately before physical activity had a negative impact on performance. However, recent evidence indicates that for most healthy, active people, the effects of eating carbohydrates are more beneficial than negative. Some people find that large quantities of fructose lead to intestinal upset and diarrhea. (Sources of fructose include honey, fruit, and table sugar.) Therefore, it is wise to avoid fructose or, for that matter, any food that upsets your stomach, before engaging in physical activity.

CAFFEINE

Caffeine is a stimulant found in coffee, tea, chocolate, and carbonated beverages. Although small amounts of caffeine may benefit physical performance, too much can cause headaches, nervousness, irritability, and increased heart rate. Olympic officials have ruled that athletes' blood caffeine levels should not exceed the amount that results from drinking up to six cups of coffee.

ALCOHOL

Alcohol is a depressant drug that supplies 7 Calories per gram. However, alcoholic beverages offer little nutritional value other than energy. The depressant effects of alcohol include reductions in physical coordination, slowed reaction times, and decreased mental alertness. Alcohol also has a diuretic effect, resulting in body water losses. Therefore, it is not wise to replace water losses from physical activity by using alcoholic beverages, such as beer. Although controversial, it has been suggested that moderate alcohol consumption (the equivalent of having about two drinks a day) may be beneficial to heart health. But keep in mind that too much alcohol is harmful, destroying the liver and brain cells and potentially causing negative effects in your personal life.

HERBS

The use of herbs as natural alternatives to drugs and medicines has clearly become a trend among American consumers. Most herbs, as edible plants, are safe to take as foods, and they are claimed to have few side effects as natural medicines, although occasionally a mild allergy-type reaction may occur.

Relative to nutrition, herbs can offer the body nutrients that are reported to nourish the brain, glands, and hormones. Unlike vitamins that work best when taken with food, it is not necessary to take herbs with other foods.

Herbs in their whole form are not drugs. As medicine, herbs are essentially body balancers that work with the body functions, so that the body can heal and regulate itself. Herbal formulas can be general for overall strength and nutrient support, or specific to a particular ailment or condition.

Hundreds of herbs are widely available today at all quality levels. They are readily available at health food stores. However, unlike both food and medicine, there are no federal or governmental controls to regulate the sale and ensure the quality of the products being sold. Thus extreme caution must be exercised by the consumer of herbal products.

Table 8-4 lists the most popular and widely used herbal products sold in health food stores. Some additional potent and complex herbs, such as capsicum, lobelia, sassafras, mandrake tansy, canada snake root, wormwood, woodruff,

TABLE 8-4
Most widely used herbs and purposes for use

dong quai—to treat menstrual symptoms

echinacea—to promote wound healing and strengthen immune system

garlic—as an antibiotic, antibacterial, antifungal agent to prevent and relieve coronary-artery disease by reducing total blood cholesterol and triglyceride levels and raising HDL levels

ginkgo biloba—to improve blood circulation, especially in the brain

ginseng—to reduce impotence, weakness, lethargy, and fatigue

kava—to reduce anxiety, relax muscle tension, produce analgesic effects, act as a local anesthetic, provide antibacterial benefit

saw palmetto—to treat inflamed prostate; also used as a diuretic and as a sexual enhancement agent

St. John's wort—used as an antidepressant; also used to treat nervous disorders, depression, neuralgia, kidney problems, wounds, and burns

valerian—to treat insomnia, anxiety, stress

yohimbe—to increase libido and blood flow to sexual organs in the male

poke root, and rue may be useful in small amounts and as catalysts but should not be used alone.

PRE-EVENT MEAL

People engaging in competitive sports are often very concerned with the kinds of foods selected for pre-event meals. However, they should be more concerned with their eating patterns well before the day of the event. The purpose of the pre-event meal is to supply the competitor with enough energy and fluids for competition. The meal should be easily digestible as well. Most experts recommend a light meal (around 300 Calories) that is rich in carbohydrate about 2 to 4 hours before the event. A full stomach is uncomfortable, so avoid fatty or greasy meals that take longer to digest. Preloading on extra water is a good idea to keep well hydrated. Individuals vary in their ability to tolerate various foods, but it is advisable to avoid known gas-forming foods or any food the athlete believes contributes to intestinal upset.

SUMMARY

- The classes of nutrients are carbohydrates, fats, proteins, vitamins, minerals, and water.
- Carbohydrates, fats, and proteins provide the energy required for muscular work and also play a role in the function and maintenance of body tissues.
- Protein supplementation is not necessary.
- Vitamins are substances found in foods that have no caloric value but are necessary to regulate body processes.
- Antioxidants are nutrients that protect the body against various destructive agents.
- Minerals are also involved in regulation of bodily functions and are used to form important body structures.

- Water is the most essential nutrient and should be the drink of choice.
- A nutritious diet consists of eating a variety of foods in the amounts recommended on the Food Pyramid. If your diet meets those recommendations, you may not need nutrient supplements.
- Some people need extra iron and calcium.
- The Dietary Guidelines are designed to help you plan meals that are healthy.
- The pre-event meal should be (1) higher in carbohydrates, (2) easily digested, (3) eaten 2 to 4 hours before an event, and (4) acceptable to the athlete.
- Glycogen loading involves maximizing the stores of carbohydrate in muscle and liver before a competitive event.

SUGGESTED READINGS

Clarkson, P.M. 1998. Nutritional supplements for weight gain. *Sports science exchange* 11(1):1–8.

Coleman, E. 1997. *Eating for endurance.* Palo Alto, CA: Bull Publishing.

Foster, S. 1998. *101 medicinal herbs.* Loveland, CO: Interweave Press.

Katz, W.A., and C. Sherman. 1998. Osteoporosis: The role of exercise in optimal management. *Physician and sports medicine* 26(2):33–35, 39–42.

Larson-Duyff, R. 1998. *The American Dietetic Association's complete food and nutrition guide.* New York: John Wiley and Sons.

Lewis, R.D., and C.M. Modlesky. 1998. Nutrition, physical activity, and bone health in women. *International Journal of Sport Nutrition* 8(3):250–84.

McArdle, W., F. Katch, and V. Katch. 1999. Sports and exercise nutrition. Baltimore: Lippencott, Williams and Wilkins.

Merrick, M.A. 1999. Creatine supplements—Do they work? Are they safe? *Athletic therapy today* 4(1):59–60.

Papas, A., and J. Quillen. 1998. Antioxidant status: diet, nutrition, and health. Boca Raton, FL: CRC Press.

Peterson, D. 1998. Athletes and iron deficiency: Is it true anemia or "sport anemia"? *Physician and sports medicine* 26(2):24.

Shi, X., and C.V. Gisolfi. 1998. Fluid and carbohydrate replacement during intermittent exercise. *Sports medicine* 25(3):157–72.

U.S. Department of Agriculture and U.S. Department of Health and Human Services. 1995. *Nutrition and your health: dietary guidelines for Americans*, 4th edition. Washington, D.C.

Wardlaw, G.M., and P.M. Insel. 1996. *Perspectives in nutrition*, 3rd edition. St. Louis: Mosby.

Williams, C., and C.W. Nicholas. 1998. Nutrition needs for team sport. *Science sports exchange* 11(3):1–6.

Williams, M. 1998. *Nutrition for health, fitness, and sport*. St. Louis: WCB/McGraw-Hill.

Williams, M., R. Kreider, and D. Branch. 1999. *Creatine: The power supplement*. Champaign, IL: Human Kinetics.

SUGGESTED WEBSITES

American Dietetic Association
This site educates individuals about how making informed food choices can help them decrease the risk of heart disease, breast cancer, osteoporosis, diabetes, and obesity; it advocates nutrition research.
http://www.eatright.org/

ASNS Publications
The American Society for Nutritional Science has a nice page on all the major vitamins and minerals, their daily requirements, sources, and toxic dosages.
http://www.faseb.org/asns/publications.html

CNN's Health News: Diet & Fitness
This site presents NEWS and helpful tips on topics related to diet and nutrition.
http://cnn.com/HEALTH/diet.fitness/

Mayo Clinic Diet and Nutrition Resource Center
Mayo Clinic nutrition experts offer practical advice, creative encouragement, and healthy recipes to cut fat, cholesterol, sodium and calories and improve your diet. This site includes a Q&A section with Mayo dietitians.
http://www.mayohealth.org/mayo/common/htm/dietpage.htm

Food, nutrition, exercise fact index
This site presents 450 articles and 63 medical abstracts—and it's growing! It gives very good information on 'diets' and their health effects and lots of good stuff about fats in the diet. A lot is vitamin and mineral supplement related, but the good bits are succulent.
http://www.afpafitness.com/factindx.htm

International Food Information Council Foundation (IFIC)
The IFIC Foundation site is an industry-sponsored foundation that steers a middle road in the debates about nutrition. This useful and cautious perspective includes some very good information on diet.
http://ificinfo.health.org/

Nutrition: Arbor Nutrition Guide
This site presents the world's largest catalogue of nutrition resources on the internet: food science, clinical nutrition, ancient diets, functional foods, and much more—an absolutely outstanding links page.
http://www.arborcom.com/

The Diet Channel
Cutting edge diet information on weight loss, sports nutrition, heart disease, cancer, and preventative nutrition is presented. Request a professional diet analysis or browse through our 600 links to reliable nutrition information on the web.
http:///www.thedietchannel.com/

The Truth about Tufts Nutritional Navigator
Tufts University Nutrition Navigator is the LEAST reliable way to find sound nutrition information on the web, unless you want information provided by processed food manufacturers selling junk food. The "Nutrition Navigator" is sponsored by Kraft Foods, a division of tobacco giant Phillip Morris.
http://www.vegsource.org/tufts_navigator.htm

Lab Activity 8-1

Nutritional Knowledge Survey

Name _____   Section _____   Date _____

PURPOSE   To test your knowledge about nutrition.

PROCEDURE   Consider the following statements and answer true or false in the space to the left of the statement. Answers and an explanation are on the next page, as well as information on how to interpret your score.

_____   1.   Butter has more calories than the same amount of margarine.
_____   2.   Carbohydrates are fattening.
_____   3.   Vitamins provide energy for the body.
_____   4.   Excessive amounts of certain vitamins can cause health problems.
_____   5.   Cholesterol is dangerous and should be avoided.
_____   6.   If your serum cholesterol levels are low, you don't have to worry about heart disease.
_____   7.   Millions of Americans suffer from hypoglycemia.
_____   8.   Sugar offers no nutritional value.
_____   9.   Sugar causes hyperactive behavior and attention span disorders in children.
_____   10.   Protein supplements are unnecessary for body builders.
_____   11.   Zinc supplements will improve your sex drive.
_____   12.   Honey is more nutritious than sugar.
_____   13.   Meat is essential for a nutritious diet.
_____   14.   Fasting removes toxic wastes that build up in your body from dietary sources.
_____   15.   Organically grown foods are nutritionally superior to conventionally grown ones.

ANSWERS

1. False   Each has 100 Calories per tablespoon. The nature of the fat is different; butter contains more saturated fat than margarine. Butter also contains cholesterol; margarine does not. However, these differences do not affect the number of Calories per serving.

2. False   Carbohydrates contribute 4 Calories per gram, the same as a gram of protein. What is added to the carbohydrate-rich food to make it tasty often piles on the calories. These include fatty spreads, sauces, and gravies.

3. False   Vitamins cannot be broken apart and used for energy. However, many do participate in chemical reactions that extract energy from carbohydrate, protein, and fat.

4. True   Excesses of the fat-soluble vitamins are toxic, and vitamin B_6, niacin, and ascorbic acid can cause health problems if taken in large amounts.

5. False   Cholesterol has many important uses in the body. It is used to make steroid hormones and bile, which is needed for proper fat digestion.

203

6. False   Although a high serum cholesterol level is associated with the development of heart disease, low serum cholesterol levels are no guarantee of protection. If too much is in the LDL form, the risk of heart disease is higher than someone who has a higher total cholesterol level but more in the HDL form.

7. False   When you haven't eaten, blood sugar drops and you feel hungry. Eating raises blood sugar levels. Hypoglycemia (low blood sugar) associated with metabolic abnormalities is rare. Medical experts consider hypoglycemia a fad disease in most cases.

8. False   Refined white sugar is almost 100% carbohydrate. It is digested into very simple sugars that are used for energy by the body.

9. False   Despite many personal reports, sugar does not cause behavioral problems in children or adults. As the answer to #8 explains, it is a simple chemical that is broken down and used for energy. Often, sugar-laden foods also contain caffeine and related stimulants, which may explain the association of sugar with hyperactive behavior.

10. True   Protein supplements are unnecessary because most Americans obtain plenty of protein in their normal diet. Exercise builds muscles, not extra protein. More protein than needed is processed by the body and used for energy or converted to fat.

11. False   Severe zinc deficiency leads to poor growth and failure to develop sexually. However, this is extremely rare in the U.S.

12. False   Honey contains large amounts of the simple sugar, fructose. Fructose is one of the components of table sugar. The body converts fructose to glucose irrespective of the source. Considering how much honey is used and the tiny amounts of nutrients it contains, honey is just a more expensive choice as a sweetener.

13. False   The iron in red meat is more easily absorbed than that which is in plant foods. However, fish and chicken contribute iron, too. Thus, red meat is not essential as a food.

14. False   Fasting actually creates metabolic wastes that must be eliminated, since more body fat is burned for energy than under fed conditions. There are no health benefits derived from fasting.

15. False   Studies have demonstrated no nutritional superiority of foods grown with natural fertilizers and without pesticides.

Scoring: Give yourself one point for each correct response and total your points.
Total: _____

Score	Rating	Comments
13-15	Superior	You have sound knowledge of the subject.
9-12	Good	Good start; you may want to read reliable nutrition books to enhance your knowledge.
6-8	Fair	Read Chapter 8 again for more information.
<5	Poor	You have accumulated some misinformation about nutrition; try locating some reliable reading material and study Chapter 8.

Lab Activity 8-2

Assessing Your Nutritional Habits

Name	Section	Date

PURPOSE To identify the number that best describes the frequency of your food-related behaviors.

PROCEDURE Indicate the number that best describes the frequency of your food-related behaviors.

Point Values

0 = never   1 = rarely   2 = occasionally   3 = often   4 = always

_____ 1. Every day I eat a nutritious breakfast.

_____ 2. I try to include recommended servings from each of the food groups in my daily diet.

_____ 3. I eat food without salting it.

_____ 4. When I snack, I choose fruits, vegetables, low-fat yogurt, or cheese.

_____ 5. I try to include mostly fresh and less processed foods in my daily diet.

_____ 6. I avoid fatty foods and trim off the visible fat from meats.

_____ 7. I include foods containing fiber, such as fruits, vegetables, whole-grain products, and beans, in my diet.

_____ 8. I drink skim milk instead of whole or 2% milk.

_____ 9. I consume fish at least once a week.

_____ 10. I avoid foods that contain large amounts of honey and sugar.

_____ 11. For reliable nutrition information, I ask a qualified nutritionist instead of relying on the popular press.

_____ 12. I do not drink alcoholic beverages.

_____ 13. I keep my weight within acceptable limits.

_____ 14. I obtain my nutrients through foods rather than rely on nutritional supplements.

_____ Total Points

Modified from Allen R, Hyde R: Investigation in stress control, Minneapolis, 1981, Macmillan.

INTERPRETATION

Score

50-60	Excellent	Your food-related behaviors should contribute to your ability to maintain good health. Keep it up!
45-49	Good	If you make some minor improvements to your food-related behaviors, it should be easy to move into the excellent rating category.
39-44	Fair	Analyze the statements to determine which had the lowest scores. Then think about actions you can take to improve your nutritional behaviors.
<39	Poor	Your need to make major changes in your food related behaviors to improve your nutritional status and your overall health. Analyze your responses to the statements and read Chapter 8 carefully.

Lab Activity 8-3

7-Day Diet Analysis

Name   Section   Date

PURPOSE   To determine your eating habits during a 7-day period.

PROCEDURE   For a 7-day period, Monday through Sunday, assign yourself the points indicated when each dietary requirement is met. Record your points in the appropriate column for each day. Total your daily and weekly points. Negative points for junk food consumption should be subtracted from your daily and weekly totals.

Food	Points	Maximum Score	Daily Score						
			M	T	W	T	F	S	S
Milk and Milk Products		15							
One cup of milk or equivalent	5								
Second cup of milk or equivalent	5								
Third serving	5								
Vegetables		25							
Three to five servings deep green or yellow	5 each								
Fruits		20							
Two to four servings whole or juices	5 each								
Bread and Cereals		30							
Six or more servings of whole-grain or enriched cereals or breads	5 each								
Protein-Rich Foods		10							
One serving of egg, meat, fish, poultry, cheese, dried beans, or peas	5								
One or two additional servings of egg, meat, fish, poultry, or cheese	5								
Junk Foods (or Negative Point Value Foods)									
Sweet rolls	−5								
Fruit pies	−5								

Food	Points	Maximum Score	Daily Score						
			M	T	W	T	F	S	S
Potato chips, corn chips, or cheese twists	−5								
Candy	−5								
Nondiet sodas	−5								
Total		100							

Point Record

Weekly point total	_____
Negative point total	_____
Adjusted weekly point total	_____

Interpretation

600-700	Excellent dietary practices
450-599	Adequate dietary practices
300-449	Poor dietary practices
Below 300	Very poor dietary practices

Assessing Your Dietary Practices

1. On which day of the week was it most difficult for you to eat a balanced diet? Why?

   _____

   _____

   _____

   _____

2. Approximately what percentage of your total points was from foods purchased in a restaurant?

   _____

   _____

3. Approximately how much money did you spend on food during this 7-day period? _____

   _____

4. Was this a typical 7-day period in terms of the types of food eaten? If not, describe how a more typical 7-day period would appear. _____

   _____

   _____

5. Your instructor may prepare a dietary profile of the class against which you can evaluate your personal 7-day diet assessment.

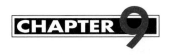

CONSUMER

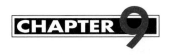
OBJECTIVES

After completing this chapter, you should be able to do the following:

- Describe what is necessary to be a careful consumer of health and fitness products.
- Discuss the various types of exercise equipment that may be used in a health and fitness program.
- Explain how clothing should be selected for exercising in hot or cold environments.
- Identify special considerations for selecting a health or fitness club.
- Discuss what you should look for in health and fitness books and magazines.

ARE YOU A WISE CONSUMER OF FITNESS PRODUCTS?

To say that the emphasis on health and fitness in American society has increased significantly during the past decade is a gross understatement. The consumer of health and fitness products has become the target of an unprecedented media advertising blitz. The

stereotypical image of the healthy and fit body appears in countless magazines at newsstands, on television, in newspaper ads and on the internet. Advertising includes everything from health foods and vitamins to exercise equipment, fitness centers, and weight-loss centers.

Further evidence of the magnitude of the interest in fitness and exercise is seen in the expenditures for sporting goods and exercise equipment. These expenditures have reached an all-time high. The sale of sporting goods has become big business. Sales of about $20 billion were recorded in the late 1990's. The athletic shoe business alone has become a $2 billion-a-year business. Recent sales figures show that close to $4 billion is being spent on athletic clothing annually. Sales of home exercise equipment have skyrocketed to about $3 billion today as individuals seek the convenience of being able to work out at home. Stationary bicycles, rowing machines, treadmills, stair climbers, and weight systems are the most popular items. Sales of diet and exercise books continue to rise. Corporate fitness programs and commercial health clubs have attracted a record number of members. The list goes on and on. There is little doubt that a significant amount of misinformation is being disseminated in an effort to merchandise a lucrative health and fitness industry.

Marketing experts are extremely sensitive to the vulnerability of American consumers when it comes to buying products that promise to make them look and feel better. How can the consumer separate fact from hype? It is essential for consumers to educate themselves by taking a critical look at a product or service to be purchased. For example, if you are going to buy a new automobile, perhaps you begin by looking at advertisements. You may wish to consult an independent consumer magazine to look at performance specifications, maintenance record, and so on. Then you go to the dealers to find who can offer the best price along with a reputation for good service. Chances are that you will buy your new car from that dealer.

The point is that most people shop around and are careful when making a choice about a large purchase such as an automobile. They take the time necessary to learn everything they can about the product. The wise consumer will take a similar approach when buying health and fitness products. You should realize that it is easy to be "taken in" by advertisements that project an image that seems to be in demand by consumers. Practicing **consumerism** means that wise consumers will take the time to analyze the entire product and to decide if the outlay of money is necessary to reap the benefits they desire.

> **consumerism:** taking the time to analyze the entire product and to decide if the outlay of money is necessary to reap the desired benefits

WHAT DO YOU NEED TO CONSIDER WHEN BUYING FITNESS EQUIPMENT?

The extent and variety of fitness and exercise equipment available to the consumer are at times mind-boggling. Prices of equipment can range from between $2 for a jump rope or Frisbee to $60,000 for certain computer-driven isokinetic devices. It is certainly not necessary to purchase expensive exercise equipment to see good results. You will achieve many of the same physiological benefits from using a $2 jump rope that result from running on a $10,000 treadmill. The following discussion identifies some of the more popular pieces of exercise equipment.

FREE WEIGHTS VS. WEIGHT MACHINES

Various types of exercise equipment can be used with progressive resistive exercise including free weights (barbells and dumbbells) or weight machines (such as Universal, Nautilus, Cybex, Eagle, DP, Soloflex, and Body Master) Figure 9-1. Dumbbells and barbells require the use of iron plates of varying weights that can be easily changed by adding or subtracting equal amounts of weight to both sides of the bar. Most of the weight machines have a stack of weights that are lifted through a series of levers or pulleys. The stack of weights slides up and down on a pair of bars that restrict the movement to only one plane. Weight can be increased or decreased simply by changing the position of a weight key.

There are advantages and disadvantages to both the free weights and weight machines. The machines are relatively safe to use in comparison with free weights. For example, if you are doing a bench press with free weights, it is essential to have someone "spot" you (help you lift the weights back onto the support racks if you don't have enough strength to complete the lift); otherwise you may end up dropping the weight on your chest. With the weight machines you can easily and safely drop the

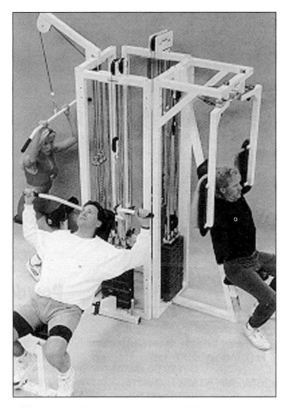

Figure 9-1. Multistation exercise machines.

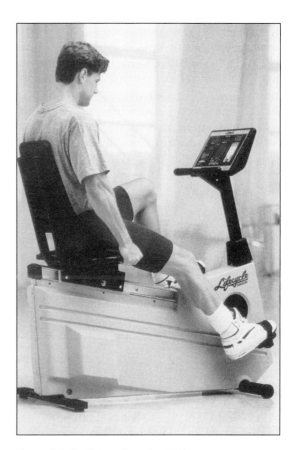

Figure 9-2. Stationary Exercise Bike.

weight without fear of injury. It is also a simple process to increase or decrease the weight by moving a single weight key with the weight machines, although changes can generally be made only in increments of 10 or 15 pounds. With free weights, iron plates must be added or removed from each side of the barbell.

Costs of purchasing free weights are substantially lower than the weight machines. Regardless of which type of equipment is used, the same principles of isotonic training may be applied.

STATIONARY EXERCISE BIKES

Many different exercise bikes are available to the consumer (Figure 9-2). Bicycle companies such as Schwinn or Ross, as well as Tun-

turi and Vitamaster, which specifically manufacture exercise equipment, are well-known name brands. Exercise bikes priced below $150 tend to be somewhat unstable. Most good models range between $150 and $700. Computerized exercise bikes used in health clubs may cost between $1500 and $3500.

There are essentially two types of exercise bikes. When you pedal a "single-action" model, resistance is created from a device such as a flywheel. With the flywheel you can change the resistance with a twist of a knob. The "dual-action" models also let you pump the handlebars back with your arms. Most of these bikes use a fan to create resistance, which can be increased by pumping the arms and legs faster. The dual-action models allow you to rest your feet on coaster pedals and exercise only your arms. Obviously, those models that work both the upper and lower extremities require a higher energy expenditure. Most models have you sitting on a bicycle seat in a standard position. Some design variations allow you to sit in a recumbent position. This position exercises the hamstring muscles to a greater degree and is useful for individuals who have back problems or poor balance.

Training stands hook a resistance device to your regular bicycle, allowing you to convert it to a stationary bike at relatively low cost. Features that are important to look for include a comfortable padded seat and some type of monitor that tells you how far you have pedaled or the time. Models with pedal straps will work your legs on the upstroke in addition to the downstroke.

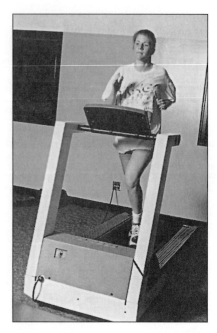

Figure 9-3. Treadmill.

TREADMILLS

An exercise treadmill is a belt stretched between two rollers (Figure 9-3). The belt may be driven manually in the least expensive models or by a motor in more expensive ones. Sears, Tunturi, Vitamaster, Voit, DP, Precor, and Proform are among the more common brands of treadmills manufactured for home use. Costs range from $400 to $1000. More expensive machines have a bigger motor, a wider belt, and a faster top speed (up to about 5 mph). It is difficult to find a good motor-driven treadmill for under $500. Treadmills subjected to high use in health clubs cost between $1000 and $12,000. Most of the more expensive motor-driven treadmills allow you to adjust both the speed of the belt and the incline angle to alter intensity.

Machine motors vary in both type and size. The type of motor can be either AC or DC. AC motors run at full speed, all the time relying on a transmission-like pulley system to regu-

late speed. This means most models start up at full speed and can be somewhat dangerous when getting on. Treadmill motors that are DC can be run at different speeds, thus start-up is not much of a problem. All models come with some type of speed control. Motor size varies from ½ horsepower to more than 1 horsepower. Bigger motors can handle heavier loads and higher speeds. A running gait requires that the treadmill is able to go at least 5 mph.

STAIR CLIMBERS

Stair climbers have become one of the more popular types of exercise machines (Figure 9-4). They are essentially a set of levers attached to some resistance device. Your legs pump the levers as if you are climbing stairs. Models vary in how they apply resistance, using either a flywheel, a hydraulic piston, a drive train, or

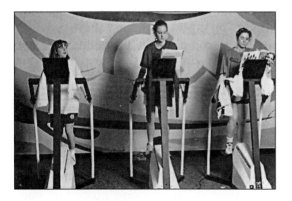

Figure 9-4. Stair Climbers.

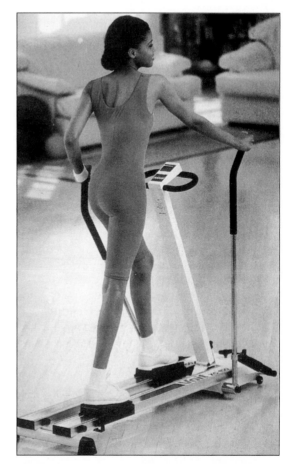

Figure 9-5. Ski Machine.

wind resistance. In some models, the stairs are linked. As one goes down, the other automatically goes up. Dual-action models allow you to work both the arms and the legs simultaneously. The more expensive models have a series of stairs that rotate as if you were climbing the wrong direction on an escalator. Monitors on many models display information such as time, steps per minute, and energy expenditure. Some may be programmed to vary both the speed and the amount of resistance during the course of a workout. Sears, Tunturi, DP, and Precor are brand names of the typical home models. Stairmaster makes most of the more expensive units for commercial use. Stair-climbing machines cost between $200 and $3000. Most of the home models are around $500. Programmable units cost a minimum of $800.

SKI MACHINES

A ski machine offers many of the aerobic benefits of cross-country skiing without having to worry about the snow. These machines have two flat boards, one for each foot, that slide back and forth in a groove on rollers. The arms are also involved, using either telescoping poles or a rope and pulley instead of the ski

poles. The design of these machines allows you to simultaneously exercise both the upper and lower extremities. (Figure 9-5)

Ski machines have either dependent or independent leg motion. With a dependent machine, the leg boards are connected. As one goes forward, the other goes backward. On independent machines, the leg boards slide independently, making them somewhat more difficult to master but also affording you a better workout. Resistance on the ski machine comes from either an electromagnetic flywheel or from a belt wrapped around a flywheel that provides friction. Some models do not have variable resistance. More expensive models may also incline, increasing the stress on the quadriceps muscles in the front of the thigh. Most machines have some type of monitor that can show heart rate, resistance, speed, calories expended, etc. Most of these machines can be folded and require little space for storage.

There are several manufacturers of ski machines, including NordicTrack, Precor, Proform, DP, Vitamaster, and Tunturi. Ski machines range in price from $300 to as high as $2000 for health club models.

ELLIPTICAL EXERCISERS

Elliptical machines provide a new mode of cardiovascular exercise that makes use of a no-impact, elliptical-shaped stride. (Figure 9-6) When using the machine, you stand upright while striding in a forward or reverse motion and holding handrails. An electronically adjustable ramp allows you to raise or lower ramp incline, adjust resistance, and use both forward and reverse motion. These options let exercisers simulate no-impact versions of their favorite exercise activities, such as walking, running, cycling, cross-country skiing, and stairclimbing. Lower ramp levels can simulate cross-country skiing or the walking or running options of a treadmill. Higher ramp levels can produce a safe, comfortable cycling or stair-climbing motion. Elliptical machines are manufactured by Vision Fitness, Life Fitness, Star Trac, Precor, NordicTrack, ICON Health and Fitness, Inc., Guthy-Renker, and Quantum Television. They range in price from $200 for home models to $3500 for more sophisticated commercial models.

ROWING MACHINES

Rowing machines are designed to mimic the action of rowing a boat or sculling. Most brands have some type of movable handles, which are similar to oars, and a sliding seat. Exercise involves pressing against stationary footplates with the legs while sliding backward on the seat and simultaneously pulling on the handles to create a rowing motion. Rowing machines are similar to stair climbers in terms of their resistance mechanisms, which may include a flywheel, a hydraulic piston, or wind resistance. (Figure 9-7)

Sears, DP, and Tunturi are the most common home models of rowing machines. Costs range between $200 and $800 for home models. Rowing machines for health clubs range between $1000 and $3000.

PASSIVE EXERCISE DEVICES AND TECHNIQUES

Unfortunately, many consumers of health and fitness products are lured into thinking that there is some easy way to achieve physical

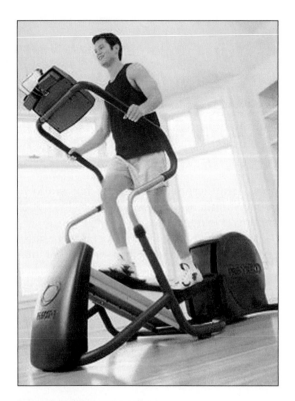

Figure 9-6. Elliptical Exerciser.

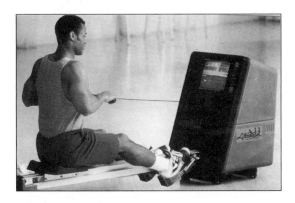

Figure 9-7. Rowing Machine.

fitness with little or no physical effort. The marketing of a variety of devices such as rubberized suits that let you sit around and sweat off weight, electrical devices that make muscles contract, and mechanical devices that shake, vibrate, or roll fat off can seem to be very appealing shortcuts to getting fit. There are, however, no shortcuts.

▶ Passive Motion Machines

These machines have only been introduced into the health and fitness market in recent years. Passive motion machines are designed to exercise individual body parts by moving them for you with no effort on your part. You are simply required to lie or sit still while the machine does all the work. For example, one machine is designed to flex and extend your trunk and lower back, while another may flex and extend your hip and your knee. Manufacturers claim that these machines will help improve muscular endurance since a particular body part is moving repeatedly, improve flexibility by using slow continuous movement, and burn off fat while reducing cellulite in the exercised areas. All of these claims are totally ludicrous. The only potential benefit offered to healthy individuals by these machines may be relaxation. However, similar passive exercise devices, referred to as constant passive motion (CPM) machines, are widely and effectively used in rehabilitation

for postsurgical patients to minimize development of scar tissue.

▶ Motor-Driven Exercise Bikes

Stationary exercise bikes or rowing machines that are motor driven may have some value in increasing circulation, particularly around joints. However, they are totally ineffective in elevating heart rate and thus stressing the cardiovascular system.

▶ Vibrating Belts and Rolling Machines

Vibrating belts placed around the trunk or the extremities that shake fat and muscle tissue or rolling machines that use movable wooden rollers to compress fat and muscle tissue in a rolling fashion have been promoted to break up fat tissue, thus making it easier to burn off. They also claim to increase muscle tone and improve posture. The truth is that they do not "break up" fat, but they may damage connective tissue around joints and within a muscle. The rollers may also cause bruising of the skin and fat from repeated compression. Use of these machines should definitely be avoided by people with low back pain and by pregnant women.

▶ Massage

Massage can be an extremely effective therapeutic technique. It is most typically used for stimulating circulation, for inducing relaxation, and for loosening up muscles. However, as in the case of rolling machines, it will not selectively rub fat away from a specific spot.

▶ Rubberized Inflatable Suits

Rubberized inflatable suits are also called sauna shorts or sauna sleeves. Promoters claim that the pressure created by the garment will help to break down fat tissue by squeezing it and that the rubber garment will help you "sweat off" fat. Once again these claims are ridiculous. Fat cannot be "squeezed off." Furthermore, sweating does not burn off a significant amount of fat.

Wearing rubberized suits may help you lose body weight fairly quickly, but the weight loss represents the water weight of perspiration rather than loss of fat tissue. Elevation of body core temperature by wearing rubberized suits may predispose an individual to various forms of heat stress.

▶ Electrical Stimulating Devices

In general, electrical stimulating devices use low-amperage electrical current of sufficient intensity to cause involuntary muscle contraction. The technique involves connecting the electrodes to specific areas of the body and generating a weak electrical current to contract the muscles. (Promoters claim that the muscle contraction requires energy, thus calories will be used from stored fat to supply energy.) Once again, there is no credibility to the value of this technique for weight loss or fitness.

Electrical stimulating currents are routinely used by qualified rehabilitation specialists for treating many different musculoskeletal and neurological problems. When appropriate treatment limits are selected, electrical currents can be effectively used for pain control and muscle reeducation after injury, as well as to decrease muscle spasm and to reduce muscle atrophy. The indiscriminant use of electrical currents by untrained individuals is strongly discouraged and in many states is against the law.

SPAS, STEAM BATHS, SAUNAS

In the health and fitness industry, the use of spas (hot tubs), steam baths, and saunas is widespread. Most health and fitness clubs offer the use of at least one form of these to their members. Hot tubs and whirlpool baths are increasingly being installed in private homes. Of all their therapeutic benefits, perhaps none is more important than the relaxation factor. Relaxation seems to be the primary reason why so many people are interested in using them. However, claims that sitting in either water or air at high temperatures will cause fat loss are again totally unfounded. Whatever weight is lost is due to a loss of water. Water loss should be immediately replaced through proper rehydration from beverages.

Saunas are likely to produce the greatest amount of body water loss because the air is hot and extremely dry. Thus significant amounts of water will be lost through the rapid evaporation of sweat. Temperatures in a sauna should not be higher than 180° F. You should limit yourself to no more than 15 minutes in the sauna at that temperature.

Steam baths, which should be no higher than 120° F., have a much lower temperature than saunas. However, the humidity in a steam bath is 100 percent. Thus individuals will appear to be sweating more heavily in a steam bath. Under humid conditions, sweat cannot evaporate to dissipate body heat, and body temperature rises rapidly. It is necessary to limit time in a steam bath to no longer than 10 minutes.

Spas or hot tubs involve full-body immersion in a whirlpool at a temperature that should be no higher than 100° F. for no longer than 10 minutes.

Certain precautions should be taken when using any of these units:

1. If you have a heart condition or skin infection or are pregnant, you should avoid their use.
2. Do not use any of these without cooling down after exercise.
3. Wash off all oils or lotions before use.
4. Never drink alcohol before use.
5. If you feel faint for any reason, get out immediately.
6. Always have someone with you when using any of these.

TANNING BEDS

For years, having a deep, golden-brown tan was associated with being fit and healthy. During the past decade, artificial tanning beds have become very popular in the health and fitness club industry. These tanning salons, beds, and booths usually consist of an array of long tubes that produce ultraviolet light. The lights are positioned in some type of frame that allows for exposure of the entire body.

We now know beyond any doubt that prolonged or continuous exposure to ultraviolet light rays predisposes an individual to the development of skin cancer. Manufacturers of artificial tanning devices claim the ultraviolet light produced by tanning devices is safe. The Food and Drug Administration (FDA) has warned the public that sunlamps are dangerous. Besides the risk of skin cancer, long-term exposure to a form of ultraviolet light (UVA) causes premature aging of the skin with wrinkling and sagging. Production of UVA tanning beds is largely unregulated. Furthermore, there is generally no standard of training for people who operate these machines. Their knowledge of the tanning process and the danger of exposure to ultraviolet radiation may be limited at best. Therefore, extreme caution should be exercised whenever you are exposed to ultraviolet radiation, either from sunlight or from artificial sources.

HOW SHOULD YOU CHOOSE APPROPRIATE CLOTHING AND SHOES FOR EXERCISE?

CLOTHING FOR EXERCISING IN HOT, HUMID WEATHER

Guidelines for selecting clothing for exercising in hot, humid weather are relatively simple and straightforward. Clothing chosen should allow for maximal dissipation of body heat while minimizing the heat gained from the environment. By far the most effective means of heat loss involves the process of evaporation. If sweat remains on the skin, it will not produce heat loss. Thus the material worn must be lightweight and dry very quickly by permitting sweat to evaporate. The body area that has the greatest number of sweat glands is the upper back and shoulders. Consequently a tank top will allow for greatest exposure for evaporation. Radiation of heat from the sun or other hot surfaces such as pavement will cause the body to gain heat. Clothing should be a light color to reflect as much radiant heat energy as possible.

It may also be advisable to wear a hat, which will help block some of the radiant heat energy from the sun. However, it is critical that the hat be made of some type of mesh fabric to allow heat to be dissipated from the head. About 40 percent of the heat lost from the body is from the head.

CLOTHING FOR EXERCISING IN COLD WEATHER

In situations where the weather is cold, the goal of wearing clothing is to create a "semitropical microclimate" for the body and to prevent chilling. The clothing should not restrict movement and should be as lightweight as possible. The material should permit free passage of sweat and body heat. Otherwise, sweat would accumulate on the skin or in the clothing and provide a chilling effect when activity ceases. This dampness, in combination with cold and wind, plays a critical role in the development of hypothermia. Individuals should routinely dress in thin layers of clothing that can be easily added or removed when the temperature increases or decreases. Constant adjustment of these layers will reduce sweating and the likelihood that clothing will become damp or wet.

Before exercise, during activity breaks, and after exercise, a warm-up suit or sweat clothes should be worn to prevent chilling. Activity in cold, wet, or windy weather poses some problem because such weather reduces the insulating value of the clothing. Consequently, the individual may be unable to achieve a level of metabolic heat production sufficient to keep pace with body heat loss. In cold weather, a hat should be worn to minimize excessive heat loss from the head.

SHOE SELECTION

The athletic and fitness shoe manufacturing industry has become extremely sophisticated and offers a number of options when it comes to purchasing shoes for different activities. Terms like forefoot varus support or rearfoot valgus wedge are confusing to a person who simply wants to buy a pair of good running, aerobic, or court shoes. Most people are simply interested in finding a long-lasting shoe that will provide good support and comfort. Figure 9-8 shows the major parts of a shoe. For the average individual, the following guidelines can help you select the most appropriate shoe to fit your needs.

▶ **Toe Box**

There should be plenty of room for your toes in the fitness shoe. Most experts recommend a ½- to ¾-inch distance between toes and the front of the shoe. A few fitness shoes are made in varying widths. If you have a very wide or narrow foot, most shoe salespersons can recommend a specific shoe for your foot. The best way to make sure there is adequate room in the toe box is to have your foot measured and then try on the shoe.

▶ **Sole**

The sole should possess two qualities. First, it must provide a shock-absorptive function; second, it must be durable. Most shoes have three layers on the sole: a thick spongy layer, which absorbs the force of the

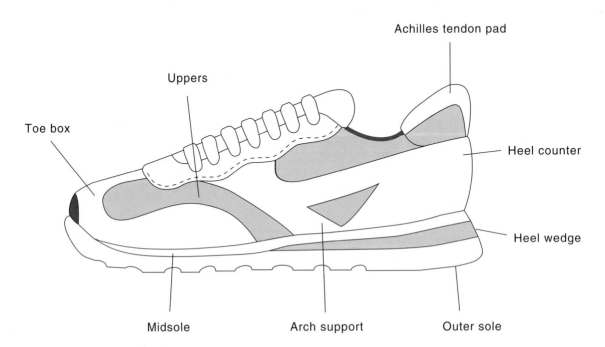

Figure 9-8. Parts of a Well-Designed Shoe.

foot strike under the heel; a midsole, which cushions the midfoot and toes; and a hard rubber layer, which comes in contact with the ground. The average runner's feet strike the ground between 1500 and 1700 times per mile. Thus it is essential that the force of the heel strike be absorbed by the spongy layer to prevent overuse-type injuries from occurring in the ankles and knees. "Heel wedges" are sometimes inserted on either the inside or the outside surface of the sole underneath the heel counter to accommodate and correct for various structural deformities of the foot that may alter normal biomechanics of the running gait. A flared heel may be appropriate for running shoes but is not recommended in aerobic or court shoes. The sole must provide good traction and must be made of a tough material that is resistant to wear. Most of the better-known brands of shoes tend to have well-designed, long-lasting soles.

▶ Heel Counters

The heel counter is the portion of the shoe that prevents the foot from rolling from side to side at heel strike. The heel counter should be firm but well fitted to minimize movement of the heel up and down or side to side. A good heel counter may prevent ankle sprains and painful blisters.

▶ Shoe Uppers

The upper part of the shoe is made of some combination of nylon and leather. The uppers should be lightweight, capable of quick drying, and well ventilated. The uppers should have some type of extra support in the saddle area, and there should also be some extra padding in the area of the Achilles tendon just above the heel counter.

▶ Arch Support

The arch support should be made of some durable yet soft supportive material and should smoothly join with the insole. The support should not have any rough seams or ridges inside the shoe, which may cause blisters.

▶ Price

Unfortunately, for many people price is the primary consideration in buying running shoes. Both running shoes and court shoes range between $40 and $160 per pair. Aerobic shoes tend to be less expensive, in the $30 to $80 range. When buying fitness shoes, remember that in many fitness activities, shoes are important for performance and prevention of injury. Thus it is worth a little extra investment to buy a quality pair of shoes.

WHAT DO YOU LOOK FOR WHEN SHOPPING FOR A HEALTH CLUB?

It's easy to get caught up in a desire to join a health club. You walk in the front door and may immediately be greeted by an attractive, energetic receptionist who quickly introduces you to an attractive, energetic "fitness consultant," which is the term frequently used in fitness centers to label the salesperson. You may be escorted into a large exercise room with plush carpeting on the floor, mirrors on every wall, chrome-plated exercise equipment, and high-energy music coming from the stereo system. Your eyes tend to ignore the overweight gentleman or the frail lady working on machines in the corner and go straight to the Adonis or Aphrodite working out in the center of the room. It is easy to think, "Hey, this place is beautiful, and if it can make me feel comfortable and look like that at the same time, I want to join—NOW." Unfortunately, in this situation the consumer has already decided to purchase the hype without investigating the facts.

Certainly it is possible to find health clubs that offer good quality instruction and guidance (Figure 9-9) in addition to an aesthetically pleasing environment in which to work out.

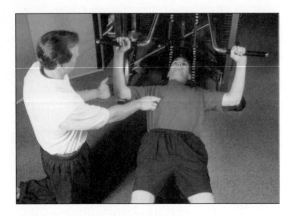

Figure 9-9. Health Club Instruction.
Well-qualified instructors are an important factor to consider when selecting a health club.

The guidelines described here are important for those individuals who are considering joining a health or fitness club.

TYPES OF FACILITIES

Familiarize yourself with the many different types of facilities available, including spas, gyms, YMCA/YWCAs, and facilities at universities or high schools. Many times local schools or colleges will offer excellent facilities for public use at little or no cost. You can most often find a listing of facilities in the telephone book. It is important to contact all the available sources to get the most detailed information.

LOCATION OF FACILITY

Certainly the location of the facility is an important factor in deciding whether to join.
- Is it close or easily accessible to your home or apartment?
- Will you be stopping to exercise on your way to or from work or school?
- What is the traffic like near the facility at the times of day you are most likely to go?

EQUIPMENT AVAILABLE

Check the type of equipment available.
- Do they have weight equipment (free weights, exercise machines)?
- Is there a pool, whirlpool, sauna, steam room, running track, racquetball court, and aerobic exercise room?
- Is there sufficient available locker space, with showers and changing areas?
- Do they have the type of equipment necessary for your fitness program?

PROGRAMS OFFERED

Check the type and quality of programs offered, such as individualized and supervised weight training, aerobic exercise classes, spinning classes, kick boxing classes, jogging classes, yoga, weight control programs, and cardiac rehabilitation programs. Do any of these cost extra?

HOURS OF OPERATION

- What are the hours of operation of the facility?
- Are they open 7 days per week?
- Is it a co-ed facility?
- Can both males and females work out there 7 days a week?
- What are the most crowded times?

QUALIFICATIONS OF PERSONNEL

You must be careful to consider the qualifications of the instructors. Many health and fitness clubs employ attractive, fit individuals whose primary function is to sell memberships to the club. Ask the salesperson the following questions:
- What is the background of the personnel who will be supervising your program?

- Do they have a background in physical education, exercise physiology, athletic training, or physical therapy?
- Are they certified by the American College of Sports Medicine as Exercise Leaders, Health/Fitness Instructors, or Exercise Specialists?
- Are they certified as aerobics instructors by the Aerobics and Fitness Association of America (AFAA), American Council on Exercise (ACE), Cooper Institute for Aerobics Research, or Exercise Safety Association (ESA)?
- Are they certified as personal trainers by the Aerobics and Fitness Association of America (AFAA), American Council on Exercise (ACE), Cooper Institute for Aerobics Research, Exercise Safety Association (ESA), International Fitness Institute, or the National Strength and Conditioning Association (NSCA)?

TYPES OF MEMBERSHIP CONTRACTS

Health and fitness clubs tend to offer a wide range of membership contract options, ranging from pay-by-the-visit to lifetime memberships. It is a good idea to avoid long-term contracts, especially in the beginning. Health clubs sell a lot of memberships because people tend to get caught up by the aesthetics of the facility and are manipulated by some very good salespeople. The firm commitment to consistently use the facility three to four times per week that is made in the sales office tends to become less important for most people over time. If all the people who bought memberships in a club were to show up at one time, it is likely that you would not be able to get in the door. If you do decide to join, check on various payment options that best suit your budget. Also check on additional fees that you may have to pay for extras, such as reserving racquetball courts or enrolling in aerobics classes.

TRIAL PERIODS

Before signing a contract, it is a good idea to spend several sessions working out at the club, talking with the instructors and with other club members. Current members can answer specific questions about the quality of the facility as well as identify its deficiencies. If there is some objection to doing this on the part of the management, then you should exercise extreme caution about signing a contract.

BE KNOWLEDGEABLE ABOUT FITNESS

It is probably wise to avoid the clubs or organizations that advertise programs, classes, equipment, or techniques that claim to result in "overnight" strength gains, weight loss, or improvements in appearance. You must realize that reaching your fitness goals requires selecting an activity you enjoy. The activity should not overload the body but progress within your individual limitations. Furthermore, by being consistent in your training program, you will accomplish your goals safely by paying attention to the basic principles outlined within this text.

WHAT TO LOOK FOR IN FITNESS MAGAZINES, BOOKS, AND VIDEOS

As with the various types of exercise equipment, consumer demand for literature and other media dealing with health and fitness issues makes publication in this area an extremely lucrative enterprise.

It is difficult, if not totally impossible, to pick up a popular magazine that does not contain at least one article about health and fitness. It is reasonable to assume that the majority of people in the United States obtain most of their health and fitness information while standing in line at the grocery store.

This is certainly not to say that grocery store sources of health and fitness information are unreliable, but there is a tremendous amount of misinformation relative to health and fitness issues routinely spread through the popular media. Often, the articles in magazines are written by individuals with little or no health or fitness expertise who may interview fitness experts. Occasionally, you will find experts writing the articles. The same is true for so-called experts who appear on television or radio talk shows. These people have charming personalities but often lack reliable credentials.

A trip to the local bookstore, public library, or internet booksellers, to locate books dealing with health, wellness, fitness, exercise, sports, diet, and nutrition can be overwhelming. Many excellent, accurate books are available. These books are written by health and fitness experts. Unfortunately, the majority of the best-selling books, and certainly the best-marketed ones, are written by celebrities who look fit and attractive. Some of these books contain excellent information. Others include some facts along with misinformation and border on being dangerous.

For anyone who has ventured into a video store, it is easy to see that celebrities also like to star or be featured in exercise videos. Again the available choices can be overwhelming. Many consumers choose to purchase exercise videos as an alternative to joining a health club. The convenience of having someone lead you through a workout at home certainly appeals to some people who have neither the time nor the motivation to leave home to participate in an exercise program. As is the case with books and magazines, the consumer must make informed choices when it comes to purchasing exercise videos. Remember, they don't always do exactly what the infomercials tell you they can do.

How do you know whether information presented in the popular media is reliable?

Simply by being an informed consumer. The information presented in this text is accurate and up-to-date. The knowledge you have obtained from this text should make you a more informed consumer.

THE BOTTOM LINE FOR THE CONSUMER

Regardless of the type of exercise equipment, the aesthetics of a health club, or the claims of nutritional products, the bottom line is that the responsibility for getting fit and healthy ultimately lies with you. Remember, a commitment to a fitness program is first and foremost a commitment to yourself. Being cautious, asking a number of questions, and being well informed will help you make the best choice possible. Basing your physical activity program on the facts rather than on marketing techniques is the way to get fit. If you find that joining a health club or buying expensive exercise equipment in some way motivates you to adhere to your program, then by all means, do so. But never neglect the basic principles.

SUMMARY

- Be a conscientious and well-informed consumer when selecting products related to health and fitness.
- Don't be afraid to ask questions and fully investigate a health and fitness club before joining.
- There is an incredible amount and diversity of exercise equipment available to the consumer.
- Deciding what type of equipment is best for you to use or purchase should be based primarily on individual interests and the goals of your physical activity program.
- Remember, there is no shortcut to fitness. Passive exercise devices are essentially use-

less when it comes to improvement in fitness levels.

- Spas, saunas, and steam baths should be used for relaxation and are not effective in reducing percentage body fat.
- The use of tanning beds and tanning booths is generally not recommended.
- Select appropriate clothing for exercising in either hot or cold environments to prevent heat stress or hypothermia.
- Selecting and purchasing a quality fitness shoe can reduce the likelihood of injury.
- Fitness books, magazine articles, and videos should be critically analyzed by the informed and educated consumer of health and fitness products.

SUGGESTED READINGS

Burke, E. 1996. *Complete Home Fitness Handbook*. Champaign, IL: Human Kinetics.

Cardio commitments: a serious workout area offers a variety of cardiovascular/aerobic equipment, including the latest in cross-training machines, treadmills, steppers, stationary cycles, rowers, testing equipment and climbing walls. 1998. *Athletic business* 22(3):69–75.

Consumer Reports. 1999. *Consumer Reports 1999 Buying Guide*. New York: Consumer Reports.

Grantham, W., R. Patten, and T. York. 1998. *Health fitness management: A comprehensive resource for managing and operating programs and facilities*. Champaign, IL: Human Kinetics.

Hamilton, A. 1998. 16 of the best: Home gym equipment review. *Ultrafit* 8(8):29–52.

Herbert, D.L. 1998. New standards for health and fitness facilities from the American Heart Association (AHA) and the American College of Sports Medicine (ACSM). *Exercise standards and malpractice reporter* 12(3):46–47.

Kreighbaum, E., and M.A. Smith (eds.). 1996. *Sports and fitness equipment design*. Champaign, IL: Human Kinetics.

Kuntzleman, C.T., and R. Wilkerson. 1997. A primer to recommending home aerobic equipment. *American College of Sports Medicine Health and Fitness Journal* 1(6):24(32).

Napolitano, F. 1999. The American College of Sports Medicine health/fitness facility standards, what they mean and how to apply them to your facility: Part 1. *American College of Sports Medicine Health and Fitness Journal*. 3(1):39–39.

O'Brien, T.S. 1997. *The personal trainer's handbook*. Champaign, IL: Human Kinetics.

Peterson, J. 1997. *American College of Sports Medicine health/fitness facility standards and guidelines*. Champaign, IL: Human Kinetics.

Stamford, B. 1997. Choosing and using exercise equipment. *Physician and sports medicine* 25(1):107–8.

Wischnia, B., and P. Carrozza. 1999. The Runner's World 1999 shoe buyer's guide. *Runner's World* 34(3):49–79.

SUGGESTED WEBSITES

Exercise Equipment At Beyond Moseying
Exercise equipment with club quality! This site features exercise equipment, fitness machines, athletic equipment, gym apparatus, treadmills, ellipticals, versaclimbers, homegyms, bikes, steppers and body building equipment.
http://www.fitnessstore.net/

Fitness Brokers
This site specializes in genuine Nautilus exercise equipment.
http://www.fitnessbrokers.com

Fitness Factory Outlet
This is America's best source for aerobic, strength training, and fitness equipment. It includes fitness tips, exercise charts, and the lowest prices on the highest quality health and fitness products available.
http://www.fitnessfactory.com/

Healthrider
Find great treadmill deals, check your fitness age, buy equipment like treadmills, and check the weekly fitness special. Enjoy relaxation therapy, massage chairs, hydrotherapy and spas.
http://www.healthrider.com/

Nellies Exercise Fitness Equipment
This site presents a complete line of treadmills, home gyms, bikes, pulse & heart monitors. We carry free weights and strength training and more.
http://www.nellies.com/

NordicTrack Exercise Equipment Site
This site features the leading manufacturer of high-quality treadmill, cycle, skier, strength training, and other fitness equipment products. Purchase conveniently online.
http://www.nordictrack.com

Precor USA
This is the industry leader in high quality fitness equipment.
http://www.precor.com/

4Sneakers
This is a shopping directory of sneakers and athletic shoes.
http://www.4sneakers.com/

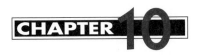

CHAPTER 10

PRACTING SAFE
FITNESS

OBJECTIVES

After completing this chapter, you should be able to do the following:

- Realize that participation in physical activity sometimes creates situations in which injuries may occur.
- Discuss the principles and guidelines of injury prevention.
- Describe fractures, contusions, ligament sprains, muscle strains, muscle soreness, tendinitis, and bursitis.
- Identify the causes of low back pain and describe how such pain can best be avoided.
- Describe the RICE approach to the initial treatment of injuries.
- Identify exercises that may be dangerous or contraindicated.
- Discuss the precautions that should be exercised when working out in either a hot or a cold environment.

HOW CAN YOU PREVENT INJURIES?

Certainly, you don't participate in physical activities with the idea that you are going to be injured. Ironically, the nature of par-

Key Terms

low back pain
RICE
heat-related illness
hypothermia

ticipation in any type of physical activity increases the possibility that injury will occur. Fitness programs will hopefully make you more fit and should ultimately reduce the possibility of injury. The overload demands placed on the body during exercise enable it to handle added stresses and strains that occur during physical activity. Thus the first step in practicing "safe fitness" and in preventing injuries associated with physical activity involves designing a well-planned fitness program based on the principles of overload, progression, consistency, individuality, and safety.

If you are involved in some physical activity and realize that a specific part of your body is causing discomfort or pain that affects your performance, it is strongly recommended that this problem be evaluated immediately. Injuries should be evaluated by persons experienced in dealing with sport-related injuries, such as physicians, physical therapists, or athletic trainers. The sooner an injury is diagnosed and treatment begun, the less chance there is that continued activity will make the problem worse. The popular quote "no pain, no gain" holds no credibility with regard to an activity program.

Pain indicates that something is wrong. You should stop activity immediately and determine what is producing the pain. There is a great difference between overloading the system while you are working hard during exercise and pushing yourself to exercise when you are hurt. When you are dealing with injuries, common sense is of prime importance. Injuries are to a large extent preventable, and paying attention to some simple guidelines can make exercise safer and more enjoyable.

Perhaps the biggest mistake that people make when beginning a physical activity program is starting at a level that is too advanced and then trying to progress too quickly. If you are physically inactive, you must begin at a

Safe Tip

Injury Prevention

- Always warm up properly before engaging in any activity.
- Do not neglect the cool-down period after exercise.
- Make certain that muscles are stretched sufficiently. Use full range-of-motion static stretching during an active warm-up period and vigorous stretching during the cool-down period.
- Avoid passive overstretching to reduce the possibility of injury to the ligaments or joint capsule.
- Avoid any movements, exercises, or activities that produce compression or impingement of joint motion.
- Begin at a low intensity and progress within your individual limits to higher intensities. Do not try to do too much too soon.
- Avoid holding your breath and straining too hard during intense activity.
- Choose a level of intensity that is compatible with your abilities in terms of strength, power, and endurance.
- Select the appropriate clothing for exercising in hot or cold environments.
- Make sure you are acclimated to the environment in which you are exercising, regardless of whether it is extremely hot or cold.
- Select and use high-quality equipment when engaging in any physical activity. Breakdown of cheap or low-quality equipment may prove to be more expensive in the long run should injury occur.
- Listen to what your body is telling you. If you experience pain during activity, stop immediately.
- Do not engage in any activity that you think may have the potential to result in injury.

much lower level and gradually increase your level of activity. Some people stop exercising for a variety of reasons, and when they start exercising again, there is a tendency to try to begin where they left off. They do too much, too fast, too soon. The Safe Tip on page 226 provides you with some tips for practicing "safe fitness."

WHAT TYPES OF INJURIES MIGHT OCCUR IN AN EXERCISE PROGRAM?

Several different types of injuries typically occur through participation in physical activity. These injuries are briefly identified here.

Fractures—Cracks or breaks in bones that usually require some type of immobilization in a cast.
Contusions—A bruise of the skin, fat, or muscle tissue.
Sprains—Damage to a ligament, which connects bone to bone, thus providing a support to a joint.
Strains—Separation or tearing of muscle fibers.
Muscle soreness—Delayed onset pain in muscle following physical activities that you are not accustomed to.
Tendinitis—Inflammation of a tendon, which connects muscle to bone.
Bursitis—Inflammation of a bursa, which is a membrane that functions to reduce friction between bone and muscle, ligament and bone, muscle and ligament, etc.

A detailed discussion of the many injuries, both acute and chronic, that can occur with participation in physical activity is beyond the scope of this text. However, a few injuries seem to occur frequently with physical activity. Table 10-1 provides a brief description of the causes and signs of the more common injuries.

LOW BACK PAIN

There is no question that low back pain is one of the most common, annoying, and disabling

> **low back pain:** pain in the lower back caused by muscle imbalances, muscle strain, ligament sprain, or disk degeneration

ailments known. Many causes and cures for low back pain have been proposed. However, so many different things can cause pain in the lower back that no single incriminating cause or absolute cure can be identified.

▶ Causes of Low Back Pain

Of all the causes of low back pain, none is more common than imbalances between the strength and flexibility of the various muscle groups associated with the lower back. In most cases, the abdominal muscles are weak and stretched out, the spinal muscles are tight and inflexible, and the hamstring muscles are also tight. Therefore an exercise program that attempts to increase the strength and the tone of the abdominal muscles, improve the flexibility of the spinal muscles in the lower back, and stretch the tight hamstring muscles may alleviate many complaints of low back pain. The Health Link on page 229 details some of the causes.

▶ Prevention of Low Back Pain

Some knowledge of the source of low back pain is important to treat the injury, but it is more important to understand how low back pain can be avoided. To prevent low back pain, the practice of avoiding unnecessary stresses and strains should be integrated into your daily life. The back is subjected to these stresses and strains when one is standing, lying, sitting, lifting, and exercising. Care should be taken to avoid postures and positions that can cause injury. Figure 10-1 shows examples of safe postures.

TABLE 10-1

Summary of Common Injuries Associated with Physical Activity

Injury	Cause/Signs and Symptoms
Shoulder impingement	Chronic irritation and inflammation of muscle tendons and a bursa underneath the tip of the shoulder, which results from repeated forceful overhead motions of the shoulder such as in swimming, throwing, spiking a volleyball, or a tennis serve. Pain is felt when the arm is extended across the body above shoulder level.
Tennis elbow	Chronic irritation and inflammation of the lateral or outside surface of the arm just above the elbow at the attachment of the muscles that extend the wrist and fingers. It results from any activity that requires forceful extension of the wrist. This typically occurs in tennis players who are using faulty techniques hitting backhand ground strokes. Pain is felt above the elbow after forcefully extending the wrist against resistance or applying pressure over the muscle attachment above the elbow.
Racquetball or golfer's elbow	Similar to tennis elbow, except the pain is located on the medial or inside surface of the arm just above the elbow at the attachment of the wrist and finger flexor muscles. It occurs in those activities that involve repeated forceful flexion of the wrist, such as hitting a forehand stroke in racquetball. Golfers also develop this inflammation in the trailing arm from too much wrist flexion in a golf swing.
Groin pull	A muscle strain that occurs in the muscles located on the inside of the upper thigh just below the pubic area resulting either from an overstretch of the muscle or from a contraction of the muscle that meets excessive resistance. Pain will be produced by flexing the hip and leg across the body or by stretching the muscles in a groin stretch position.
Quadriceps contusion, "charlie horse"	A deep bruise of the muscles in the front part of the thigh caused by a forceful impact or by some object that results in severe pain, swelling, discoloration, and difficulty flexing the knee or extending the hip. Small calcium deposits may develop in the muscle without adequate rest and protection from additional trauma.
Hamstring pull	A muscle strain of the muscles of the back of the upper thigh that most often occurs while sprinting. In most cases, severe pain is caused simply by walking or in any movement that involves knee flexion or extension of the hamstring muscle. Some swelling, tenderness to touch, and possibly some discoloration extending down the back of the leg may occur in severe strains.
Patellofemoral knee pain	Nonspecific pain occurring around the knee, in particular the front part of the knee, or kneecap (patella). Pain can result from many causes, including improper movement of the kneecap in knee flexion and extension; tendinitis of tendon just below the kneecap caused by repetitive jumping; bursitis (swelling) either above or below the kneecap; osteoarthritis (joint surface degeneration) between the kneecap and thigh bone. This may possibly involve inflammation with swelling, tenderness, warmth, and pain with movement.

TABLE 10-1
Summary of Common Injuries Associated with Physical Activity—*Cont.*

Injury	Cause/Signs and Symptoms
Shin splints	A "catch-all" term used to refer to any pain that occurs in the front part of the lower leg or shin, most often caused by excessive running on hard surfaces. Pain is usually caused by muscle strains of those muscles that move the ankle and foot at their attachment points in the skin. It is usually worse during activity. In more severe cases it may be caused by stress fractures of the long bones in the lower leg, with the pain being worse after activity is stopped.
Achilles tendinitis	A chronic tendinitis of the "heel cord" or muscle tendon located on the back of the lower leg just above the heel. It may result from any activity that involves forcefully pushing off of the foot and ankle, such as running and jumping. This inflammation involves swelling, warmth, tenderness to touch, and pain during walking and especially running.
Ankle sprains	Stretching or tearing of one or several ligaments that provide stability to the ankle joint. Ligaments on the outside or lateral side of the ankle are more commonly injured by rolling the sole of the foot downward and to the inside. Pain is intense immediately after injury followed by considerable swelling, tenderness, loss of joint motion, and some discoloration over a 24- to 48-hour period.
Plantar fascitis or arch pain	Chronic inflammation and irritation of the broad ligament that runs from the heel to the base of the toes, forming part of the long arch on the bottom of the foot. It most often occurs in runners or walkers. It is frequently caused by wearing shoes that do not have adequate arch support. At first, pain is localized at the attachment on the heel; it then tends to move more onto the arch. It is most painful when you first get out of bed and then in the evening when you have been on your feet for long periods.

Health Link

Causes of Low Back Pain

Low back pain may result from the following associated problems:
1. Disk degeneration and rupture (herniation).
2. A sprain of the intervertebral ligaments in the lumbosacral region of the spine.
3. A sprain of the ligaments in the sacroiliac region.

TREATMENT AND MANAGEMENT OF INJURIES

Initial first-aid and management techniques for most fitness injuries associated with physical activity are fairly simple and straightforward. Regardless of which type of injury we are talking about, there is one problem they all have in common—swelling. Swelling is most likely during the first 72 hours after an injury. Once swelling has occurred, the healing process is significantly retarded. The injured area cannot return to normal until all the swelling is gone. Therefore everything that is done in terms of first-aid management of any of these conditions should be directed toward controlling the

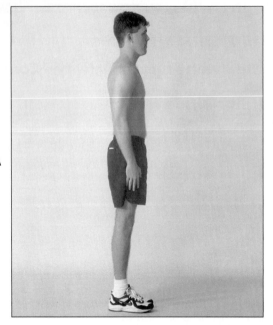
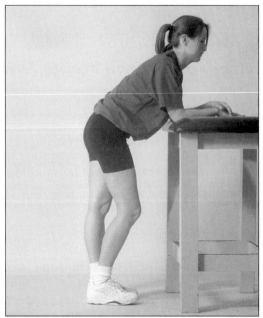
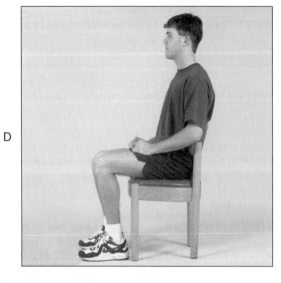
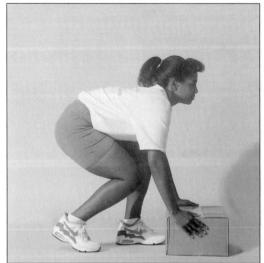

Figure 10-1. Examples of Safe Postures

A, Ideal standing posture. B, Correct leaning posture. C, Correct sleeping position. D, Ideal sitting position. E, Correct lifting position.

230

swelling. If the swelling can be controlled initially in the acute state of injury, it is likely that the time required for rehabilitation will be significantly reduced.

To control and severely limit the amount of swelling, the **RICE** principle can be applied. RICE stands for Rest, Ice, Compression, and Elevation (Figure 10-2). Each factor plays a critical role in limiting swelling, and all four methods should be used simultaneously.

Rest—You should rest the injured body part for approximately 72 hours before a rehabilitation program is begun.
Ice—Ice should be applied to the injured area in a plastic bag to slow bleeding and for analgesia.
Compression—The purpose of compression is to reduce the amount of space available for swelling by applying pressure around the injured area using an elastic wrap (such as an Ace bandage).
Elevation—The injured part, particularly an extremity, should be elevated to eliminate the effects of gravity on blood pooling in the extremities.

RICE: initial first-aid technique for treating injuries including rest, ice, compression, and elevation

The goal of rehabilitation should be to return the person to the usual physical activities as quickly and as safely as possible. Long-term rehabilitation programs require the supervision of a trained professional if they are going to be safe and effective. An injury that is not given proper rehabilitation may continue to cause many problems with increasing age.

WHAT EXERCISES SHOULD BE AVOIDED?

Throughout this text, an effort has been made to recommend specific exercises that are both effective and safe. Over the years, other sources have recommended and widely used a number of exercises that place abnormal stresses, strains, or compression forces on particular muscles or joints. Such exercises potentially predispose these structures to injury. Appropriate stretching, strengthening, conditioning, and in some cases corrective exercises are described in detail within individual chapters. Figures 10-3 through 10-14 identify a series of exercises that for one reason or another are *not* recommended as being safe and may potentially result in injury.

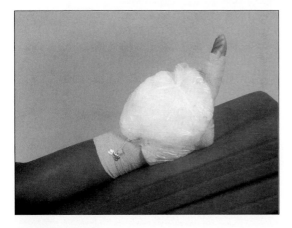

Figure 10-2. RICE.
Rest, ice, compression, elevation technique for treatment of a sprained ankle.

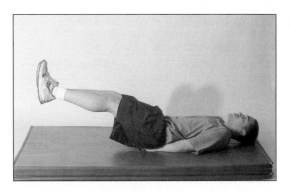

Figure 10-3. Straight Leg Lifts.
Used for strengthening abdominal muscles and hip flexors. Tends to tilt the pelvis forward, thus causing hyperextension of the lower back, which compresses the intervertebral disks.

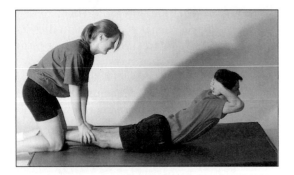

Figure 10-4. Back Hyperextensions.
Used to strengthen lower back muscles and stretch abdominal muscles. Causes compression of inter-vertebral disks with possible disk herniation or spinal nerve impingement.

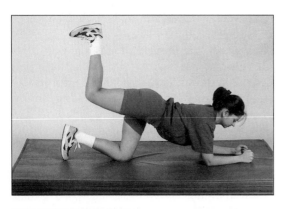

Figure 10-5. Donkey Kicks.
Used to develop extensor muscles of the lower back. Involves a ballistic backward and upward kick with the leg and an extension of the neck. Causes com-pression of intervertebral disks and possible disk herniation or spinal nerve impingement.

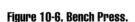

Figure 10-6. Bench Press.
Used for strengthening pectoral and triceps muscles. This lift, when done with the feet on the floor and an arched back, hyperextends the lower back.

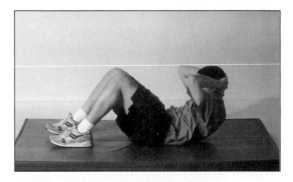

Figure 10-7. Sit-Ups with Hands Behind Neck.
Used for strengthening abdominal muscles. Pulls head and neck into hyperflexed position, stretching the intervertebral joint ligaments of the cervical spine.

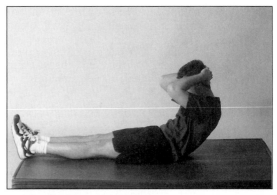

Figure 10-8. Straight-Leg Sit-Ups.
Causes a forward tilt of the pelvis, placing the lower back in a hyperextended position, thus adding unnecessary compression forces.

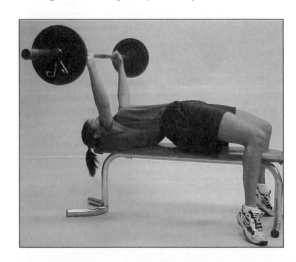

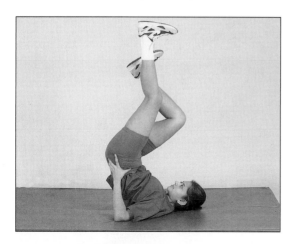

Figure 10-9. Up-Right Bicycling.
Used for strengthening abdominal muscles. Places the cervical and upper thoracic regions of the spine in a hyperflexed position, creating increased compression forces on intervertebral disks and stretching intervertebral ligaments.

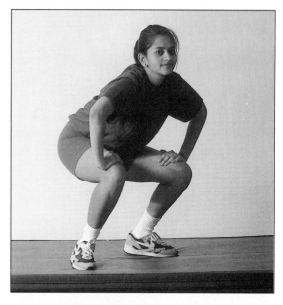

Figure 10-11. Deep Knee Bends.
Used for strengthening hip and knee extensors. Places extreme compressive forces on the knee joint, stressing ligaments, joint capsule, and cartilage (menisci).

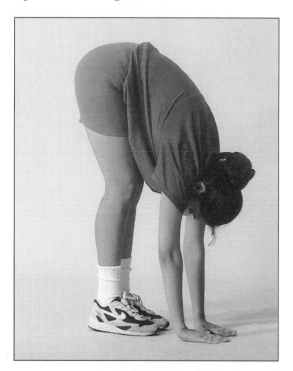

Figure 10-10. Standing Toe-Touches.
Used to stretch the hamstring muscles. Causes hyperextension of the knees and also pressure in the lower back, especially if the hamstring muscles are tight.

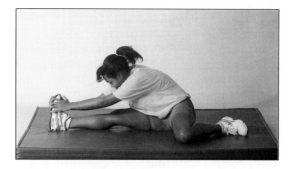

Figure 10-12. Hurdlers' Stretch.
Used for stretching the quadriceps muscle. Rotation of the tibia with compression of the knee joint causes stress to the medial ligaments and compression of the medial cartilage.

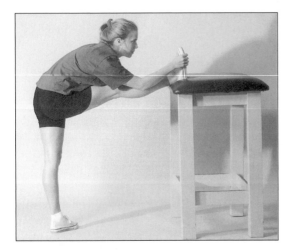

Figure 10-13. Bar Stretch.
Used for stretching hamstring muscles. Hyperextends the knee, placing stress on the posterior joint capsule and ligaments. Also stretches and may irritate the sciatic nerve, which innervates most of the muscles in the posterior leg.

WHAT PRECAUTIONS SHOULD YOU TAKE WHEN EXERCISING IN HOT OR COLD ENVIRONMENTS?

EXERCISING IN THE HEAT

Regardless of your level of physical conditioning, extreme caution must be taken when exercising in extreme environmental climates. Prolonged exposure to extreme heat can result in heat stress. Heat stress is certainly preventable, but each year many people will suffer illness or perhaps death from some heat-related cause. People who exercise in the heat are particularly vulnerable to heat stress. Body temperature must be maintained within a normal range. Maintaining a normal temperature in a hot environment depends on the ability of the body to eliminate heat. It should be obvious that heat-related problems have

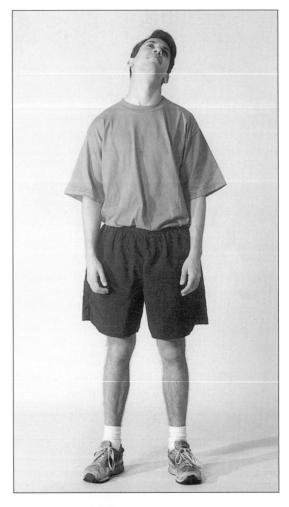

Figure 10-14. Neck Circles.
Used for range of motion in the cervical spine. Requires hyperextension of the cervical spine, which causes unnecessary compression of the cervical intervertebral disks.

the greatest chance of occurring on those days when the sun is bright and the temperature and relative humidity are high. But it is certainly true that various forms of heat stress, including heat cramps, heat exhaustion, or heatstroke, can occur whenever the body's ability to dissipate heat is impaired.

▶ Heat Cramps

Heat cramps are extremely painful muscle spasms that most commonly occur in the calf and abdomen, although any muscle can be involved. Heat cramps may be prevented by adequate replacement of water. The immediate treatment for heat cramps is ingestion of large quantities of water and mild stretching with ice massage of the muscle in spasm. Ingestion of salt tablets is not recommended. Various "sport drinks" have been recommended but are no more effective than water in preventing heat cramps.

▶ Heat Exhaustion

Like heat cramps, heat exhaustion results from inadequate replacement of fluids lost through sweating. Clinically, the victim of heat exhaustion will collapse and manifest profuse sweating, pale skin, mildly elevated temperature, dizziness, rapid breathing, and rapid pulse. Immediate treatment of heat exhaustion requires ingestion of large quantities of cool water. If possible, the person should be placed in a cool environment, although it is more essential to replace fluids.

▶ Heatstroke

Unlike heat cramps and heat exhaustion, heatstroke is a serious, life-threatening emergency. The specific cause of heatstroke is unknown; however, there is a breakdown of the sweating mechanism, and the body loses the ability to sweat. It is characterized by sudden collapse with loss of consciousness; red, relatively dry skin; and most important, a very high body temperature. Heatstroke can occur suddenly and without warning. Usually, the victim will not experience signs of heat cramps or heat exhaustion. Every first-aid effort should be directed to lowering body temperature. It is imperative that the victim be transported to a hospital as quickly as possible. The possibility of death from heatstroke can be significantly reduced if body temperature is lowered to normal within 45 minutes.

▶ Prevention of Heat-Related Illness

To a large extent heat-related illness can be prevented by simply paying attention to the following recommendations.

Acclimatization. It is most important to acclimate yourself to the existing heat and humidity conditions. This is the process of gradually preparing your body to be able to work in heat by slowly exposing the system to the stresses of a hot, humid environment. Heat dramatically reduces performance capabilities, and abrupt exposure to these conditions can predispose a person to heat-related illness. Acclimatization to heat generally occurs rapidly, usually within 5 to 7 days of gradually increasing periods of exercise in the heat. It is enhanced by being in good physical condition and by adequate fluid replacement.

Replacing Water. During hot weather it is essential to continually replace fluids lost through evaporation by drinking large quantities of fluid, regardless of whether you are thirsty. There is little question that adequate replacement of fluids is the best defense against heat stress. Water is undoubtedly the best form of fluid replacement during exercise. Fluids should be replenished as often and in as great a quantity as necessary during exercise.

Clothing. When exercising in the heat, wear as little clothing as possible to allow maximal evaporation. Light-colored, 100 percent cotton material allows maximal evaporation. Caution should be used when wearing a hat because about 40 percent of all heat lost from the body is lost through the head. Thus a hat tends to interfere with keeping cool. The use of sunscreens and sunglasses is also recommended to reduce the long-term effects of exposure to the sun.

heat-related illness: exercising in a hot environment may cause heat cramps, heat exhaustion, or heatstroke

Exercise Your Common Sense When Exercising. If possible, do not exercise during the hottest parts of the day—between 11:00 AM and 4:00 PM. The temperature is usually highest at about 4:00 PM. Try to avoid exercising on surfaces such as asphalt, concrete, or Astroturf, which tend to absorb and hold heat. If you experience any of the heat-related problems, stop the activity immediately, get into a cool environment, and drink large quantities of cool water. Common sense is the best prevention for heat stress.

EXERCISING IN THE COLD

Although being able to dissipate heat is a problem in hot, humid weather, conserving heat becomes a major concern when exercising in cold weather. It is essential to consider the environmental factors that may combine to significantly lower body temperature or produce hypothermia. These major factors are temperature, dampness, and wind, which collectively can be a real problem. Most cases of hypothermia occur when the temperature is in the 50° to 60° F range and when it is also damp and windy. Hypothermia results when the body's temperature drops below 35° C (95° F). Essentially it is a breakdown in the body's ability to produce heat. Initially there is shivering followed by loss of coordination and difficulty speaking. As the body's temperature continues to drop, shivering stops, the muscles stiffen, and the person becomes unconscious. People who have hypothermia should be taken to the hospital for treatment, and all efforts should be directed toward elevating body temperature. The Safe Tip above provides recommendations that may help reduce the chances of hypothermia.

hypothermia: exercising in cold can cause a lowered body temperature

Safe Tip

Hypothermia Prevention

- Use common sense, and be aware of the environmental conditions that predispose to hypothermia.
- Wear a hat to reduce loss of body heat through the head.
- Dress in layers of clothing, which can be removed layer by layer to prevent sweating. Remember that dampness is one of the more critical factors. If possible, wear materials such as Gortex, which allow moisture to escape from the body while keeping out moisture from the environment.
- Wear sufficiently protective clothing on the feet, hands, ears, and neck to prevent frostbite.
- Gradually acclimate yourself to exercising in the cold. Acclimatization to exercising in the cold is just as important as acclimatization when exercising in a hot, humid environment.

SUMMARY

- Listen to what your body is telling you. The "no pain, no gain" mentality will likely worsen an existing injury. The best way to prevent injury is to pay close attention to the basic principles of training and conditioning.
- Low back pain can have many causes, but the most common are herniated disks, lumbosacral strains, sacroiliac sprains, excessive tightness of the hamstrings, and weak abdominal muscles.
- Low back pain can be prevented by paying attention to standing, lying, sitting, and

lifting posture to prevent the lower back from being placed in potentially injurious positions.

- All injuries should be initially managed using rest, ice, compression, and elevation (RICE) to control swelling and thus reduce the time required for rehabilitation.
- It is important to understand the dangers involved in exercising in extreme environmental conditions.

SUGGESTED READINGS

Arnheim, D., and W.E. Prentice. 1999. *Essentials of athletic training.* St. Louis: McGraw-Hill.

Arnheim, D., and W.E. Prentice. 2000. *Principles of athletic training.* St. Louis: McGraw-Hill.

Boyle, D. 1999. *The sports medicine handbook for parents and coaches.* Washington, D.C.: Georgetown University Press.

Burruss, P. et al. 1998. Winter sports: risks during cold exposure. *Sports science exchange-roundtable* 9(4):1–6.

Carpenter, D.M., and B.W. Nelson. 1999. Low back strengthening for the prevention and treatment of low back pain. *Medicine and science in sports and exercise* 31(1):18–24.

Casa, D. 1999. Exercise in the heat II. Critical concepts in rehydration, exertional heat illnesses, and maximizing athletic performance. *Journal of Athletic Training* 34(3):253–62.

Gallaspie, J., and D. May. 1996. *Signs and symptoms of athletic injuries.* St. Louis: Mosby.

Galloway, S.D.R. et al. 1997. Exercise in the heat: Factors limiting exercise capacity and methods for improving heat tolerance. *Sports exercise and injury* 3(1):19–24.

Mellion, M. (ed.). 1998. *Sports medicine secrets.* Philadelphia: Hanley and Belfus.

Micheli, L., and M. Jenkins. 1995. *The sports medicine bible.* New York: Harper Perennial.

Morris, A. 1992. *Sports medicine: prevention of athletic injuries.* Dubuque: W.C. Brown.

Pfeiffer, R., and B. Magnus. 1998. *Concepts of athletic training.* Boston: Jones and Bartlett.

Porterfield, J., C. Derosa, and M. Bilbas. 1998. *Mechanical low back pain: perspectives in functional anatomy.* Philadelphia: W.B. Saunders.

Prentice, W. 1999. Rehabilitation techniques in sports medicine. St. Louis: WCB/McGraw-Hill.

SUGGESTED WEBSITES

American Orthopaedic Society for Sports Medicine
This site has a directory of doctors, publications, links to other sites, an ask the doctor section, and the *Sports Medicine Journal.*
http://www.sportsmed.org/

Common Sports Injuries
This site presents background information and Quick Time movies on injuries such as ankle sprain, pulled hamstring, and others.
http://www.southflorida.digitalcity.com/ DCSports/s...

ESPN.com: Training Room
This site has articles about fitness and conditioning, sports injuries, and sports nutrition.
http://espn.go.com/trainingroom/

Hughston Sports Medicine Hospital
This is the nation's first hospital specifically designed to treat patients suffering from activity related injuries and disorders. It is in Columbus, Georgia.
http://www.mindspring.com/~hughston/~

National Athletic Trainers' Association
Links to injury information, news about the organization, research and education, the *Journal of Athletic Training,* and other related topics are presented.
http://www.nata.org/

SportsDoc
Be the doctor to virtual patients. Reference information includes an extensive medical library.
http://www.medfacts.com/sprtsdoc.htm

Sports Injuries: Health World Online
Information on prevention, sports herbs, homeopathic medicine, and more is presented.
http://www.healthy.net/clinic/dandc/sportinj/

Sports Science, Sport Medicine & Physical Education
Sports Science Directory on SPORTQuest provides links to sport science/medicine and related topics.
http://www.sportquest.com/sportscience.html

Sportsmedicine.com
The sports medicine network offers information on education, organizations, and topics about sports medicine, plus a chat room, mail list, and message board to connect people interested in sports medicine.
http://www.sportsmedicine.com/

The Female Athlete
This site presents information about typical women's sports health issues like knee injuries, osteoporosis, and strength training.
http://www.sportsmed.org/d/answers/jan97.htm

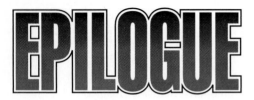

NOW DO YOU SEE WHY YOU SHOULD CARE ABOUT GETTING FIT?

Throughout this text, I have tried to emphasize the value of establishing lifelong patterns of healthy living and physical activity. I have tried to provide you with facts and principles that establish the basis for motivating you to incorporate some form of physical activity into your daily life. The text has also identified the exercises, activities, resources, and assessment instruments that can be used in developing an individualized, well-rounded physical activity program. Although there are many different approaches that will ultimately lead to being physically fit, following certain principles and guidelines makes the pursuit of a healthy lifestyle safer and more effective. How, where, or what you choose to do or use to get yourself fit and healthy is of little consequence as long as you pay attention to the basic principles that have been detailed in each of the chapters in this text.

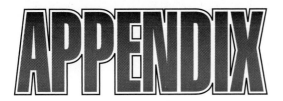

Appendix A
Food Composition Table

Food Name	Serving	KCAL Kc	PROT Gm	CARB Gm	FAT Gm	CHOL Mg	SAFA Gm	FIBD Gm
BABY FOODS								
Baby-carrots	ounce	8	0.2	1.7	0	0	0	0.7
Baby-teething biscuits	item	43	1.2	8.4	0.5	0	-	0.1
Baby-mixed cereal/milk	ounce	32	1.3	4.5	1	0	-	0.25
Baby-oatmeal cereal/milk	ounce	33	1.4	4.3	1.2	0	-	0.7
Baby-rice cereal/milk	ounce	33	1.1	4.7	1	0	-	0.25
Baby-beef lasagna	ounce	22	1.2	2.8	0.6	-	-	0.1
Baby-beef stew	ounce	14	1.4	1.5	0.3	3.55	0.16	0.34
Baby-mixed vegetables	ounce	11	0.3	2.7	0.028	0	0	0.25
Baby-turkey & rice	ounce	14	0.5	2.1	0.4	2.84	0.12	0
Baby-veal & vegetables	ounce	20	1.7	1.7	0.8	-	-	0.1
Baby-apple blueberry	ounce	17	0.1	4.6	0.1	0	0	0.1
Baby-applesauce	ounce	12	0.1	3.1	0	0	0	0.7
Baby-peaches	ounce	20	0.1	5.4	0	0	0	0.7
Baby-pears	ounce	12	0.1	3.1	0	0	0	0.55
Baby-apple juice	fl oz	14	0	3.6	0	0	0	0.25
Baby-apple peach juice	fl oz	13	0	3.2	0	0	0	0.25
Baby-orange juice	fl oz	14	0.2	3.2	0.1	0	0	0.25
Baby-beef	ounce	30	3.9	0	1.5	-	0.73	0
Baby-chicken	ounce	37	3.9	0	2.2	-	0.58	0
Baby-egg yolks	serving	58	2.8	0.3	4.9	223	1.47	0
Baby-ham	ounce	32	3.9	0	1.6	-	0.55	0
Baby-lamb	ounce	29	4	0	1.3	0	0.66	0
Baby-liver	ounce	29	4.1	0.4	1.1	52	0.39	0
Baby-pork	ounce	35	4	0	2	-	0.68	0
Baby-turkey	ounce	32	4	0	1.7	-	0.54	0
Baby-beans-green	ounce	7	0.4	1.7	0	0	0	0.39
Baby-cookie-arrowroot	item	24	0.4	4.3	0.9	0	0.2	0.1
Baby-garden vegetables	ounce	11	0.7	1.9	0.1	0	0	0.7
Baby-peas	ounce	11	1	2.3	0.1	0	0	0.7
Baby-squash	ounce	7	0.2	1.6	0.1	0	0	0.7
Baby-sweet potatoes	ounce	16	0.3	3.7	0	0	0	0.7
Baby-pretzels	item	24	0.7	4.9	0.1	0	0	0
Baby-Zwieback	piece	30	0.7	5.2	0.7	1.46	0.28	0
Baby-cereal & egg yolks	ounce	15	0.5	2	0.5	18	0.17	0

Appendix A
Food Composition Table—cont'd

Food Name	Serving	KCAL Kc	PROT Gm	CARB Gm	FAT Gm	CHOL Mg	SAFA Gm	FIBD Gm
Baby-apple betty	ounce	20	0.1	5.6	0	0	0	0.1
Baby-beef & egg noodles	ounce	15	0.6	2	0.5	-	-	0.1
Baby-beans-green-buttered	ounce	9	0.3	1.9	0.2	0	0	0.7
Baby-beets	ounce	10	0.4	2.2	0	0	0	0.4
Baby-corn-creamed	ounce	16	0.4	4	0.1	0	0	0.9
Baby-peas-creamed	ounce	15	0.6	2.5	0.5	0	-	0.7
Baby-spinach-creamed	ounce	11	0.7	1.6	0.4	0	-	1.12
BEVERAGES								
Carn inst break-choc-env	item	130	7	23	1	-	-	-
Choc bev drink-no milk-dry	ounce	99.1	0.937	25.6	0.88	0	0.521	-
Beer-regular	fl oz	12.2	0.089	1.1	0	0	0	0.07
Whis/gin/rum/vod-80 proof	fl oz	64	0	0	0	0	0	0
Whis/gin/rum/vod-86 proof	fl oz	69.5	0	0.028	0	0	0	0
Whis/gin/rum/vod-90 proof	fl oz	72.9	0	0	0	0	0	0
Wine-dessert	fl oz	45.9	0.06	3.54	0	0	0	0
Wine-red-table	fl oz	21	0.059	0.502	0	0	0	0
Club soda	fl oz	0	0	0	0	0	0	0
Coffee-brewed	fl oz	0.592	0.03	0.118	0	0	0.001	0
Coffee-instant-prepared	cup	4.78	0.239	0.956	0	0	0.005	0
Tea-brewed	fl oz	0.296	0	0.089	0	0	0.001	0
Tea-instant-prep-unsweet	cup	2.37	0	0.474	0	0	0	0
Tea-instant-prep-sweetened	cup	88.1	0.259	22.1	0	0	0.008	0
Cordials/liqueur-54 proof	fl oz	97	-	11.5	0	0	0	0
Brandy-cognac-pony	item	73	-	-	0	0	0	0
Cider-fermented	fl oz	11.8	-	0.3	0	0	0	0
Whis/gin/rum vod-94 proof	fl oz	76.5	0	0	0	0	0	0
Whis/gin/rum vod-100 proof	fl oz	82	0	0	0	0	0	0
Champagne-domestic-glass	item	84	0.2	3	0	0	0	0
Wine-vermouth-dry-glass	item	105	0	1	0	0	0	0
Wine-vermouth-sweet-glass	item	167	0	12	0	0	0	0
Beer-light	fl oz	8.26	0.059	0.384	0	0	0	0
Hot cocoa-prep/milk-home	cup	218	9.1	25.8	9.05	33.3	5.61	3
Cream soda	fl oz	15.8	0	4.1	0	0	0	0
Perrier-mineral water	cup	0	0	0	0	0	0	0
Ovaltine-choc-prep/milk	cup	227	9.53	29.2	8.79	-	-	-
Coffee substitute-prepared	fl oz	1.52	0.03	0.303	0	0	0.002	0
Postum-inst grain bev-dry	ounce	103	1.93	24.1	0.028	0	0	0
Tang-inst drink-orange-dry	ounce	104	0	26.1	0	0	0	-
Wine-white-table	fl oz	20.1	0.03	0.236	0	0	0	0
Fruit punch drink-can	fl oz	14.6	0	3.69	0	0	0.001	0
Wine-cooler-white wine-7UP	serving	54.9	0.05	5.72	0	0	0	0

Food Name	Serving	KCAL Kc	PROT Gm	CARB Gm	FAT Gm	CHOL Mg	SAFA Gm	FIBD Gm
Water	cup	0	0	0	0	0	0	0
Lemon lime soda-7UP	fl oz	12.3	0	3.19	0	0	0	0
Tea-herb-brewed	fl oz	0.296	0	0.059	0	0	0.001	0
Gatorade-thirst quencher	fl oz	7.53	0	1.9	0	0	0	0
Tonic water-quinine soda	fl oz	10.4	0	2.68	0	0	0	0
Wine-rosé-table	fl oz	20.9	0.059	0.413	0	0	0	0

Breads

Food Name	Serving	KCAL Kc	PROT Gm	CARB Gm	FAT Gm	CHOL Mg	SAFA Gm	FIBD Gm
Bagel-egg	item	163	6.02	30.9	1.41	8	-	1.16
Bagel-water	item	163	6.02	30.9	1.41	0	0.2	1.16
Biscuits-prepared/mixed	item	104	1.63	13	5.05	1.4	3.31	0.504
Breadcrumbs-dry-grated	cup	390	13	73	5	0	1	3.65
Bread-cracked wheat	slice	65.5	2.32	12.5	0.868	0	0.1	1.33
Bread-french-enriched	slice	98	3.33	17.7	1.36	0	0.2	0.805
Bread-raisin-enriched	slice	69.5	2.05	13.2	0.99	0	0.2	0.55
Bread-rye-American-light	slice	65.5	2.12	12	0.913	0	-	1.55
Bread-pumpernickel	slice	81.6	2.93	15.4	1.1	0	-	1.89
Bread-white-firm	slice	61.4	1.9	11.2	0.902	0	0.2	0.437
Bread-white-firm-toasted	slice	65	2	12	1	0	0.2	0.5
Bread-whole wheat-firm	slice	61.3	2.41	11.3	1.09	0	0.1	2.83
Bread-wheat-firm-toasted	slice	59	2.31	10.9	1.05	0	0.1	2.38
Crackers-graham-plain	item	27.5	0.5	5	0.5	0	0.1	0.224
Crackers-rye wafers	item	22.5	1	5	0	0	0	1.05
Crackers-saltines	item	12.5	0.25	2	0.25	0.75	0.1	0.072
Muffin-blueberry-home rec	item	110	3	17	4	21	1.1	0.85
Muffin-bran-home rec	item	112	2.96	16.7	5.08	21	1.2	2.52
Muffin-corn-home rec	item	125	3	19	4	21	1.2	0.95
Muffin-plain-home rec	item	120	3	17	4	21	1	0.85
Pancakes-buckwheat-mix	item	55	2	6	2	20	0.8	0.621
Pancakes-plain-home recipe	item	60	2	9	2	20	0.5	0.45
Pancakes-plain-mix	item	58.9	1.85	7.87	21.7	20	0.7	0.394
Roll-brown & serve-enr	item	85	2	14	2	0	0.4	0.988
Roll-hamburger/hotdog	item	114	3.43	20.1	2.09	0	0.5	1.01
Roll-hard-enriched	item	155	5	30	2	0	0.4	1.5
Roll-submarine/hoagie-enr	item	390	12	75	4	0	0.9	3.75
Waffles-enr-home recipe	item	245	6.93	25.7	12.6	45	2.3	1.05
Muffin-English-plain	item	133	4.43	25.7	1.09	0	-	1.29
Muffin-English-plain-toast	item	154	5.13	29.8	1.26	0	-	1.49
Bread-corn-home rec	slice	108	2.21	15.6	3.94	0	-	1.17
Crackers-cheese	item	5.38	0.091	0.52	0.327	-	0.09	0.025
Crackers-graham-sug/honey	item	30.1	0.519	5.4	0.732	0	0.1	0.119
French toast-home recipe	slice	153	5.67	17.2	6.73	-	-	2.02
Waffles-frozen	item	103	2.15	15.9	3.52	0	-	0.888
Bread-mixed grain	slice	64.3	2.49	11.7	0.93	0	-	1.58
Bread-whole wheat-home rec	slice	66.5	2.25	11.6	1.16	0	-	2.83

Appendix A
Food Composition Table—cont'd

Food Name	Serving	KCAL Kc	PROT Gm	CARB Gm	FAT Gm	CHOL Mg	SAFA Gm	FIBD Gm
Bread-pita	item	105	3.95	20.6	0.57	0	-	0.608
Crackers-Rykrisp-natural	item	7.5	0.25	1.67	0.033	0	0	0.34
Crackers-animal	item	8.67	0.127	1.47	0.2	0	-	0.027
Crackers-cheddar snacks	item	7.22	0.144	1.11	0.261	-	-	0.056
Crackers-triscuits	item	21	0.4	3.1	0.75	0	-	0.155
Crackers-wheat thins	item	9	0.125	1.25	0.35	0	-	0.099
Roll-whole wheat-homemade	item	90	3.5	18.3	1	0	-	1.83
Croissant-roll-Sara Lee	item	109	2.3	11.2	6.1	-	-	0.56
Muffin-soy	item	119	3.9	16.7	4.4	0	-	0.835
Bread stick-vienna type	item	106	3.3	20.3	1.1	0	-	1.02
Crackers-Ritz	item	18	0.233	21.3	0.967	0	-	0.107
BREAKFAST CEREALS								
Cereal-corn grits-enriched	cup	145	3.39	31.5	0.484	0	0.073	0.6
Cereal-farina-cook-enr	cup	117	3.26	24.7	0.233	0	0.023	3.26
Cereal-wheat-rolled-cooked	cup	180	5	41	1	0	0.182	2.87
Cereal-wheat-wholemeal	cup	110	4	23	1	0	0.182	1.61
Cereal-frost flake-Kellogg	cup	133	1.75	31.7	0.07	0	0	0.77
Cereal-corn-shredded sugar	cup	95	2	22	0	0	0	1.54
Cereal-oats-puffed-sugar	cup	100	3	19	1	0	0.185	2.65
Cereal-rice-puffed-plain	cup	56.3	0.882	12.6	0.07	0	0	0.1
Cereal-rice-puffed-sugar	serving	115	1	26	0	0	0	0.2
Cereal-wheat-flakes-sugar	cup	105	3	24	0	0	0	2.7
Cereal-wheat-puffed plain	cup	43.7	1.76	9.55	0.144	0	0	0.4
Cereal-wheat-puffed sugar	serving	138	5.59	30.2	0.456	0	-	2.11
Cereal-wheat-shred-biscuit	item	83	2.6	18.8	0.3	0	0	2.2
Cereal-wheat germ-toasted	cup	432	32.9	56.1	12.1	0	2.07	14.6
Cereal-cream/wheat-packet	item	132	2.5	28.9	0.4	0	0	2.02
Cereal-oatmeal-inst packet	item	104	4.4	18.1	1.7	0	0.289	1.62
Cereal-Ralston-cooked	cup	134	5.57	28.2	0.8	0	0	4.2
Cereal-All Bran	cup	212	12.2	63.4	1.53	0	-	25.5
Cereal-Alpha Bits	cup	111	2.2	24.6	0.6	0	-	0.3
Cereal-Bran Buds	cup	220	11.8	64.8	2.04	0	-	23.6
Cereal-Bran Chex	cup	156	5.05	39	1.37	0	-	7.9
Cereal-C.W. Post-plain	cup	432	8.7	69.4	15.2	0.184	11.3	2.2
Cereal-Cheerios	cup	88.8	3.42	15.7	1.45	0	0.27	0.863
Cereal-corn bran	cup	125	2.45	30.3	1.26	0	-	6.84
Cereal-Corn Chex	cup	111	2.02	24.9	0.114	0	0	0.5
Cereal-cornflakes-Kellogg	cup	88.3	1.84	19.5	0.068	0	0	0.454
Cereal-Cracklin Bran	cup	229	5.52	41.2	8.76	0	-	9.1
Cereal-Crispy rice	cup	112	1.82	25.2	0.114	0	0	1
Cereal-fortified oat flake	cup	177	8.98	34.8	0.72	0	0	1.2

Food Name	Serving	KCAL Kc	PROT Gm	CARB Gm	FAT Gm	CHOL Mg	SAFA Gm	FIBD Gm
Cereal-bran flakes-Kellogg	cup	127	4.91	30.5	0.741	0	0	5.5
Cereal-Frosted Mini Wheats	item	25.5	0.731	5.86	0.071	0	0	0.54
Cereal-granola-homemade	cup	594	15	67.3	33.2	0	5.84	12.8
Cereal-Grape Nuts	cup	407	13.3	93.5	0.456	0	0	5.47
Cereal-Grape Nuts Flakes	cup	116	3.48	26.6	0.358	0	0	2.08
Cereal-Heartland Natural	cup	499	11.6	78.5	17.7	0	-	5.4
Cereal-Honey Nut Cheerios	cup	125	3.63	26.5	0.759	0	0.132	1.3
Cereal-Honey Bran	cup	119	3.08	28.6	0.735	0	0	3.9
Cereal-Life-plain/cinnamon	cup	162	8.1	31.5	0.836	0	0	1.4
Cereal-Lucky Charms	cup	125	2.91	26.1	1.22	0	0.224	0.6
Cereal-granola-Nature Val	cup	503	11.5	75.5	19.6	0	13	4.2
Cereal-Nutri Grain-barley	cup	153	4.47	33.9	0.328	0	0	2.4
Cereal-Nutri Grain-corn	cup	160	3.36	35.4	0.966	0	-	2.6
Cereal-Nutri Grain-rye	cup	144	3.48	33.9	0.28	0	0	2.56
Cereal-Nutri Grain-wheat	cup	158	3.83	37.2	0.44	0	0	2.8
Cereal-100% bran	cup	178	8.25	48.1	3.3	0	0.587	19.5
Cereal-Product 19	cup	126	3.23	27.4	0.231	0	0	0.4
Cereal-Raisin Bran-Kellogg	cup	154	5.31	37.1	0.984	0	-	5.31
Cereal-Rice Chex	cup	99.5	1.34	22.5	0.101	0	0	0.151
Cereal-Rice Krispies	cup	112	1.93	24.8	0.199	0	0	0.1
Cereal-Special K	cup	83.1	4.2	16	0.085	0.028	0	0.17
Cereal-Sugar Corn Pops	cup	108	1.42	25.7	0.085	0	0	0.2
Cereal-Sugar Smacks	cup	141	2.65	33	0.72	0	0	0.531
Cereal-Team	cup	164	2.69	36	0.756	0	0	0.7
Cereal-Toasties	cup	87.8	1.84	19.5	0.045	0	0	0.386
Cereal-Total	cup	116	3.3	26	0.693	0	0.099	2.4
Cereal-Trix	cup	109	1.53	25.2	0.398	0	0	0.32
Cereal-Wheat Chex	cup	169	4.55	37.8	1.15	0	-	3.4
Cereal-wheat germ-sugar	cup	426	24.6	68.7	9.04	0	1.57	5.7
Cereal-Wheaties	cup	101	2.8	23.1	0.5	0	0.07	2
Cereal-cream/wheat-reg-hot	cup	133	3.8	27.7	0.5	0	0	1.94
Cereal-cream/wheat instant	cup	153	4.4	31.6	0.6	0	0	2.21
Cereal-malt o meal-cook	cup	122	3.6	25.9	0.24	0	0	0.6
Cereal-Maypo-cook-hot	cup	170	5.8	31.8	2.4	0	-	1.2
Cereal-Roman Meal-cooked	cup	147	6.51	33	0.964	0	-	2.31
Cereal-Wheatena-cooked	cup	136	4.86	28.7	1.22	0	-	2.6
Cereal-whole wheat natural	cup	150	4.84	33.2	0.968	0	-	2.7
Cereal-oatmeal-raw	cup	311	13	54.2	5.1	0	0.9	4.6
COMBINATION FOODS								
Beef-Raviolios-canned	ounce	27.5	1.14	4.26	0.568	-	0.11	0.23
Salad-three-bean-Del Monte	ounce	22.4	0.71	5.06	0.056	0	0	1.52
Salad-tuna	cup	350	30	7	22	68	4.3	1.03
Beef-vegetable stew	cup	220	16	15	11	72	4.9	3.19
Beef potpie-home recipe	slice	515	21	39	30	44	7.9	3.9

Appendix A
Food Composition Table—cont'd

Food Name	Serving	KCAL Kc	PROT Gm	CARB Gm	FAT Gm	CHOL Mg	SAFA Gm	FIBD Gm
Chili concarne/beans-can	cup	340	19	31	16	38	7.5	5
Chicken a la king-home rec	cup	470	27	12	34	186	12.9	1.2
Chicken chow mein-canned	cup	95	7	18	0	98	0	0.9
Chicken potpie-baked-home	slice	545	23	42	31	72	11	4.2
Macaroni & cheese-enr-can	cup	230	9	26	10	42	4.2	1.44
Macaroni & cheese-enr-home	cup	430	17	40	22	42	8.9	1.2
Pizza-cheese-baked	slice	140	7.68	20.5	3.21	9	1.54	1.59
Spaghetti/tom/che-home rec	cup	260	9	37	9	4	2	2.5
Spaghetti/tom/che-can	cup	190	6	39	2	4	0.5	2.5
Spaghetti/tom/meat-home	cup	330	19	39	12	75	3.3	2.73
Spaghetti/tom/meat-can	cup	260	12	29	10	39	2.2	2.75
Beans/pork/frankfurter-can	cup	365	17.3	39.6	16.9	15.4	6.05	12.8
Beans/pork/tom sauce-can	cup	248	13.1	49.1	2.61	17	0.999	13.8
Beans/pork/sweet sauce/can	cup	281	13.4	53.1	3.69	17.7	1.42	14
Salad-potato	cup	358	6.7	27.9	20.5	170	3.57	5.25
Vegetables-mixed-froz-boil	cup	107	5.21	23.8	0.273	0	0.056	6.92
Salad-fruit-can/juice	cup	125	1.27	32.5	0.075	0	0.01	1.64
Salad-coleslaw	tbsp	5.52	0.103	0.993	0.209	1	0.031	0.297
Taco	item	370	20.7	26.7	20.6	57	11.4	2.67
Pizza-pepperoni-baked	slice	181	10.1	19.9	6.96	14	2.24	1.48
Sand-bac/let/tom/mayo	item	282	6.8	28.8	15.6	-	-	2.88
Sandwich-club	item	590	35.6	41.7	20.8	-	-	4.17
Salad-macaroni	serving	50.7	0.7	5.3	3	-	-	0.29
Salad-carrot raisin-home	cup	306	3.8	55.8	11.6	-	-	16.7
Salad-mandarin orange gel	serving	22.7	0.4	5.7	0	0	0	0.57
Salad-chicken	cup	502	26	17.4	36.2	-	-	-
Chili with beans-canned	cup	286	14.6	30.4	14	43.4	6	6.93
Salad-green salad-tossed	serving	32	2.6	6.67	0.16	0	0.021	2.11
Meat loaf-celery/onions	serving	213	15.8	5.23	13.9	107	5.29	0.11
Salad-chef salad-ham/chees	serving	196	13.4	7.42	12.7	46	6.98	2.39
DAIRY PRODUCTS								
Cheese-blue	ounce	100	6.06	0.659	8.14	21	5.29	0
Cheese-camembert-wedge	item	114	7.52	0.18	9.22	27	5.8	0
Cheese-cheddar-shredded	cup	455	28.1	1.45	37.5	119	23.8	-
Cheese-cottage-4% lar curd	cup	232	28.1	6.03	10.1	33.8	6.41	0
Cheese-cream	ounce	100	2.17	0.759	10	31.4	6.31	0
Cheese-mozzarella-skim milk	ounce	72	6.88	0.78	4.51	16	2.87	0
Cheese-parmesan-grated	cup	456	41.6	3.74	30	79	19.1	0
Cheese-provolone	ounce	100	7.25	0.61	7.55	20	4.84	0
Cheese-ricotta-skim milk	cup	340	28	12.6	19.5	76	12.1	0
Cheese-romano	ounce	110	9.02	1.03	7.64	29	4.85	0

Food Name	Serving	KCAL Kc	PROT Gm	CARB Gm	FAT Gm	CHOL Mg	SAFA Gm	FIBD Gm
Cheese-Swiss	ounce	107	8.06	0.96	7.78	26	5.04	0
Cheese-American-processed	ounce	106	6.28	0.45	8.86	27	5.58	0
Cheese-swiss-processed	ounce	95	7.01	0.6	7.09	24	4.55	0
Cheese food-American-proc	ounce	93	5.56	2.07	6.97	18	4.38	0
Cheese-spread-processed	ounce	82	4.65	2.48	6.02	16	3.78	0
Cream-half & half-fluid	cup	315	7.16	10.4	27.8	89	17.3	0
Cream-coffee-table-light	cup	469	6.48	8.78	46.3	159	28.9	0
Cream-whipping-heavy	cup	821	4.88	6.64	88.1	326	54.8	0
Cream-whip-pressurized	cup	154	1.92	7.49	13.3	46	8.3	0
Cream-sour-cultured	cup	493	7.27	9.82	48.2	102	30	0
Cream-whip-imit-froz	cup	239	0.94	17.3	19	0	16.3	0
Cream-whip-imit-pressurize	cup	184	0.69	11.3	15.6	0	13.2	0
Milk-whole-3.3% fat-fluid	cup	150	8.03	11.4	8.15	33	5.07	0
Milk-2% fat-lowfat-fluid	cup	121	8.12	11.7	4.68	18	2.92	0
Milk-2% milk solids added	cup	125	8.53	12.2	4.7	18	2.93	0
Milk-1% fat-lowfat-fluid	cup	102	8.03	11.7	2.59	10	1.61	0
Milk-buttermilk-fluid	cup	99	8.11	11.7	2.16	9	1.34	0
Milk-evaporated-whole can	cup	338	17.2	25.3	19.1	73.1	11.6	0
Milk-evaporated-skim can	cup	199	19.3	28.9	0.51	10.2	0.309	0
Milk-condensed-sweet can	cup	982	24.2	166	26.6	104	16.8	0
Milk-chocolate-whole	cup	208	7.92	25.9	8.48	30	5.26	0.15
Milk-eggnog-commercial	cup	342	9.68	34.4	19	149	11.3	0
Milkshake-chocolate-thick	item	356	9.15	63.5	8.1	32	5.04	0.75
Milkshake-vanilla-thick	item	350	12.1	55.6	9.48	37	5.9	0.2
Yogurt-fruit flavor-lowfat	cup	231	9.92	43.2	2.45	10	1.58	0.8
Yogurt-plain-low-fat	cup	144	11.9	16	3.52	14	2.27	0
Yogurt-plain-nonfat	cup	127	13	17.4	0.41	4	0.264	0
Yogurt-plain-whole	cup	139	7.88	10.6	7.38	29	4.76	0
Cheese-feta	ounce	75	4.03	1.16	6.03	25	4.24	0
Cheese-gouda	ounce	101	7.07	0.63	7.78	32	4.99	0
Cheese-limburger	ounce	93	5.68	0.14	7.72	26	4.75	0
Cheese-monterey	ounce	106	6.94	0.19	8.58	25.2	5.41	0
Cheese-roquefort	ounce	105	6.11	0.57	8.69	26	5.46	0
Cream-sour-half & half	tbsp	20	0.44	0.64	1.8	6	1.12	0
Cream-sour-imitation	ounce	59	0.68	1.88	5.53	0	5.04	0
Milk-whole-low sodium	cup	149	7.56	10.9	8.44	33	5.26	0
Milk-human-whole-mature	cup	171	2.53	17	10.8	34	4.94	0

DESSERTS

Food Name	Serving	KCAL Kc	PROT Gm	CARB Gm	FAT Gm	CHOL Mg	SAFA Gm	FIBD Gm
Ice cream-van-hard-10% fat	cup	269	4.8	31.7	14.3	59	8.92	0
Ice cream-van-soft serve	cup	377	7.04	38.3	22.5	153	13.5	0
Ice milk-van-soft-2.6% fat	cup	223	8.03	38.4	4.62	13	2.88	0
Sherbet-orange 2% fat	cup	270	2.16	58.7	3.82	14	2.38	0
Custard-baked	cup	305	14	29	15	278	6.8	1.02
Pudd-tapioca cream-home	cup	220	8	28	8	80	4.1	0.56

Appendix A
Food Composition Table—cont'd

Food Name	Serving	KCAL Kc	PROT Gm	CARB Gm	FAT Gm	CHOL Mg	SAFA Gm	FIBD Gm
Pudd-choc-cooked-mix/milk	cup	320	9	59	8	32	4.3	0
Pudd-choc-inst-mix/milk	cup	325	8	63	7	28	3.6	0
Cake-angelfood-mix/prep	slice	142	4.2	31.5	0.122	0	-	0.037
Cupcake/chocolate icing	item	130	2	21	5	15	2	0.42
Cake-gingerbread-mix/prep	slice	175	2	32	4	1	1.1	1.83
Cake-yellow/icing-home rec	slice	268	2.9	40.3	11.4	36	3	0.552
Cake-fruit-dark-home rec	slice	56.9	0.72	8.96	2.3	6.75	0.48	0.313
Cake-sheet-no icing-home	slice	315	4	48	12	1	3.3	0.96
Cake-pound-home recipe	slice	160	2	16	10	68	54.9	0.08
Cake-sponge-home recipe	slice	188	4.82	35.7	3.14	162	1.1	0
Cookie-chocolate chip-mix	item	50	0.5	6.96	2.42	5.52	0.7	0.284
Cookie-choc chip-home rec	item	46.3	0.5	6.41	2.68	5.25	0.6	0.27
Cookie-macaroon	item	90	1	12.5	4.5	0	-	0.437
Cookie-oatmeal/raisin-mix	item	61.5	0.732	8.93	2.6	0	0.5	0.351
Cookie-sandwich-choc/van	item	50	0.5	7	2.25	0	0.55	0.15
Cookie-vanilla wafer	item	18.5	0.2	3	0.6	2.5	0.1	0.01
Danish pastry-plain	item	250	4.06	29.1	13.6	0	4.7	0.582
Doughnuts-cake-plain	item	104	1.28	12.2	5.77	10	1.2	0.325
Doughnuts-yeast-glazed	item	205	3	22	11.2	13	3	1.1
Pie-apple-home rec	slice	323	2.75	49.1	13.6	0	3.9	2.16
Pie-banana cream-home rec	slice	285	6	40	12	40	3.8	1.4
Pie-cherry-home rec	slice	350	4	52	15	0	4	1.08
Pie-custard-home rec	slice	285	8	30	14	-	4.8	2.08
Pie-lemon meringue-home	slice	300	3.86	47.3	11.2	0	3.7	1.44
Pie-mince-home rec	slice	365	3	56	16	0	4	1.96
Pie-peach-home rec	slice	345	3	52	14	0	3.5	1.82
Pie-pecan-home rec	slice	495	6	61	27	0	4	4.13
Pie-pumpkin-home rec	slice	275	5	32	15	0	5.4	3.51
Piecrust-mix/prep-baked	item	743	10	70.5	46.5	0	11.4	4.23
Granola bar	item	109	2.35	16	4.23	-	-	0.96
Cookie-sugar-mix	item	98.8	0.908	13.1	4.79	-	-	0.262
Cake-cheesecake-commercial	slice	257	4.61	24.3	16.3	-	-	1.79
Ice cream sundae-hot fudge	item	297	5.89	49.8	9.01	21.5	5.25	-
Turnover-apple	ounce	85.2	0.738	10.5	4.71	1.42	-	0.21
Cookie-peanut butter-mix	item	50	0.8	5.87	2.64	-	-	0.18
Pudd-rice/raisins	cup	387	9.5	70.8	8.2	-	-	1.42
Cake-strawberry shortcake	serving	344	4.8	61.2	8.9	-	-	2.14
Froz yogurt-fruit variety cup	216	7	41.8	2	-	-	-	-
Twinkie-Hostess	item	143	1.25	25.6	4.2	21	-	-

Food Name	Serving	KCAL Kc	PROT Gm	CARB Gm	FAT Gm	CHOL Mg	SAFA Gm	FIBD Gm
EGGS								
Egg-whole-raw-large	item	75	6.25	0.61	5.01	213	1.55	0
Egg-white-raw-large	item	17	3.52	0.34	0	0	0	0
Egg-yolk-raw-large	item	59	2.78	0.3	5.12	213	1.59	0
Egg-hard-large-no shell	item	77	6.29	0.56	5.3	213	1.63	0
Egg-poached-whole-large	item	74	6.22	0.61	4.99	212	1.54	0
Egg-substitute-liquid	cup	211	30.1	1.61	8.31	2.51	1.65	0
FATS/OILS								
Butter-regular-tablespoon	tbsp	100	0.119	0.008	11.4	30.7	7.07	0
Butter-whipped-tablespoon	tbsp	64.5	0.077	0.005	7.3	19.7	4.54	0
Shortening-vegetable-soy	cup	1812	0	0	205	0	51.2	0
Margarine-diet Mazola	tbsp	50	0	0	5.7	0	1	0
Margarine-veg spray-Mazola	serving	6	0	0	0.72	0	0.08	0
Margarine-reg-hard-stick	item	812	1.02	1.02	91	0	17.9	0
Vegetable oil-corn	cup	1927	0	0	218	0	27.7	0
Vegetable oil-olive	cup	1909	0	0	216	0	29.2	0
Sal dress-blue cheese	tbsp	77.1	0.7	1.1	8	2.6	1.5	0.05
Sal dress-blue che-low cal	tbsp	10	0	1	1	4	0.5	0
Sal dress-French	tbsp	67	0.1	2.7	6.4	1.95	1.5	0.1
Sal dress-French-low cal	tbsp	21.9	0.033	3.5	0.9	0.978	0.13	0.09
Sal dress-Italian	tbsp	68.7	0	1.5	7.1	0	1	0.05
Sal dress-Italian-low cal	tbsp	15.8	0	0.7	1.5	1	0.2	0.09
Sal dress-mayonnaise type	tbsp	57.3	0.132	4.91	4.91	3.82	0.72	0
Sal dress-mayo-low cal	tbsp	20	0	2	2	2	0.4	0
Sal dress-Thousand Island	tbsp	58.9	0.14	2.4	5.6	4.9	0.9	0.6
Sal dress-Thous Isl-low cal	tbsp	24.3	0.1	2.5	1.6	2	0.2	0.3
Animal fat-cooking-chicken	tbsp	115	0	0	12.8	11	3.8	0
Margarine-corn-reg-hard	tsp	33.8	0	0	3.8	0	0.6	0
Margarine-corn-reg-soft	tsp	33.7	0	0	3.8	0	0.7	0
Mayonnaise-imitation-soy	tbsp	34.7	0.045	2.4	2.9	3.6	0.495	0
Sal dress-Russian-low cal	tbsp	23	0.082	4.5	0.652	1	0.1	0.2
Sal dress-Russian	tbsp	76	0.2	1.6	7.8	0	1.1	0
Sal dress-vinegar/oil-home	tbsp	70	0	0.39	7.81	0	1.42	0
Sandwich spread-commercial	tbsp	59.5	0.1	3.4	5.2	12	0.8	0.02
Mayonnaise-light-low-cal	tbsp	40	0	1	4	5	-	0
Miracle Whip-light-low cal	tbsp	45	0	2	4	5	-	0
Sal dress-Caesar	tbsp	70	0	1	7	-	-	0.04
Sal dress-ranch style	tbsp	54	0.4	0.6	5.7	-	-	0
FISH								
Fish-bluefish-baked/butter	item	246	40.6	0	8.1	108	1.83	0
Fish-clams-raw-meat only	serving	62.9	10.9	2.18	0.83	28.9	0.08	0
Fish-clam-can-solid/liquid	ounce	12.8	2.33	0.667	0.333	17.7	0.067	0

Appendix A
Food Composition Table—cont'd

Food Name	Serving	KCAL Kc	PROT Gm	CARB Gm	FAT Gm	CHOL Mg	SAFA Gm	FIBD Gm
Fish-crab meat-king-can	cup	135	24	1	3.2	135	0.6	0
Fish-stick-bread-froz-cook	ounce	77.2	4.44	6.75	3.47	31.8	0.894	0.665
Fish-perch-breaded-fried	piece	195	16	6	11	32	2.7	0.05
Fish-oysters-raw-meat only	cup	171	17.5	9.7	6.14	136	1.56	0
Fish-salmon-pink-can	serving	118	16.8	0	5.14	46.8	1.3	0
Fish-sardines-can/oil	item	25	2.95	0	1.37	17	0.184	0
Fish-shad-bake/marg/bacon	serving	201	23.2	0	11.3	69.4	2.45	0
Fish-shrimp-meat-can	cup	154	29.5	1.32	2.51	221	0.477	0
Fish-shrimp-french fried	serving	206	18.2	9.75	10.4	150	1.77	0.48
Fish-tuna-can/oil-drained	serving	168	24.8	0	6.98	15.3	1.3	0
Fish-tuna-white can/water	serving	116	22.7	0	2.09	35.7	0.556	0
Fish-tuna-diet-low sodium	ounce	35.5	7.67	0.011	0.54	9.94	0.09	0
Fish-tuna-light-can/water	serving	111	25.1	0	0.525	15.3	0.136	0
Fish-anchovy-fillet can	item	8.4	1.16	0	0.388	3.4	0.088	0
Fish-cod-cooked-dry heat	piece	189	41.1	0	1.55	99	0.302	0
Fish-crab cake	item	93	12.1	0.288	4.51	90	0.89	0.03
Fish-crab-steamed pieces	cup	150	30	0	2.39	82.2	0.206	0
Fish-sole/flounder-baked	serving	148	30.7	0	1.94	86	0.461	0
Fish-haddock-cook-dry heat	serving	95.2	20.6	0	0.79	62.9	0.142	0
Fish-mackerel-Atlantic-can	cup	296	44.1	0	12	150	3.53	0
Fish-rockfish-ckd-dry heat	serving	121	24	0	2.01	44	0.474	0
Fish-roe-raw-eggs	ounce	39.4	6.34	0.426	1.82	106	0.414	0
Fish-salmon-smoked	serving	117	18.3	0	4.32	23	0.929	0
Fish-scallops-steamed	ounce	31.8	6.59	0.511	0.398	15.1	-	0
Fish-swordfish-broil/marg	serving	174	28	0	6	4	-	0
Fish-trout-brook-cooked	serving	196	23.5	0.4	11.2	-	-	0
Fish-whitefish-bake/stuff	serving	215	15.2	5.8	14	-	-	0.58
Fish-white perch-fri-fillet	item	108	12.5	0	5.3	-	-	0
Fish-carp-cooked-dry heat	serving	138	19.4	0	6.1	71.4	1.18	0
Fish-catfish-fried-breaded	serving	195	15.4	6.83	11.3	68.9	2.79	0.8
Fish-flatfish-ckd-dry heat	serving	99.5	20.5	0	1.3	58	0.309	0
Fish-grouper-ckd-dry heat	serving	100	25.7	0	1.11	40	0.254	0
Fish-mackerel-ckd-dry heat	serving	223	20.3	0	15.1	63.8	3.55	0
Fish-ocean perch-ckd-dry	serving	103	20.3	0	1.78	45.9	0.266	0
Fish-perch-cooked-dry heat	serving	99.5	21.1	0	1	98	0.201	0
Fish-pollock-ckd-dry heat	serving	96.1	20	0	0.952	81.6	0.196	0
Fish-pompano-ckd-dry heat	serving	179	20.1	0	10.3	54.4	3.82	0
Fish-salmon-ckd-moist heat	serving	157	23.3	0	6.41	41.7	1.19	0
Fish-sea-bass-ckd-dry heat	serving	105	20.1	0	2.18	45.1	0.557	0
Fish-smelt-cooked-dry heat	serving	105	19.2	0	2.64	76.5	0.492	0

Food Name	Serving	KCAL Kc	PROT Gm	CARB Gm	FAT Gm	CHOL Mg	SAFA Gm	FIBD Gm
Fish-red snapper-ckd-dry	serving	109	22.4	0	1.46	40	0.31	0
Fish-surimi	serving	84.2	12.9	5.82	0.765	25.5	0.153	0
Fish-pollock-Atlantic-raw	serving	78.2	16.5	0	0.833	60.4	0.115	0
Fish-swordfish-cooked-dry	serving	132	21.6	0	4.37	42.5	1.2	0
Fish-trout-rainbow-ckd-dry	serving	128	22.4	0	3.66	62.1	0.707	0
Fish-tuna-yellowfin-raw	serving	91.8	19.9	0	0.81	38.3	0.2	0
Fish-whiting-ckd-dry heat	serving	98	20	0	1.43	71.4	0.269	0
Fish-crab-imitation-surimi	serving	86.7	10.2	8.69	1.11	17	0.221	0
Fish-crayfish-ckd-moist	serving	96.9	20.3	0	1.15	151	0.197	0
Fish-lobster-ckd-moist	ounce	27.8	5.82	0.364	0.168	20.4	0.03	0
Fish-shrimp-ckd-moist heat	serving	84.2	17.8	0	0.918	166	0.246	0
Fish-clams-breaded-fried	serving	172	12.1	8.78	8.78	51.9	2.28	0.32
Fish-clams-ckd-moist heat	serving	126	21.7	4.36	1.65	57	0.16	0
Fish-mussel-blue-ckd-moist	serving	147	20.2	6.28	3.81	47.6	0.723	0
Fish-oyster-Eastern-canned	cup	171	17.5	9.7	6.14	136	1.57	0
Fish-oyster-East-ckd-moist	serving	117	12	6.65	4.21	92.7	1.07	0
Fish-oysters-Pacific-raw	serving	68.9	8.03	4.21	1.96	42.5	0.434	0
Fish-squid-cooked-fried	serving	149	15.3	6.62	6.36	221	1.6	0.3
Fish-halibut-broiled-dry	serving	119	22.7	0	2.5	34.9	0.354	0
FROZEN DINNERS								
Fish divan-Lean Cuisine	item	270	31	16	10	85	-	-
Fettucini alfredo-Stouffer	item	270	8	19	18	-	-	-
Turkey pie-Stouffer	item	460	20	35	26	-	-	-
Meatballs/noodles-Stouffer	item	475	25	33	27	-	-	-
Beef/green peppers-Stouf	item	225	10	18	11	-	-	-
Lasagna-Stouffer	item	385	28	36	14	-	-	-
Chicken cacciatore-Stouf	item	310	25	29	11	-	-	-
Veal parmigiana-froz din	item	296	24	17	14	-	-	-
Cabbage roll/tom sauc-Horm	ounce	23	1.1	3.2	0.7	3	0.281	-
Chicken kiev-Le Menu	item	500	21	35	30	-	-	-
Vegetable lasagna-Le Menu	item	400	15	30	24	-	-	-
Beef sirloin tips-Le Menu	item	400	29	27	19	-	-	-
Chicken parmigiana-Le Menu	item	390	26	28	19	-	-	-
Manicotti-cheese-Le Menu	item	310	18	29	13	-	-	-
Sole-light-Van de Kamps	item	293	16	17	18	-	-	-
Mexican dinner-Swanson	item	590	20	64	29	-	-	-
Beef dinner-Swanson	item	320	25	34	9	-	-	-
Turkey dinner-Swanson	item	340	20	42	10	-	-	-
Chicken dinner-Swanson	item	660	26	64	33	-	-	-
Egg roll-beef/shrimp/froz	item	27	0.9	3.5	1	-	-	0.12
Fish & chips-Van de Kamps	item	500	16	45	30	-	-	-
Meatloaf-froz din-Banquet	item	412	20.9	29	23.7	-	-	-
Ham-froz din-Banquet	item	369	16.8	47.7	12.2	-	-	-
Salisbury steak din-Banq	item	390	18.1	24	24.6	-	-	-

Appendix A
Food Composition Table—cont'd

Food Name	Serving	KCAL Kc	PROT Gm	CARB Gm	FAT Gm	CHOL Mg	SAFA Gm	FIBD Gm
FRUITS								
Apples-raw-unpeeled	item	81	0.262	21.1	0.497	0	0.08	3.04
Apple-juice-canned/bottled	cup	116	0.15	29	0.28	0	0.047	0.52
Applesauce-can-sweetened	cup	194	0.459	50.8	0.47	0	0.077	3.06
Applesauce-can-unsweetened	cup	105	0.415	27.6	0.12	0	0.02	3.66
Apricot-raw-without pit	item	16.9	0.494	3.93	0.138	0	0.01	0.67
Apricots-dried-uncooked	cup	309	4.75	80.3	0.6	0	0.042	10.1
Apricots-dried-cooked-unsw	cup	213	3.24	54.8	0.4	0	0.028	19.5
Avocado-raw-California	item	306	3.65	12	30	0	4.48	6.13
Bananas-raw-peeled	item	105	1.17	26.7	0.547	0	0.211	1.82
Blackberries-raw	cup	74.9	1.04	18.4	0.562	0	0.07	8.93
Blueberries-raw	cup	81.2	0.972	20.5	0.551	0	0.07	3.34
Cherries-sweet-raw	item	4.9	0.082	1.13	0.065	0	0.015	0.1
Cranberry sauce-can-sweet	cup	418	0.554	108	0.416	0	0.06	3.2
Dates-natural-dried-chop	cup	490	3.51	131	0.801	0	0.05	15.5
Grapefruit-raw-pink & red	item	74	1.36	18.5	0.246	0	0.034	3.2
Grapefruit-raw-white	item	78	1.63	19.3	0.236	0	0.033	2.5
Grapefruit juice-raw	cup	96.3	1.24	22.7	0.247	0	0.035	0.5
Grapefruit juice-can-uns	cup	93.9	1.28	22.1	0.247	0	0.032	0.442
Grapefruit juice-can-sweet	cup	115	1.45	27.8	0.225	0	0.03	0
Grapefruit juice-froz-dilu	cup	101	1.36	24	0.321	0	0.047	0
Grape juice-can & bottle	cup	154	1.42	37.8	0.202	0	0.063	0
Grape juice-froz-diluted	cup	128	0.475	31.9	0.225	0	0.073	0
Grape drink-canned	cup	154	1.42	37.8	0.202	0	0.063	0
Lemons-raw-peeled	item	16.8	0.638	5.41	0.174	0	0.023	0.58
Lemon juice-raw	cup	61	0.927	21.1	0	0	0	0.732
Lemon juice-can & bottle	cup	51.2	0.976	15.8	0.708	0	0.093	0.732
Lemonade-froz-diluted	cup	105	0	28	0	0	0	0.56
Lime juice-raw	cup	66.4	1.08	22.2	0.246	0	0.027	0
Lime juice-can & bottle	cup	51.7	0.615	16.5	0.566	0	0.064	0
Melons-cantaloupe-raw	cup	56	1.41	13.4	0.448	0	0	1.28
Melons-honeydew-raw	cup	59.5	0.782	15.6	0.17	0	0	1.53
Oranges-raw-all varieties	item	61.6	1.23	15.4	0.157	0	0.02	3.14
Orange juice-raw	cup	111	1.74	25.8	0.496	0	0.06	1.98
Orange juice-can	cup	104	1.47	24.5	0.349	0	0.045	0.26
Orange juice-froz-diluted	cup	112	1.69	26.8	0.149	0	0.017	0.498
Papayas-raw	cup	54.6	0.854	13.7	0.196	0	0.06	1.27
Peaches-raw-whole	item	37.4	0.609	9.66	0.078	0	0.009	1.39
Peaches-raw-sliced	cup	73.1	1.19	18.9	0.153	0	0.017	2.72
Peaches-can/water pack	cup	58.6	1.07	14.9	0.146	0	0.015	1.08
Peaches-dried-uncooked	cup	382	5.78	98.1	1.22	0	0.131	14

Food Name	Serving	KCAL Kc	PROT Gm	CARB Gm	FAT Gm	CHOL Mg	SAFA Gm	FIBD Gm
Peaches-dried-cooked-uns	cup	199	2.99	50.8	0.645	0	0.067	6.7
Peaches-froz-sliced-sweet	cup	235	1.58	60	0.33	0	0.035	5.99
Pears-raw-Bartlett-unpeeled	item	97.9	0.647	25.1	0.664	0	0.037	4.32
Pineapple-raw-diced	cup	76	0.605	19.2	0.667	0	0.05	1.88
Pineapple juice-can	cup	140	0.8	34.5	0.2	0	0.013	0.25
Plums-raw-prune type	item	20	0	6	0	0	0	0.588
Prunes-dried-uncooked	cup	385	4.2	101	0.837	0	0.066	11
Prune juice-can & bottle	cup	182	1.56	44.7	0.077	0	0.008	2.56
Raisins-seedless	cup	435	4.67	115	0.667	0	0.218	7.69
Raisins-seedless-packet	item	42	0.451	11.1	0.064	0	0.021	0.742
Raspberries-raw	cup	60.3	1.12	14.2	0.677	0	0.023	5.5
Rhubarb-raw-cooked-sugar	cup	380	1	97	0	0	0	5.4
Strawberries-raw-whole	cup	44.7	0.909	10.5	0.551	0	0.03	3.87
Tangerines-raw-peeled	item	37	0.53	9.4	0.16	0	0.018	1.68
Watermelon-raw	cup	51.2	0.992	11.5	0.688	0	-	0.64
Apples-raw-peeled-boiled	cup	90.6	0.45	23.3	0.61	0	0.099	4.1
Apple juice-frozen-diluted	cup	112	0.34	27.6	0.239	0	0.043	0.55
Apricots-can/juice	cup	119	1.56	30.6	0.09	0	0.007	2.81
Blackberries-frozen-unsw	cup	96.6	1.78	23.7	0.649	0	-	7.55
Blueberries-frozen-unsweet	cup	79.1	0.651	18.9	0.992	0	-	4.94
Boysenberries-frozen-unsw	cup	66	1.45	16.1	0.343	0	-	5.15
Figs-dried-uncooked	cup	507	6.07	130	2.33	0	0.466	18.5
Fruit cocktail-can/juice	cup	114	1.14	29.4	0.025	0	0.005	1.51
Kiwifruit-raw	item	46.4	0.752	11.3	0.334	0	0	2.58
Limes-raw	item	20.1	0.469	7.06	0.134	0	0.015	0.353
Melons-casaba-raw	cup	44.2	1.53	10.5	0.17	0	0	2
Nectarines-raw	item	66.6	1.28	16	0.626	0	-	2.18
Papaya nectar-can	cup	143	0.425	36.3	0.375	0	0.118	1.2
Pears-can/juice	cup	124	0.843	32.1	0.174	0	0.01	4.71
Pineapple-can/juice	cup	150	1.05	39.3	0.2	0	0.015	1.88
Pineapple juice-froz-dilu	cup	130	1	31.9	0.075	0	0.005	0.3
Pomegranates-raw	item	105	1.46	26.4	0.462	0	-	1.1
Strawberries-froz-unsweet	cup	52.2	0.641	13.6	0.164	0	0.009	3.9
Cranapple juice-can	cup	170	0.253	43.3	0	0	0	0
Fruit roll up-cherry	item	50	0	12	1	0	-	-
GRAINS								
Cornmeal-degerm-enr-cooked	cup	878	20.4	186	3.96	0	0.54	1.9
Macaroni-cooked-firm-hot	cup	183	6.2	36.9	0.871	0	0.124	2.08
Noodles-egg-enr-cooked	cup	200	7	37	2	50	-	3.52
Popcorn-popped-plain	cup	25	1	5	0	0	0	0.4
Popcorn-popped-sugar coat	cup	135	2	30	1	0	0.5	1.35
Pretzel-thin-stick	item	1.19	0.028	0.242	0.011	0	0	-
Rice-white-instant-hot	cup	162	3.4	35.1	0.264	0	0.073	1.32
Rice-white-long grain-cook	cup	264	5.51	57.2	0.574	0	0.158	2.13

Appendix A
Food Composition Table—cont'd

Food Name	Serving	KCAL Kc	PROT Gm	CARB Gm	FAT Gm	CHOL Mg	SAFA Gm	FIBD Gm
Rice-white-parboil-cooked	cup	199	4.01	43.3	0.473	0	0.128	0.875
Spaghetti-cooked-tender-hot	cup	155	5	32	1	0	-	2.24
Flour-wheat-enr-sifted	cup	419	11.9	87.7	1.12	0	0.178	3.11
Corn chips	ounce	155	1.7	16.9	9.14	0	1.5	1.66
Taco shells	item	49.8	0.967	7.24	2.15	0	-	0.88
Tortilla-corn	item	67.2	2.15	12.8	1.14	0	-	1.56
Rice-brown-Uncle Ben's	cup	220	5	46.4	1.82	0	0.462	2.48
Shake'n Bake	ounce	116	2.44	17.7	4.26	-	-	-
Bisquick mix-dry	cup	480	8	76	16	-	-	3.02
Tortilla chips-Doritos	ounce	139	2	18.6	6.6	0	1.43	1.85
Croutons-herb seasoned	cup	100	4.29	20	0	0	0	1.41
Tortilla-flour	item	95	2.5	17.3	1.8	0	-	0.778
Rice-Spanish-home recipe	cup	213	4.4	40.7	4.2	0	-	1.83
Stuffing-mix-dry form	cup	111	3.9	21.7	1.1	-	-	-
Stuffing-mix-prepared	cup	501	9.1	49.8	30.5	-	-	-
Rice cake-regular	item	35	0.7	7.6	0.28	0	-	0.158
Noodles-Ramen-oriental	cup	207	5.9	30.7	8.6	-	-	2.04
MEATS								
Bacon-pork-broiled/fried	slice	36.3	1.92	0.037	3.1	5.36	1.1	0
Roast beef-rib lean/fat	slice	308	18.3	0	25.5	73.1	10.8	0
Roast beef-rib-lean	slice	122	13.9	0	7.03	41.3	2.96	0
Steak-sirloin-lean/fat	item	238	23.3	0	15.3	76.5	6.38	0
Steak-sirloin-lean/broiled	item	116	17	0	4.89	49.8	2	0
Steak-round-lean/fat	slice	179	26.2	0	7.5	72	2.8	0
Corned beef hash-canned	cup	400	19	24	25	50	11.9	-
Lamb-chop-lean/fat-broiled	serving	307	18.8	0	25.2	84.2	10.8	0
Lamb-chop/rib-lean-broiled	serving	134	15.8	0	7.38	51.9	2.65	0
Lamb-leg-lean/fat-roasted	slice	219	21.7	0	14	79	5.85	0
Beef-liver-fried/marg	slice	184	22.7	6.67	6.8	410	2.4	0
Ham-reg-roasted-pork	cup	249	31.7	0	12.6	82.6	4.37	0
Ham-reg-lunch meat-11% fat	slice	52	4.98	0.88	3	16.2	0.962	0
Pork-chop-lean/fat-broiled	item	284	19.3	0	22.3	77	8.06	0
Pork-chop-lean/broiled	item	169	18.4	0	10.1	63	3.48	0
Pork-loin-lean/fat-roast	item	268	22.4	0	19.1	80	6.92	0
Pork-loin-lean-roasted	slice	173	20.5	0	9.42	65.5	3.25	0
Pork-tenderloin-lean-roast	ounce	47.1	8.18	0	1.37	26.3	0.471	0
Bologna-pork	slice	56.8	3.52	0.168	4.57	13.6	1.58	0
Braunschweiger-saus-pork	slice	64.6	2.43	0.56	5.78	28.1	1.96	0
Sausage-patty-pork-cooked	item	100	5.31	0.28	8.41	22.4	2.92	0
Deviled ham-canned	tbsp	45	2	0	4	10	1.5	0
Frankfurter-hot dog-no bun	item	183	6.43	1.46	16.6	28.5	6.13	0

Food Name	Serving	KCAL Kc	PROT Gm	CARB Gm	FAT Gm	CHOL Mg	SAFA Gm	FIBD Gm
Sausage-link-pork-cooked	item	48	2.55	0.13	4.05	10.8	1.41	0
Salami-dry or hard-park	slice	40.7	2.26	0.16	3.37	7.9	1.19	0
Salami-cooked-beef	slice	60.3	3.46	0.646	4.76	15	2.07	0
Italian sausage-pork-link	item	216	13.4	1.01	17.2	52	6.05	0
Canadian bacon-pork-grill	slice	43	5.64	0.315	1.96	13.5	0.66	0
Liverwurst/liver saus-pork	slice	59	2.54	0.4	5.14	28	1.91	0
Polish sausage-pork	item	740	32	3.71	65.2	159	23.4	0
Kielbasa-pork/beef	slice	80.6	3.45	0.56	7.06	17.4	2.58	0
Knockwurst-pork/beef-link	item	209	8.08	1.2	18.9	39.4	6.94	0
Mortadella-pork/beef	slice	46.7	2.46	0.458	3.81	8.4	1.43	0
Bacon bits	tbsp	26.6	1.92	1.72	1.55	0	-	-
Spareribs-pork-braised	ounce	113	8.25	0	8.61	34.4	3.34	0
Steak-chicken fried	item	389	17.9	12.3	30	-	-	0
Pot roast-arm-beef-cooked	slice	231	33	0	9.98	101	3.79	0
Steak-rib-cooked	item	221	28	0	11.2	80	4.75	0
Hamburger-ground-reg-baked	serving	244	19.6	0	17.8	74	6.99	0
Hamburger-ground-reg-fried	serving	260	20.3	0	19.2	75.7	7.53	0
MISCELLANEOUS								
Pickle/hot dog relish	ounce	35	0	8	0	0	0	-
Pickle/hamburger relish	ounce	30	0	7	0	0	0	-
Baking powder-home use	tsp	3.87	0.003	0.936	0	0	0	-
Baking powder-low sodium	tsp	7.4	0.004	1.79	0	0	0	-
Gelatin-dry envelope	item	25	6	0	0	0	0	0
Gelatin dessert-prep	cup	140	4	34	0	0	0	0
Olives-green-pickled-can	item	3.75	0.1	0.1	0.5	0	0.05	0.104
Olives-mission-rice-can	item	5	0.1	0.1	0.667	0	0.067	0.09
Pickle-dill-cucumber-med	item	5	0	1	0	0	0	0.78
Pickle-fresh pack-cucumber	item	5	0	1.5	0	0	0	0.09
Pickle-sweet-gherkin-small	item	20	0	5	0	0	0	0.165
Pickle relish-sweet	tbsp	20	0	5	0	0	0	-
Popsickle	item	70	0	18	0	0	0	-
Vinegar-cider	tbsp	0	0	1	0	0	0	0
Yeast-baker-dry-act-packet	serving	20	3	3	0	0	0	2.21
Yeast-brewers-dry	tbsp	25	3	3	0	0	0	-
Baking soda	tsp	0	0	0	0	0	0	0
Jello-gel-sugar free-prep	cup	16	2	0	0	0	0	0
Gel-D Zerta-low-cal-prep	cup	16	4	0	0	0	0	0
Chewing gum-Wrigleys	item	10	0	2.3	-	0	0	-
Vinegar-distilled	cup	29	0	12	0	0	0	0
Chewing gum-candy coated	item	5	-	1.6	-	0	0	-
NUTS/SEEDS								
Nuts-almond-shelled-sliver	cup	677	22.9	23.5	60	0	5.69	10.7
Nuts-Brazil-dried-shelled	cup	918	20.1	17.9	92.7	0	22.6	10.8
Nuts-filbert-hazel-dri-chop	cup	727	15	17.6	72	0	5.29	9.77

Appendix A
Food Composition Table—cont'd

Food Name	Serving	KCAL Kc	PROT Gm	CARB Gm	FAT Gm	CHOL Mg	SAFA Gm	FIBD Gm
Nuts-peanuts-oiled roasted	cup	837	37.9	27.3	71	0	9.85	12.8
Peanut-butter-smooth type	tbsp	94.1	3.94	3.32	8	0	1.53	0.96
Nuts-pecans-dried-halves	cup	720	8.37	19.7	73.1	0	5.85	7.02
Nuts-walnut-black-dri-chop	cup	759	30.4	15.1	70.7	0	4.54	8.08
Nuts-walnut-Persian/English	cup	770	17.2	22	74.2	0	6.7	5.76
Nuts-cashew-dry roasted	cup	786	21	44.8	63.5	0	12.5	10
Nuts-macadamia-dried	cup	941	11.1	18.4	98.8	0	14.8	12.4
Nuts-mixed-dry roasted	cup	814	23.7	34.7	70.5	0	9.45	11.6
Nuts-mixed-oiled roasted	cup	876	23.8	30.4	80	0	12.4	12.8
Nuts-peanuts-Spanish-dried	cup	828	37.7	23.6	71.9	0	9.98	11.7
Nuts-pecans-oil roasted	cup	754	7.65	17.7	78.3	0	6.27	8.47
Nuts-pistachio-dried	cup	739	26.3	31.8	61.9	0	7.84	13.8
Nuts-pistachio-dry roasted	cup	776	19.1	35.2	67.6	0	8.56	13.8
Seeds/pumpkin/squash-roast	cup	285	11.9	34.4	12.4	0	2.35	29.4
Seeds-sesame-roasted-whole	ounce	161	4.82	7.31	13.6	0	1.91	5.32
Seeds-sunflower-oil roast	cup	830	28.8	19.9	77.6	0	8.13	9.18
Peanut butter-low sodium	tbsp	95	5	2.5	8.5	0	1.36	1.7
Nuts-peanuts-oil-salted	cup	837	37.9	27.3	71	0	9.85	12.8
Peanut butter-chunk style	tbsp	94.8	3.87	3.48	8.04	0	1.54	1.06
Peanut butter-old fashion	tbsp	95	4.2	2.7	8.1	0	1.5	1.06
POULTRY PRODUCTS								
Chicken-breast-fried/flour	item	436	62.4	3.22	17.4	176	4.8	0.07
Chicken-drumstick-fried	item	120	13.2	0.8	6.72	44	1.79	0
Chicken-breast-fri/batter	item	728	69.6	25.2	36.9	238	9.86	-
Turkey-dark meat-no skin	cup	262	40	0	10.1	119	3.39	0
Turkey-light-no skin-roast	cup	219	41.9	0	4.5	97	1.44	0
Turkey-light/dark-no skin	cup	238	41	0	6.95	107	2.29	0
Turk-breast-no skin-roast	item	826	184	0	4.5	508	1.47	0
Chicken-giblets-fri/flour	cup	402	47.2	6.31	19.5	647	5.5	-
Chicken-giblets-simmered	cup	228	37.5	1.37	6.92	570	2.16	0
Chicken-liver-simmered	cup	219	34.1	1.23	7.63	883	2.58	0
Chicken-breast-roasted	item	386	58.4	0	15.3	166	4.3	0
Chicken-breast-stewed	item	404	60.3	0	16.3	166	4.58	0
Chicken-breast-no skin-fri	item	322	57.5	0.88	8.1	156	2.22	0
Chicken-breast-no skin-roast	item	284	53.4	0	6.14	146	1.74	0
Chicken-leg roasted	item	265	29.6	0	15.4	105	4.24	0
Chicken-leg-no skin-roast	item	182	25.7	0	8.01	89	2.18	0
Chicken-leg-no skin-stewed	item	187	26.5	0	8.14	90	2.22	0
Chicken-thigh-fried/flour	item	162	16.6	1.97	9.29	60	2.54	0.04
Chicken-thigh-no skin-roast	item	109	13.5	0	5.66	49	1.57	0
Chicken-wing-fried/flour	item	103	8.36	0.76	7.09	26	1.94	0

Food Name	Serving	KCAL Kc	PROT Gm	CARB Gm	FAT Gm	CHOL Mg	SAFA Gm	FIBD Gm
Chicken-wing-roasted	item	99	9.13	0	6.62	29	1.85	0
Chicken-wing-stewed	item	100	9.11	0	6.73	28	1.88	0
Duck-flesh & skin-roasted	item	2574	145	0	217	640	73.9	0
Duck-no skin-roasted	item	890	104	0	49.5	396	18.4	0
Chicken-frankfurter	item	116	5.82	3.06	8.76	45.5	2.49	0
Chicken-liver pate-can	tbsp	26	1.75	0.85	1.7	-	-	0.01
Chicken roll-light	slice	45	5.54	0.695	2.09	14.2	0.574	0
Chicken spread-canned	tbsp	25	2	0.7	1.52	-	-	-
Turk ham-cured thigh meat	slice	36.5	5.37	0.105	1.44	15.9	0.483	0
Turkey loaf-breast	serving	31.2	6.39	0	0.449	11.6	0.136	0
Turkey pastrami	slice	40	5.21	0.47	1.76	15.3	0.514	0
Turkey roll-light	ounce	41.7	5.31	0.15	2.05	12.2	0.574	0
SAUCES/DIPS								
Sauce-chili-bottled	tbsp	16	0.4	3.7	0	0	0	-
Sauce-Heinz 57	tbsp	15	0.4	2.7	0.2	0	0	-
Sauce-tartar-regular	tbsp	75	0	1	8	9	1.5	-
Dip-guacamole-Kraft	tbsp	25	0.5	1.5	2	0	-	-
Dip-French onion-Kraft	tbsp	30	0.5	1.5	2	0	-	-
Sauce-taco-canned	fl oz	11	0.4	2.2	0.7	0	-	-
Sauce-salsa/chilies-canned	fl oz	10	0.4	2	0.7	0	0	-
Sauce-picante-canned	fl oz	9	0.3	1.9	0.5	0	0	-
Tomato catsup	tbsp	15	0	4	0	0	0	-
Sauce-barbecue	cup	188	4.5	32	4.5	0	0.675	2.3
Mustard-yellow-prepared	tsp	5	0.1	0.1	0.1	0	0	0.06
Sauce-bearnaise-mix/milk	cup	701	8.34	17.5	68.3	189	41.8	0.09
Sauce-cheese-mix/milk	cup	307	16	23.2	17.1	53	9.32	0.1
Sauce-curry-mix/milk	cup	269	10.7	25.7	14.7	35.4	6.04	0.9
Sauce-mushroom-mix/milk	cup	227	11.3	23.8	10.3	34	5.39	0.5
Sauce-sweet/sour-mix/prep	cup	294	0.751	72.7	0.063	0	0	-
Sauce-soy	tbsp	9.54	0.931	1.53	0.014	0	0.002	-
Gravy-beef-canned	cup	123	8.74	11.2	5.49	6.99	2.69	0.093
Gravy-chicken-canned	cup	188	4.59	12.9	13.6	4.76	3.36	-
Gravy-turkey-canned	cup	121	6.2	12.2	5.01	4.76	1.48	-
Sauce-marinara-canned	cup	170	4	25.5	8.38	0	1.2	-
Sauce-tomato-can-salt add	cup	73.5	3.26	17.6	0.417	0	0.059	3.68
Sauce-tomato-Spanish-can	cup	80.5	3.51	17.7	0.659	0	0.092	3.66
Sauce-spaghetti-canned	cup	271	4.53	39.7	11.9	0	1.7	-
Sauce-sour cream-mix/milk	cup	509	19.1	45.4	30.2	91	16.1	-
Sauce-Teriyaki-bottled	tbsp	15.1	1.07	2.87	0	0	0	-
Horseradish-prepared	tbsp	6	0.2	1.4	0	0	0	-
Sauce-Worcestershire	tbsp	12	0.3	2.7	0	0	0	-
Sauce-tabasco	tsp	0	0.1	0.1	0	0	0	0
Mustard-brown-prepared	cup	228	14.8	13.3	15.8	0	-	-
Sauce-tomato-can-low sod	cup	90	4	18	0	0	0	3.39

Appendix A
Food Composition Table—cont'd

Food Name	Serving	KCAL Kc	PROT Gm	CARB Gm	FAT Gm	CHOL Mg	SAFA Gm	FIBD Gm
SOUPS								
Soup-cream/chick-can-milk	cup	191	7.46	15	11.5	27.3	4.64	0.5
Soup-cream/mushroom-milk	cup	203	6.05	15	13.6	19.8	5.13	-
Soup-tomato-can-milk	cup	161	6.1	22.3	6	17.4	2.9	0.8
Soup-bean/bacon-can-water	cup	173	7.89	22.8	5.94	2.53	1.52	3.2
Soup-beef broth-can-ready	cup	16.8	2.74	0.096	0.528	0	0.264	0
Soup-clam-Manhattan-water	cup	78.1	2.2	12.2	2.22	2.44	0.383	-
Soup-minestrone-can-water	cup	81.9	4.26	11.2	2.51	2.41	0.554	1.9
Soup-pea-split-can-water	cup	189	10.3	28	4.4	7.59	1.77	-
Soup-tomato-can-water	cup	85.4	2.05	16.6	1.92	0	0.366	0.9
Soup-vegetable beef-can	cup	78.4	5.61	10.2	1.91	4.9	0.858	0.98
Soup-vegetarian-can-water	cup	72	2.1	12	1.93	0	0.289	1.21
Soup-beef-broth-dehy-cubed	item	6.12	0.62	0.58	0.14	0.144	0.072	-
Soup-onion-dehy-packet	serving	115	4.52	20.9	2.33	1.95	0.538	2.2
Soup-cream/celery-can-milk	cup	164	5.68	14.5	9.7	32.2	3.94	0.77
Soup-cheese-can-milk	cup	230	9.46	16.2	14.6	47.7	9.11	-
Soup-chick broth-can/water	cup	39	4.93	0.93	1.39	0	0.39	0
Soup-chicken noodle-can	cup	74.7	4.05	9.35	2.46	7.23	0.65	1.45
Soup-clam-New England-milk	cup	163	9.47	16.6	6.6	22.3	2.95	-
Soup-cream/potato-can-water	cup	148	5.78	17.2	6.45	22.3	3.77	-
Soup-black bean-can-water	cup	116	5.63	19.8	1.51	0	0.395	-
Soup-beef-chunky-can	cup	170	11.7	19.6	5.14	14.4	2.55	-
Soup-chicken-chunky-can	cup	178	12.7	17.3	6.63	30.1	1.98	-
Soup-chicken/rice-can	cup	127	12.3	13	3.19	12	0.96	1.44
Soup-onion-can-water	cup	57.8	3.75	8.17	1.74	0	0.265	-
Soup-pea-green-can-water	cup	165	8.6	26.5	2.94	0	1.4	-
Soup-tomato rice-can-water	cup	119	2.11	21.9	2.72	2.47	0.519	1.7
Soup-turkey-chunky-can	cup	135	10.2	14.1	4.41	9.44	1.23	2.5
Soup-turkey noodle-can	cup	68.3	3.9	8.63	1.99	4.88	0.561	0.7
Soup-turkey vegetable-can	cup	72.3	3.09	8.63	3.04	2.41	0.892	0.964
SUGARS/SWEETS								
Nuts-coconut-dri-flake-can	cup	341	2.58	31.5	24.4	0	21.6	4.4
Icing-cake-white-boiled	cup	295	1	75	0	0	0	0
Icing-cake-white/coco-boil	cup	605	3	124	13	0	11	-
Icing-cake-choc-mix/prep	cup	1035	9	185	38	0	23.4	-
Icing-cake-fudge-mix/water	cup	830	7	183	16	0	5.1	-
Icing-cake-white-uncooked	cup	1200	2	260	231	0	12.7	0
Candy-caramels-plain/choc	ounce	115	1	22	3	0	1.6	0.784
Candy-milk chocolate-plain	ounce	145	2	16	9	0	5.5	-
Candy-chocolate-semisweet	cup	860	7	97	61	0	36.2	-
Candy-choc coated peanuts	ounce	160	5	11	12	0	4	-

Food Name	Serving	KCAL Kc	PROT Gm	CARB Gm	FAT Gm	CHOL Mg	SAFA Gm	FIBD Gm
Candy-fondant-uncoated	ounce	105	0	25	1	0	0.1	0
Candy-fudge-choc-plain	ounce	115	1	21	3	0	1.3	-
Candy-gum drops	ounce	00	0	25	0	0	0	0
Candy-hard	ounce	110	0	28	0	0	0	0
Marshmallows	ounce	90	1	23	0	0	0	0
Honey-strained/extracted	tbsp	65	0	17	0	0	0	0.06
Jams/preserves-regular	tbsp	55	0	14	0	0	0	0.2
Molasses-can-light	tbsp	50	0	13	-	0	-	0
Molasses-cane-blackstrap	tbsp	45	0	11	-	0	-	0
Sugar-brown-pressed down	cup	820	0	212	0	0	0	0
Sugar-white-granulated	tbsp	45	0	12	0	0	0	0
Sugar-white-powder-sifted	cup	385	0	100	0	0	0	0
Nuts-coconut-dried-shred	cup	466	2.68	44.3	33	0	29.3	3.9
Nuts-coconut-cream-raw	cup	792	8.7	16	83.2	0	73.8	1.6
Candy-milk choc/peanuts	ounce	154	4	12.6	10.8	-	5.22	-
Candy-milk choc/almonds	ounce	151	2.6	14.5	10.1	-	4.06	-
Sugar-Sweet & Low-packet	item	4	-	0.9	-	0	-	-
Sugar-Equal-packet	item	4	0	1	0	0	0	-
Candy-Life Savers	item	7.8	0	1.94	0.02	0	0	0
Candy-M & M's package	item	220	3	31	10	-	-	-
Candy-Snickers bar	item	270	6	33	13	-	4.73	-
Candy-Milky Way bar	item	260	3	43	9	-	5.05	-
Candy-Kit Kat bar	item	210	3	25	11	-	5.6	-
Candy-Bit O Honey	ounce	121	0.9	21.2	3.6	-	1.65	-
Candy-Almond Joy	ounce	151	1.7	18.5	7.8	-	1.74	-
Candy-jelly beans	item	6.6	0	2.64	0	0	0	0
Candy-peanut brittle	ounce	123	2.4	20.4	4.4	-	1.85	-
Candy-peanut butter cup	piece	92	2.2	8.7	5.35	2.5	2.8	-
Candy-lollipop	item	108	0	28	0	0	0	0
VEGETABLES								
V-8 veg juice-low sodium	cup	51	0	9.72	0	0	0	2.7
Tomato juice-low sodium	cup	41.5	1.85	10.3	0.146	0	0.02	2.8
Beans-garbanzo-can	serving	27.8	1.31	4.66	0.511	0	0.07	1.4
Beans-navy pea-dry cooked	cup	225	15	40	1	0	-	9.31
Beans-red kidney-can	cup	230	15	42	1	0	-	12.5
Peas-split-dry-cooked	cup	230	16	42	1	0	-	10.5
Asparagus-froz-boil-spears	cup	50.4	5.31	8.77	0.756	0	0.171	2.16
Beans-lima-froz-boil-drain	cup	170	10.3	32	0.578	0	0.131	8.33
Beans-snap-green-raw-boil	cup	43.8	2.36	9.86	0.35	0	0.08	2.25
Beans-green-froz-French	cup	35.1	1.84	8.26	0.189	0	0.41	2.16
Beans-snap-green-can-cuts	cup	27	1.55	6.08	0.135	0	0.03	1.76
Beans-snap-wax-raw-boil	cup	43.8	2.36	9.86	0.35	0	0.08	2.25
Beans-snap-yellow/wax-can	cup	27.2	1.56	6.12	0.136	0	0.03	1.77
Beans-mung-sprouted-boil	cup	26.3	2.54	5.24	0.113	0	0.031	2.7

Appendix A
Food Composition Table—cont'd

Food Name	Serving	KCAL Kc	PROT Gm	CARB Gm	FAT Gm	CHOL Mg	SAFA Gm	FIBD Gm
Beets-can-sliced-drain	cup	52.7	1.55	12.2	0.238	0	0.039	2.89
Cowpeas-blackeye-raw-boil	cup	160	5.23	33.5	0.627	0	0.158	11
Cowpeas-blackeye-froz-boil	cup	224	14.4	40.4	1.12	0	0.298	9.8
Broccoli-raw	cup	24.6	2.62	4.61	0.308	0	0.048	2.46
Broccoli-raw-boil-drain	cup	43.4	4.62	7.84	0.543	0	0.084	4.03
Cabbage-white mustard-raw	cup	9.1	1.05	1.53	0.14	0	0.018	0.7
Broccoli-froz-boil-drain	cup	51.8	5.74	9.85	0.21	0	0.033	7.3
Cabbage-common-raw-shred	cup	21.6	1.09	4.83	0.162	0	0.021	1.8
Cabbage-common-boil-drain	cup	30.5	1.39	6.92	0.363	0	0.046	4
Cabbage-red-raw-shredded	cup	18.9	0.973	4.28	0.182	0	0.024	1.4
Cabbage-celery-raw	cup	12.2	0.912	2.45	0.152	0	0.033	0.76
Cabbage-white mustard-boil	cup	20.4	2.65	3.03	0.272	0	0.036	2.72
Carrot-raw-whole-scraped	item	31	0.74	7.3	0.137	0	0.022	2.3
Carrot-raw-shred-scraped	cup	47.3	1.13	11.2	0.209	0	0.033	3.52
Carrots-boil-drain-sliced	cup	70.2	1.7	16.3	0.28	0	0.053	5.77
Carrots-can-sliced-drain	cup	33.6	0.934	8.08	0.277	0	0.052	2.19
Cauliflower-raw-chopped	cup	24	1.99	4.92	0.18	0	0.027	2.4
Cauliflower-raw-boil-drain	cup	30	2.32	5.74	0.22	0	0.046	27.3
Cauliflower-froz-boil	cup	34.2	2.9	6.75	0.396	0	0.059	3.24
Celery-Pascal-raw-stalk	item	6.4	0.3	1.46	0.056	0	0.015	0.64
Celery-Pascal-raw-diced	cup	19.2	0.9	4.38	0.168	0	0.044	1.92
Collards-raw-boil-drain	cup	34.6	1.73	7.85	0.243	0	-	2.1
Collards-frozen-boil-drain	cup	61.2	5.05	12.1	0.697	0	-	5.2
Corn-kernels from 1 ear	item	83.2	2.56	19.3	0.986	0	0.152	2.85
Corn-kernels & cob-froz-boil	item	117	3.92	28.1	0.932	0	0.144	2.65
Corn-froz-boil-kernels	cup	134	4.98	33.9	0.116	0	0.018	3.47
Corn-sweet-cream style-can	cup	184	4.45	46.4	1.08	0	0.166	3.07
Corn-sweet-can-drained	cup	134	4.32	30.7	1.65	0	0.254	2.31
Cucumber-raw-sliced	cup	13.5	0.562	3.03	0.135	0	0.034	1.04
Endive-raw-chopped	cup	8.5	0.625	1.68	0.1	0	0.024	-
Lettuce-butterhead-leaves	slice	1.95	0.194	0.348	0.03	0	0.004	0.15
Lettuce-iceberg-raw-leaves	piece	2.61	0.202	0.418	0.038	0	0.005	0.2
Lettuce-iceberg-raw-chop	cup	7.15	0.556	1.15	0.105	0	0.014	0.55
Lettuce-looseleaf-raw	cup	9.9	0.715	1.93	0.165	0	0.022	0.76
Mushrooms-raw-chopped	cup	17.5	1.46	3.26	0.294	0	0.039	0.91
Onions-mature-raw-chopped	cup	60.8	1.86	13.8	0.256	0	0.042	2.56
Carrots-frozen-boil-drain	cup	52.6	1.74	12	0.161	0	0.031	5.4
Onions-mature-boil-drain	cup	92.4	2.86	21.3	0.399	0	0.065	1.68
Onions-young green	item	1.25	0.087	0.278	0.007	0	0.001	0.12
Parsley-raw-chopped	tbsp	1.32	0.088	0.276	0.03	0	0.005	0.176
Peas-green-can-drained	cup	117	7.51	21.4	0.595	0	0.105	5.78

Food Name	Serving	KCAL Kc	PROT Gm	CARB Gm	FAT Gm	CHOL Mg	SAFA Gm	FIBD Gm
Peas-green-froz-boil-drain	cup	125	8.24	22.8	0.432	0	0.078	6.08
Peppers-hot-red-dried	tsp	5	0	1	0	0	0	0.685
Potato-French fried-raw	item	13.5	0.2	1.8	0.7	0	0.17	0.16
Potato-French fried-froz	item	11.1	0.173	1.7	0.438	0	0.208	0.16
Potato-hashed brown-froz	cup	340	4.93	43.8	17.9	0	7.01	1.5
Potato-mashed-milk/butter	cup	223	3.95	35.1	8.88	4.2	2.17	3.15
Potato-mashed-dehy-prep	cup	166	4.2	27.5	4.62	4	1.43	1.2
Potato chips-salt added	item	10.5	0.128	1.04	0.708	0	0.181	0.029
Radishes-raw	item	0.765	0.027	0.162	0.024	0	0.001	0.1
Sauerkraut-canned	cup	44.8	2.15	10.1	0.33	0	0.083	6.06
Spinach-raw-chopped	cup	12.3	1.6	1.96	0.196	cup	0.032	1.46
Spinach-raw-boil-drain	cup	41.4	5.35	6.75	0.468	0	0.076	3.96
Spinach-froz-boil-chopped	cup	57.4	6.44	10.9	0.431	0	0.068	4.51
Squash-summer-boil-sliced	cup	36	1.64	7.76	0.558	0	0.115	2.52
Squash-winter-bake-mash	cup	80	1.82	17.9	1.29	0	0.267	5.74
Sweet potato-bake-peel	item	117	1.96	27.7	0.125	0	0.027	3.42
Sweet potato-boil-mashed	cup	344	5.41	79.6	0.984	0	0.21	9.84
Sweet potato-candied	piece	144	0.914	29.3	3.41	0	1.42	1.1
Sweet potato-can-mashed	cup	258	5.05	59.2	0.51	0	0.11	4.59
Tomato-raw-red-ripe	item	25.8	1.05	5.71	0.406	0	0.056	1.6
Tomato-red-can-whole	cup	48	2.23	10.3	0.576	0	0.084	1.93
Tomato juice-can	cup	41.5	1.85	10.3	0.146	0	0.02	2.9
Tomato powder	ounce	85.8	3.67	21.2	0.125	0	0.018	-
Alfalfa seeds-sprouted-raw	cup	9.57	1.32	1.25	0.228	0	0.023	0.726
Artichokes-boil-drain	item	60	4.18	13.4	0.192	0	0.044	4
Beans-lima-can	cup	186	11.3	34.4	0.744	0	0.168	10.4
Beans-pinto-froz-boil	ounce	46	2.64	8.77	0.136	0	0.016	1.39
Beans-shelled-can	cup	73.5	4.31	15.2	0.466	0	0.056	12
Chives-raw-chopped	tbsp	0.75	0.084	0.114	0.018	0	0.003	0.096
Eggplant-boiled-drained	cup	26.9	0.8	6.37	0.221	0	0.042	2.69
Garlic-raw-cloves	item	4.47	0.191	0.992	0.015	0	0.003	-
Leeks-boil-drain	item	38.4	1.01	9.45	0.248	0	0.033	3.97
Mushrooms-boil-drain	item	3.24	0.26	0.617	0.056	0	0.007	0.264
Mushrooms-can-drain	item	2.88	0.224	0.595	0.035	0	0.005	0.216
Onion rings-froz-prep-heat	item	40.7	0.534	3.82	2.67	0	0.858	0.382
Peppers-jalapeno-can-chop	cup	32.6	1.09	0.664	0.816	0	0.084	-
Potato-skin-baked	item	115	2.49	26.7	0.058	0	0.015	3.02
Potato-au gratin-home rec	cup	323	12.4	27.6	18.6	56.4	11.6	4.41
Potato-hash brown-prep-raw	cup	239	3.77	11.6	21.7	-	8.48	3.12
Potato-scallop-home rec	cup	211	7.03	26.4	9.02	29.4	5.52	4.41
Potato-scallop-mix-prep	ounce	26.4	0.602	3.63	1.22	-	0.748	0.54
Potato pancakes-home rec	item	495	4.63	26.4	12.6	93.5	3.42	-
Pumpkin pie mix-can	cup	281	2.94	71.3	0.351	0	0.176	-
Rutabagas-boil-drain	cup	57.8	1.87	13.2	0.323	0	0.042	2.5

Appendix A
Food Composition Table—cont'd

Food Name	Serving	KCAL Kc	PROT Gm	CARB Gm	FAT Gm	CHOL Mg	SAFA Gm	FIBD Gm
Seaweed-wakame-raw	ounce	12.8	0.861	2.6	0.182	0	0.037	1.2
Squash-zucchini-raw-sliced	cup	18.2	1.51	3.77	0.182	0	0.038	2
Squash-zucchini-raw-boil	cup	28.8	1.15	7.07	0.09	0	0.018	2.3
Squash-zucchini-froz-boil	cup	37.9	2.56	7.94	0.29	0	0.06	3.23
Squash-zucchini-italia-can	cup	65.8	2.34	15.5	0.25	0	0.052	7.02
Succotash-boil-drain	cup	221	9.73	46.8	1.54	0	0.284	14
Tomato-red-raw-boil	cup	64.8	2.57	14	0.984	0	0.137	2.1
Tomato-stew-cook-home rec	cup	79.8	1.98	13.2	2.71	0	0.526	1.04
Tomato-red-can-stewed	cup	66.3	2.37	16.5	0.357	0	0.051	2.04
Tomato-paste-can-low sod	cup	220	9.9	49.3	2.33	0	0.333	11.3
Tomato puree-can-low sod	cup	103	4.18	25.1	0.3	0	0.04	5.75
Vegetable juice-can	cup	46	1.52	11	0.218	0	0.032	2.7
Nuts-chestnuts-roasted	ounce	67.9	1.27	14.9	0.34	0	0.05	2.19
Squash-hubbard-boil-mash	cup	70.8	3.49	15.2	0.873	0	0.179	4.2
Squash-butternut-baked	cup	82	1.84	21.5	0.185	0	0.039	3.5
Squash-acorn-baked	cup	115	2.29	29.9	0.287	0	0.059	4.3
Lettuce-romaine-raw-shred	cup	8.96	0.9	1.33	0.112	0	0.014	0.952
Soybean-dry-cooked	cup	234	19.8	19.4	10.3	0	-	-
Tofu-soybean curd	piece	86	9.4	2.9	5	0	-	1.44
Tomato-can-low sodium diet	cup	48	2.23	10.3	0.576	0	0.084	1.69
Spinach-can-solids/liquids	cup	44.5	4.94	6.83	0.866	0	0.14	5.08
Tomato paste-can-salt add	cup	220	9.9	49.3	2.33	0	0.332	11.3
Tomato puree-can-salt add	cup	103	4.18	25.1	0.3	0	0.04	5.75
Miso-fermented soybeans	cup	567	32.5	76.9	16.7	0	2.41	9.9
Beans-baked beans-canned	cup	236	12.2	52.1	1.14	0	0.295	19.6
Beans-refried beans	cup	271	15.8	46.8	2.7	0	10.4	11.6

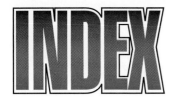